Baker's
HEALTH CARE FINANCE

Basic Tools For Nonfinancial Managers

Thomas K. Ross, PhD

Associate Professor, Department of Nutrition and
Health Care Management at Appalachian State
University, Boone, North Carolina

JONES & BARTLETT
LEARNING

World Headquarters
Jones & Bartlett Learning
25 Mall Road
Burlington, MA 01803
978-443-5000
info@jblearning.com
www.jblearning.com

Jones & Bartlett Learning books and products are available through most bookstores and online booksellers. To contact Jones & Bartlett Learning directly, call 800-832-0034, fax 978-443-8000, or visit our website, www.jblearning.com.

23321-6

Production Credits

Vice President, Product Management: Marisa R. Urbano
Vice President, Content Strategy and Implementation: Christine Emerton
Director, Content Management: Donna Gridley
Manager, Content Strategy: Carolyn Pershouse
Director, Project Management and Content Services: Karen Scott
Director, Product Management: Matthew Kane
Product Manager: Sophie Fleck Teague
Content Strategist: Tess Sackmann
Content Coordinator: Mark Restuccia
Manager, Project Management: Kristen Rogers
Project Manager: Belinda Thresher
Senior Digital Project Specialist: Angela Dooley

Director, Marketing: Andrea DeFronzo
Senior Marketing Manager: Susanne Walker
Content Services Manager: Colleen Lamy
Vice President, Manufacturing and Inventory Control: Therese Connell
Composition: Straive
Project Management: Straive
Cover and Text Design: Michael O'Donnell
Media Development Editor: Faith Brosnan
Rights & Permissions Manager: John Rusk
Rights Specialist: Maria Leon Maimone
Cover Image (Chapter Opener): © dinn/E+/Getty Images.
Printing and Binding: LSC Communications

Library of Congress Cataloging-in-Publication Data

Names: Ross, Thomas K, author. | Baker, Judith J. Health care finance.
Title: Baker's health care finance : basic tools for nonfinancial managers / Thomas K. Ross.
Other titles: Health care finance
Description: Sixth edition | Burlington, Massachusetts : Jones & Bartlett Learning, [2023] | Preceded by Health care finance / Judith J. Baker, R.W. Baker, and Neil R. Dworkin. Fifth edition. [2018]. | Includes bibliographical references and index. | Summary: "A foundation in health care finance; practical skills to manage a budget and the vocabulary to communicate effectively with staff, other managers, and the health care executive management team. For students of Nursing and other allied health professionals who are furthering their career by stepping into management roles and/or are pursuing MHA's or Nursing Leadership/Management degrees and certificates"– Provided by publisher.
Identifiers: LCCN 2021970005 | ISBN 9781284233162 (paperback)
Subjects: MESH: Financial Management | Health Facilities–economics | Health Facility Administration | United States | BISAC: MEDICAL / Administration
Classification: LCC RA971.3 | NLM W 80 | DDC 362.1068/–dc23/eng/20220214
LC record available at https://lccn.loc.gov/2021970005

LCCN: 2019947448

6048

Printed in the United States of America
26 25 24 23 22   10 9 8 7 6 5 4 3 2 1

Brief Contents

PART VIII **Case Studies** 419

Contents

PART I Healthcare Finance Overview   1

PART IV   Reporting and Measuring Financial Performance   145

CHAPTER 11 Financial Statements, Reporting Organizational Financial Performance 147

CHAPTER 12 Financial Ratios and Operating Indicators, Assessing Financial Performance 163

CHAPTER 13 Common Sizing, Trend Analysis, Compound Growth Rates, and Counts Versus Rates 179

PART V   Constructing and Evaluating Budgets   191

CHAPTER 14 Constructing an Operating Budget 193

CHAPTER 25 Creating a Business Plan. 335

CHAPTER 26 Healthcare Delivery Systems, Finance, and Reimbursement 343

New to This Edition

The major changes to the *Sixth Edition* begin with the use of Microsoft Excel. Excel is introduced in Chapter 3 and used throughout the text. Excel simplifies financial calculations and helps students understand how finance operates and what financial information means.

The second change is chapters have been reordered to improve flow. The budgeting and variance analysis chapters are together, emphasizing that managing the budget follows building the budget. They are both chapters in Part V, Constructing and Evaluating Budgets, which also includes benchmarking and Lean Six Sigma. Similarly, Part VI, Evaluating Capital Investments, pairs the time value of money chapter with the capital budgeting chapter as well as chapters on investing and borrowing, financing costs, and lease versus purchase decisions.

The third change is problems have been moved from the end of the text to the end of the chapter to emphasize completion of problems as essential to mastering financial skills.

PowerPoint slides have been updated. In the Test Bank, the number of Multiple Choice and True or False questions in most chapters has been doubled.

New Materials in the *Sixth Edition*

Chapter 1, Introduction to Healthcare Finance, includes an examination of how national health expenditures, healthcare employment, and health outcomes have changed over time to set the stage for the exploration of healthcare costs and concludes with a brief discussion of how managers can use resources more effectively, a theme that will be pursued in subsequent chapters.

Chapter 2, Five Things the Healthcare Manager Needs to Know About Financial Management Systems, introduces a section on responsibility center accounting as responsibility centers are used in future chapters.

Chapter 3, Using Excel, is a new chapter that covers using the Ribbon, mathematical operations and formulas, and graphing.

Chapter 4, Assets, Liabilities, and Net Worth, provides pie charts showing the distribution of assets in hospitals and physician practices and how the assets are financed.

Chapter 5, Revenues, provides pie charts showing the distribution of hospital and physician practice revenues by source and the distribution of U.S. revenues by care setting.

Chapter 6, Expenses, provides pie charts showing the distribution of hospital and physician practice expenses.

The inclusion of pie charts in Chapters 4, 5, and 6 is to provide readers with insight into the structure and operation of hospitals and physician practices as they account for 55% of total health expenditures.

Chapter 7, Direct and Indirect Costs, includes a new section showing how the allocation base for indirect costs affects the reported profitability of profit centers and can be utilized to encourage cost reduction.

Chapter 8, Cost Behavior and Break-Even Analysis, includes a discussion of efficient and profit-maximizing output levels and demonstrates how Excel scatter graphs with an inserted trendline can be used to calculate fixed and variable costs (extends prior discussion of scatter graph method).

Chapter 9, Managing Staffing and Salaries: Methods, Operations, and Regulations, begins with a scenario on staff scheduling that better matches staffing level to workload and reduces salary expense and includes a new section on calculating and reducing employee turnover.

Chapter 10, Managing Supplies, Equipment, and Facilities, adds calculations of inventory loss ratio and economic order quantity, incorporates depreciation methods into the chapter that were previously in the appendix, and concludes with a discussion of utilization of fixed assets.

Chapter 11, Financial Statements, Reporting Organizational Financial Performance, includes vertical and horizontal analysis and a run chart of income from operations to highlight the role of financial statements in reporting the performance of an organization.

Chapter 12, Financial Ratios and Operating Indicators, Assessing Financial Performance, adds turnover ratios and operating indicators to explore the reasons why net income is increasing or decreasing.

Chapter 13, Common Sizing, Trend Analysis, Compound Growth Rates, and Counts versus Rates, adds the calculation of compound growth rates to better understand changes occurring over multiple years and the need to calculate rates versus only counts when assessing performance.

Chapter 14, Constructing an Operating Budget, provides a step-by-step approach to creating incremental and flexible budgets and includes the process for restating the flexible budget for actual output at the end-of-the-accounting period. Forecasting, due to its critical role in budgeting, was incorporated into this chapter from another chapter.

Chapter 15, Variance Analysis and Sensitivity Analysis, combines comparative budget review and variance analysis (previously in Chapter 18) and relies more heavily on formulas than the 5th edition to calculate volume, price, and efficiency variances at a line-item level.

Chapter 16, Benchmarking, Estimates, and Measurement Tools, provides benchmarks for financial ratios and operating indicators.

Chapter 17, Using Lean Six Sigma to Improve Financial Performance, a new chapter, provides a guide to implement improvement includes identifying wastes; principles of Lean Six Sigma; Define, Measure, Analyze, Improve, and Control (DMAIC) methodology; and performance improvement cycle.

Chapter 18, The Time Value of Money, incorporates Excel functions for calculating present values and includes a new section on future value.

Chapter 19, Constructing a Capital Budget, provides steps to create a capital budget, an Excel capital budget worksheet, a capital rationing example, and a discussion of balancing financial and nonfinancial factors in a capital funding decisions.

Chapter 20, Investing, Borrowing, and Statistics, adds measures of dispersion and a graph of a frequency distribution.

Chapter 22, Purchasing Versus Leasing, compares lease and purchase decisions in a single table (reduces the number of tables from 11 to four) and adds a discussion of managed service agreements.

Chapters 21 and 23 through 30 have been updated and in most cases shortened in length.

Chapters 31 through 35, Case Studies, are all new and designed to test the reader's mastery of the concepts and tools provided in multiple chapters to extract actionable information from the provided data and convey findings effectively to others. The cases provide the issue under consideration, historical financial information and assumptions, and needed deliverables (i.e., the required analyses and the analyst's interpretations and conclusions). The case studies require a more comprehensive understanding of finance (i.e., integration of more than one chapter) to develop the inputs needed to complete them, explain the financial situation, and justify the recommended action.

To summarize, the updates to the *Sixth Edition* are designed to broaden a reader's understanding of how healthcare organizations operate and provide them with the skills to analyze financial performance, prepare and manage operating budgets, prepare capital budgets, and improve financial performance. The aim is to ensure that students become more effective healthcare managers and have more rewarding careers.

Preface

Teaching healthcare finance has always been challenging as the overwhelming majority of healthcare management students will not work in financial areas and are not motivated by the traditional approach to finance. Early in my career, I began to develop an approach that would appeal to a wider and nonfinancial audience but soon discovered that Baker, Baker, and Dworkin had pursued this idea a decade or more before me with their *Health Care Finance: Basic Tools for Nonfinancial Managers*. I was delighted to be invited to contribute to the sixth edition of the text, and after working through the text, I am more appreciative of their approach. Their emphasis on responsibility centers highlights not only what managers should be doing but also what accounting and finance should be doing for managers. Managers should control the resources at their command, and accounting and finance should provide the information managers need to understand resource use.

Many people are perplexed by the cost of health care and at a loss to understand how they can reduce expenses. Chapter 1 has been expanded to show how national health expenditures, healthcare employment, and health outcomes have changed over time to set the stage for the exploration of healthcare costs. The exploration of the costs associated with labor (Chapter 9) and supplies, equipment, and facilities (Chapter 10) will lead students to see that costs can be reduced through better staffing and use of supplies and equipment.

Chapters 11 through 13 examine the question "How is the organization performing?" Chapter 11 covers financial statements, Chapter 12 analyzes the statements using ratios to understand performance, and Chapter 13 demonstrates how performance can be compared over time and across institutions to identify where improvements can or should be made.

After discovering Baker, Baker, and Dworkin had produced a text for nonfinancial managers, my later work subsequently pursued a more technical approach focusing on budgeting and variance analysis. Budgeting and variance analysis are the two areas of finance that managers will routinely need to complete their responsibilities and are only given two chapters in most healthcare finance textbooks. A manager's career often depends upon their ability to produce and manage a budget. Chapter 14 on budgeting provides a step-by-step approach to creating incremental and flexible budgets and includes the process for restating the flexible budget for actual output at the end-of-the-accounting period. I often told my students that my job was not allowing them to answer the question "Can you prepare a budget?" with "Yes" but rather ask "What type of budget would you like prepared?" Chapter 15, Variance Analysis and Sensitivity Analysis, has been expanded and takes a different approach than the prior edition by focusing on calculating volume, price, and efficiency variances at a line-item level.

Chapters 18 through 22 cover capital assets and have been rearranged so time value of money (Chapter 18) precedes capital budgets (Chapter 19). Chapter 19 reports the steps needed to create a capital budget and provides a sample Excel worksheet for data collection and analysis. Chapters 20 through 22 introduce readers to investment terms, the costs of debt, and how to analyze lease versus purchase options.

You'll find Chapter 3, Using Excel, is entirely new as I have found that Excel instruction has given my students a step up in seeking jobs (and can be applied to fields beyond finance). Chapter 3 covers using the Ribbon, mathematical operations and formulas, and graphing. As with any quantitative subject, you must do the calculations to fully understand the subject, and students learn what finance is about by following Excel calculations and reporting information using graphs. Excel spreadsheets are provided, and students will have the opportunity to practice using Excel in many chapters. Students consistently report on end-of-course surveys that Excel was one of the most important skills or concepts they learned during the semester, plus it is my belief they also gain a sense of accomplishment from mastering Excel.

While understanding financial information is the first step toward improvement, improvement is difficult, so a new chapter on Lean Six Sigma (Chapter 17) has been added to guide people through a proven change process. Like Excel, Lean Six Sigma is applied in nonfinancial areas and provides students with tools that they can offer current or potential employers.

I hope my additions improve the text and illuminate the role of finance in health care. I have endeavored to answer *why* finance is important and *how* financial tools are employed to improve performance. It is obvious that healthcare expenditures will continue to increase and generate calls for better use of resources and outcomes. Your understanding of the U.S. healthcare system and how money flows into and out of healthcare organizations is vital to improving resource use and outcomes and leading you to a rewarding career in health care.

Acknowledgments

For Kent V. Ross, Mardell L. Remick, and Deanna M. Zaenglein for showing me how to work and providing an example.

For Judith J. Baker, R. W. Baker, and Neil R. Dworkin for their contributions to this work over the last two decades.

For all the employees of Jones & Bartlett Learning, including Sophie Teague, Susanne Walker, Faith Brosnan, Tess Sackmann, Bel Thresher, Athiyappan Manoharan, and Maria Maimone, for working with me.

About the Author

Thomas K. Ross, PhD, is an Associate Professor in the Department of Nutrition and Health Care Management at Appalachian State University where he teaches Health Care Finance and Introduction to Health System Organization. He received his PhD in Economics from Saint Louis University, and a MBA in Finance and Accounting from the University of Cincinnati.

Dr. Ross currently has four books in print, *Practical Health Care Budgeting: A Concise Guide*, © 2020, *Applying Lean Six Sigma in Health Care*, © 2019, and *A Comprehensive Guide to Budgeting for Health Care Managers*, © 2018, all published by Jones & Bartlett Learning. His first book, *Health Care Quality Management*, was published in 2014 by Jossey-Bass.

He has been a faculty member for Charlotte AHEC since 2017 where he has given workshops on Quality Improvement, Lean Six Sigma, and Excel tools. He has previously taught classes in research, quality management, strategic planning, and economics at East Carolina University, Kings College (PA), Indiana University South Bend, and Saint Louis University. Prior to entering education, Dr. Ross worked in health care finance as a director of patient accounts, manager of system support, and senior financial analyst.

Dr. Ross lives with his three dogs, three cats, and four seasonal hummingbirds on a one-acre site in Boone, North Carolina that he is trying to transform into a garden.

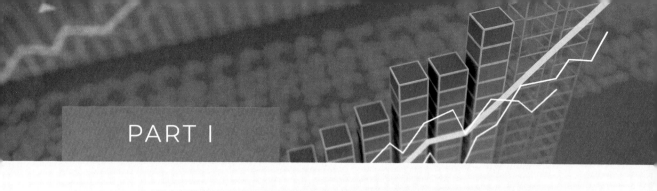

PART I

Healthcare Finance Overview

CHAPTER 1

Introduction to Healthcare Finance

PROGRESS NOTES

After completing this chapter, you should be able to

1. Explain the idea that finance is a method of getting money into and out of an organization.
2. Describe the four components of management.
3. Explain the difference between financial and managerial accounting.
4. Describe the difference between for-profit, nonprofit, and public organizations.
5. Describe the purpose of an organization chart.
6. Describe how every manager can improve the financial performance of an organization.

Overview: Healthcare Finance

Finance issues comprise a large part of the day-to-day duties of managers, yet many individuals in large organizations feel powerless to improve their financial performance. The average hospital has hundreds of millions of dollars in revenues and expenses and is subject to forces that often seem beyond the control of anyone. The belief that one is powerless is unfortunate as all managers control a set of resources and have the power to reduce costs. Failure to obtain the maximum benefit from the resources one commands can lead directly to the bankruptcy of the organization. Healthcare organizations that go out of business inflict an enormous cost on patients, employees, and the community. According to the Shep Center, 174 rural hospitals have gone bankrupt since 2005, 95 have closed, and 79 have been converted to other uses; 40 of the bankruptcies occurred in isolated areas where access to care is limited.[1]

The patients of these organizations were forced to travel longer distances for care. The recent closing of Southwest Regional Medical Center, a critical access hospital in Georgia, will require patients drive 23 miles to reach another hospital. Likewise, employees of shuttered hospitals are forced to find new work, which often requires additional travel time and causes communities to lose an economic engine. Holmes et al. found that the closure of the sole hospital in a community reduces per capita income by $703 or 4.0% and increases the unemployment rate by 1.6%. Hospital closures in communities with more than one hospital reduced income for 2 years after the closure but had no long-term economic impact.[2]

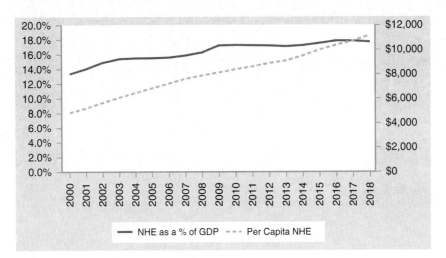

Figure 1.1 U.S. National Health Expenditures

Accounting and finance are the language of business. Accounting defines how economic transactions are recorded, and budgets establish the goals against which performance should be measured. More than 25% of hospitals in the United States lose money from operations, highlighting the need for better financial management.

The United States spends close to 18% of its gross domestic product (GDP) on healthcare services, and there is concern that we are spending too much and receiving too little from our investment. The United States more than tripled its investment in health care from 5.0% of GDP in 1960 to 17.7% in 2018. In 1960 one dollar of every $19.94 earned was spent on health care; in 2018, one in every $5.64 was spent on health care, and spending continues to increase. **Figure 1.1** shows healthcare spending from 2000 through 2018. Spending per person increased from $4,855 to $11,174, while healthcare expenditures as a percent of GDP increased from 13.4% to 17.7%.[3]

As expenditures increase, healthcare employment has increased to make health care the largest employer in the United States, and healthcare wages are higher than the average for all occupations. The median annual wage for healthcare practitioners and technical occupations such as physicians and surgeons, registered nurses, and pharmacists was $85,900 in May 2020 versus $56,310 for all occupations. Healthcare practitioners and technical occupations accounted for 8,579,180 jobs. Healthcare support occupations such as nursing assistants, medical assistants, and physical and occupational therapy assistants had a median annual wage of $32,250 and accounted for 6,440,880 jobs. Health services managers, accounting for 402,540 jobs, had an average income of $118,800.[4] As you can see, high wages are partially due to the high level of education needed to fill healthcare positions. **Table 1.1** shows the growth in employment from 2009 through 2019 and the anticipated growth from 2019 through 2029.

Table 1.1 Healthcare Employment

Employment (000)	2009	2019	2029	Growth rate 2009–2019	Growth rate 2019–2029
Total	143,036	162,796	168,835	1.3%	0.4%
Health care	16,540	20,413	23,492	2.1%	1.4%

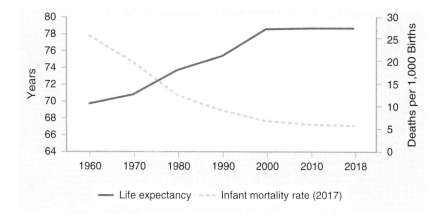

Figure 1.2 Health Outcomes

Health care was the second largest employer in 2009, accounting for 12% of total employment, second to state and federal state government, which accounted for 14%. In 2019, health care accounted for 13% of total employment, while federal and state government fell to 12%. Based on growth projections, health care will add more than 3 million positions in the next 10 years and account for 14% of all employment.[5] The increase in employment is partially due to the increase in the population and those over 65 years of age, who use more health services than younger people.

The higher investment in health care begs the question of whether outcomes are better. Figure 1.2 shows the increase in life expectancy and reduction in the infant mortality rate between 1960 and 2018.[6]

Figure 1.2 shows large increases in life expectancy between 1960 and 2000 and minimal change thereafter. It is interesting that life expectancy increased by 12.6 years between 1929 and 1960 when NHE was only 5.0% of GDP and only increased by 3.3 years between 1990 and 2018 when NHE increased from 12.1% to 17.7% of GDP. Infant mortality rates dropped significantly between 1960 and 1980, had a lesser but still large decline between 1980 and 2000, and had a modest decline thereafter. Given the small improvements in health outcomes since 2000, can we use our resources more efficiently and produce better health? The goal of the text is to provide

you with insight into financial information and tools to improve financial performance to benefit patients, yourself, and your organization. This text will introduce you to financial terms and tools so you can understand the financial performance of the organization and your area(s) of responsibility. Managers control labor, supplies, equipment, and facilities; the text will show you how to measure resource use and improve performance.

The Concept

A Method of Getting Money into and out of the Business

One of our colleagues, a nurse, talks about healthcare finance as "a method of getting money into and out of the business." It is not a bad description. As you shall see, revenues are inflows and expenses are outflows. Inflows are the value patients and payers place on the goods and services that providers deliver, and outflows are the cost of resources consumed in producing the goods and services. The goal of financial management is to ensure that revenues exceed expenses. Life is better in organizations where inflows exceed outflows, and managers have more choices when they generate more money than they spend.

Organizations with more money than they spend can use the excess to improve or expand services to patients, improve equipment and facilities, and/or increase employee compensation. On the other hand, organizations that spend more money than they bring in must reduce expenditures. Unfortunately, reducing expenditures requires decreasing patient services, working in old facilities with outdated equipment, and/or cutting employment or employee compensation. (Reductions in compensation may come from no cost of living increases or increasing employee contributions to health insurance premiums.) In many cases, poor financial management results in the closure of hospitals, physician practices, and other healthcare organizations. The successful manager, through **planning**, **organizing**, and controlling processes and **evaluating** outcomes, ensures that revenues exceed expenses to maximize the value of the organization and guarantee its continued operation.

How Does Finance Work in Health Care?

The purpose of this text is to show how the various elements of finance fit together in healthcare businesses. The key to effective financial management is understanding the various elements and their relationship to each other. If you, the manager, truly see how the elements work, you will know which elements are in your control and how they can be changed to improve financial performance. Finance provides you with one of the essential tools needed to achieve management success.

Health care is a service industry. It is not in the business of manufacturing computers, automobiles, or other physical products. The essential business of healthcare providers is improving the health of patients through the effective and efficient delivery of healthcare services such as therapies and surgeries. Healthcare providers hold inventories of medical supplies and drugs, but those inventories are necessary to service delivery rather than manufacturing. As the primary business of health care is service, the explanations and illustrations in this text focus on the practice of financial management in service industries.

Viewpoints

Managers in large healthcare organizations will generally have one of three views: (1) managerial or senior administrative including finance, (2) clinical, or (3) support. The way they manage is influenced by the view they hold. A large organization may be one with more than 20 employees where it would be extremely difficult, if not impossible, for one person to oversee all aspects of the business. In a solo physician practice, the physician may be able to understand all views and perform all functions.

1. The managerial or senior administrative view includes overseeing and directing the total operation. One of the critical activities is directing financial operations. Finance managers work with finance information on a daily basis, including collecting payment for services delivered, paying bills, budgeting, and reporting financial performance. The chief financial officer and others are often deeply involved in strategic planning (i.e., determining short- and long-term goals for the organization). Other senior-level functions include the chief executive office, human resources, and legal affairs.
2. Clinical managers are responsible for service delivery, nursing, and ancillary services including head nurses and the directors of radiology and pharmacy. They have direct interaction with the patients, supervise caregivers, and are responsible for healthcare outcomes.
3. Support services include housekeeping, groundskeeping, maintenance, material management, and medical records. Managers in support services generally work with the systems of the organization to ensure that clinical employees have the resources they need to provide quality care. Information system managers provide another support function: They are responsible for data accumulation and ensuring that clinical workers and senior managers receive information when they need it.

Managers in large organizations must, of necessity, interact with one another to produce

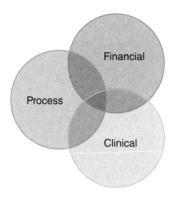

Figure 1.3 Three Views of Management Within an Organization

goods and services that will attract and retain customers and ensure the organization's continued success. Healthcare managers holding different views and skills must work together to ensure patient satisfaction. Their concerns intersect as illustrated by **Figure 1.3**, and operational excellence demands that each area supports the other two. The nonfinancial manager who understands healthcare finance will be able to interpret and negotiate successfully such interactions between and among viewpoints.

The role of financial management is to supply information to other managers to maintain or improve performance and ensure the organization has the financial resources necessary to provide care. Health care is a business that requires financial management skills to balance the inflows and outflows that are a part of the business.

Why Manage?

Businesses do not run themselves and require a variety of management activities to operate properly. Customer satisfaction, cost control, and defects vary greatly across industries, Marketing Charts reported that TV/Internet providers had the worst customer experience while retail had the fewest dissatisfied customers.[7] The job of managers is to ensure that customers receive satisfying products and the organization generates more revenue than it spends.

The Elements of Management

Management encompasses four major functions: (1) planning, (2) organizing, (3) controlling and directing, and (4) evaluating outcomes. The four functions require different skills and are needed to reach organizational goals. Senior managers and owners establish the organization's mission, values, and goals. Planning how the goals will be met includes determining what services will be provided, the quantity of services to be delivered, and what patients will be served. Lower-level managers are subsequently responsible for ensuring that goods and services are delivered to these patients at the required level of quality.

1. *Planning.* Senior managers make choices among available alternatives. All subsequent management activities—organizing, controlling, and evaluating—are designed to ensure that plans are achieved.
2. *Organizing.* When organizing, the manager decides how to use the resources of the organization to most effectively carry out the plans that have been established. They identify the resources, labor, supplies, equipment, and facilities needed to accomplish the organization's goals, (i.e., they create a budget).
3. *Controlling and directing.* After goals are set and resources are identified, managers should ensure that their area or areas are following the plans that have been established. One way to do this is to study current reports and compare them with budgets and reports from earlier periods (i.e., whether output and quality meet expectations and revenues are greater than expenses). These comparisons can show where the organization may need improvement when an area is not effective and/or efficient. The reports that the manager uses for this purpose are often called feedback. The purpose of controlling is to ensure that plans are being followed.
4. *Evaluating.* Managers are expected to modify operations in response to unanticipated events during the controlling phase.

Evaluation assesses how successful managers were in meeting organizational goals, whether outcomes were achieved and the budget was met, and whether managers took effective action when improvement was needed. Evaluation establishes accountability and incentives; when accountability or incentives are absent, managers may not be motivated to take the required steps to improve the performance of their areas and the organization.

The Organization's Structure

Who owns an organization and how authority and decision-making are delegated have a major impact on performance.

Ownership

Organizations fall into one of three basic types: for-profit, nonprofit, and public. In the United States, these designations follow the taxable status of the organizations. For-profit entities, also known as **proprietary organizations**, pay income taxes. Proprietary subgroups include individuals, partnerships, and corporations.

The nonprofit or **voluntary organizations** have tax-exempt status and do not pay income taxes. In general, voluntary nonprofits are associated with churches, private schools, or foundations. Public or government entities also do not pay taxes and include (1) federal, (2) state, (3) county, (4) city, (5) combined city and county, (6) a hospital taxing district (with the power to raise revenues through taxes), and (7) state university (perhaps with a teaching hospital affiliated with the university) entities. Ownership may also affect who makes decisions and who receives any excess revenue produced by the organization. In for-profits, any profit is the property of owners; in nonprofit or **public organizations**, any excess revenue over expenses should be used for the good of the general public. **Exhibit 1.1** summarizes the subgroups of both proprietary and **nonprofit organizations**.

Exhibit 1.1 **Types of Organizations**

For-Profit—Proprietary
  Individual
  Partnership
  Corporation
  Other

Nonprofit—Voluntary
  Church Associated
  Private School Associated
  Foundation Associated
  Other

Public—Government
  Federal
  State
  County
  City
  City–County
  Hospital District
  State University
  Other

Organization Charts

In a small organization, senior management will be able to monitor all of the activities undertaken and the outcomes produced. Extensive measures and indicators are not necessary because management can view overall operations. In large organizations, senior managers must use the management control system to understand what is going on. In other words, to view operations, management must use measures and indicators because they cannot continuously monitor all aspects of their organization's operations.

As a rule of thumb, an informal management control system is acceptable only if the manager can stay in close contact with all aspects of the operation. Otherwise, a formal system is required. In the context of health care, a one-physician practice could use an informal method (**Figure 1.4**), but a hospital system must use a formal method of management control (**Figure 1.5**).

The structure of the organization will affect its financial management. **Organization charts** are often used to illustrate the structure of the organization. Each box on an organization chart represents a particular area of management

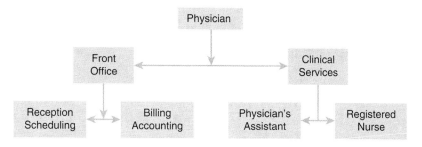

Figure 1.4 Physician's Office Organization Chart
Courtesy of Resource Group, Ltd., Dallas, Texas.

responsibility. The lines between the boxes are lines of authority.

In the health system organization chart illustrated in Figure 1.5, the president/chief executive officer oversees seven senior vice presidents. Each senior vice president has vice presidents reporting to him or her in each particular area of responsibility designated on the chart. These vice presidents, in turn, have an array of other managers reporting to them at varying levels of managerial responsibility.

The organization chart also shows the degree of decentralization within the organization. In decentralized organizations, authority for decision-making is delegated to lower-level managers; centralization limits decision-making to senior executives. Decision-making in centralized organizations is slow due to the multiple management levels that must be negotiated so decentralized structures are used when rapid decision and action are needed. Organization charts thus illustrate the pattern of how managers are allowed—or required—to make key decisions within the particular organization. The purpose of an organization chart is to indicate how authority is assigned to managers and the formal lines of communication and reporting.

Two Types of Accounting

Financial Accounting

Financial accounting is generally used to report organization performance to people outside the organization (i.e., external reporting). External reporting to third parties in health care includes government entities such as the Internal Revenue Service, Medicare, Medicaid, and other government programs; health plan payers; and the general public. For-profits may also have to report to stockholders. Financial reporting for external purposes must be in accordance with generally accepted accounting principles (GAAP). Financial reporting is usually concerned with transactions that have already occurred: that is, it is retrospective.

Managerial Accounting

Managerial accounting is generally for internal use by managers and employees. Planning, organizing, controlling, and evaluating processes all require financial performance measures. The reporting of profitability of services and the pricing of services are common uses of managerial accounting. Strategic planning and other intermediate and long-term decision-making represent an additional use of managerial accounting.

Managerial accounting intended for internal use is not bound by generally accepted accounting principles. Managerial accounting deals with transactions that have already occurred, but it is also concerned with the future in the form of projecting outcomes and preparing budgets. Thus, managerial accounting is prospective as well as retrospective.

The Role of Financial Management

The general components of management, planning, organizing, controlling, and evaluating were discussed earlier; financial management deals

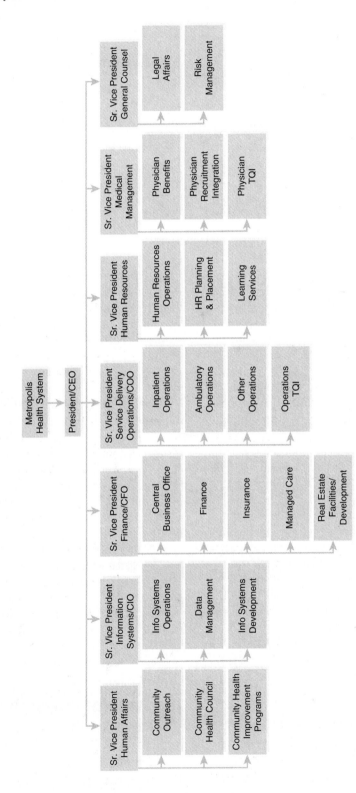

Figure 1.5 Health System Organization Chart

Courtesy of Resource Group, Ltd. Dallas, Texas.

more specifically with ensuring that revenues exceed expenses. Every manager is responsible for resources and thus can contribute to ensuring that revenues exceed expenses by using resources effectively, (i.e., using the minimum amount of resources to complete a job); eliminating or reducing unused or underutilized labor, materials, equipment, and/or facilities; and minimizing defects. Managers with responsibility over revenues should ensure that appropriate prices are set and the organization's product and patient mix are sustainable.

As you will see and will probably be called upon to perform in the future, finance encompasses analysis of revenues and expenses, labor scheduling, inventory and purchasing decisions, budgeting, variance analysis, and evaluation of capital investments. Managers have a responsibility to see that organizational resources improve patient health and that minimum resources are used to complete tasks. Thus, managers must schedule the appropriate level of personnel to complete tasks, monitor supply and equipment usage to ensure that waste or overinvestment does not occur, and minimize defects. This text provides you with the tools to effectively complete these duties.

WRAP-UP

Summary

The United States is devoting more resources to health care, and public expectations have increased. People are demanding more information on healthcare spending and outcomes, and healthcare managers will be called upon to justify their resource use. On an organizational level, the goal of financial management and managers can be summarized as ensuring that revenues (inflows) exceed expenses (outflows).

Financial management, like management in general, has four distinct phases: planning, organizing, controlling and directing, and evaluating. Planning requires establishing where an organization or department should be in the future. Organizing assembles the resources needed to reach goals. Controlling oversees the use of resources to ensure that they are effectively and efficiently employed to achieve desired outcomes and makes adjustments when outcomes are not met and/or costs are too high. Evaluating assesses organizational and departmental performance after the end of a fiscal period to determine how managers and employees performed.

Ownership and organization structure affect how employee incentives and performance.

In **for-profit organizations** where profits can be distributed to owners, there is generally more effort devoted to holding down costs than nonprofit or public organizations where the beneficiaries of any excess revenue over expenses is less clearly defined. Similarly, for-profit and nonprofit organizations dependent upon continuing patient support often seem to provide better customer service than public organizations. Managers of organizations must determine whether performance will be better under a tightly controlled centralized decision-making structure or decentralized decision-making that encourages lower-level managers to take action when they see fit.

Whether for-profit, nonprofit, or public and decentralized or centralized decision-making, managers need financial information to assess performance. The role of accounting and financial management is to highlight and improve pricing, labor scheduling, supply and inventory, and investment in equipment and facility decisions. Budgeting establishes the goals of the organization in dollars and cents, what revenue is expected, and how much it should cost to generate the revenue.

Variance analysis examines actual performance to determine if goals are being met and the actions needed to improve performance and establish accountability. Capital budgeting analysis looks to the future to determine where future investments should be made. Mastering budgeting, variance analysis, and capital budgeting will make you a more effective manager.

Key Terms

Controlling and Directing
Evaluating
Financial Accounting
For-Profit Organization (also see Proprietary Organization)
Managerial Accounting
Nonprofit Organization (also see Voluntary Organization)
Organization Chart
Organizing
Planning
Public Organization

Discussion Questions

1. Explain the idea that finance is a method of getting money into and out of an organization.
2. Describe the four components of management.
3. Explain the difference between financial and managerial accounting.
4. Describe the difference between for-profit, nonprofit, and public organizations.
5. Explain the composition and purpose of an organization chart.
6. Describe why every manager can improve the financial performance of an organization.

Notes

1. Shep Center, "Rural Hospital Closures," https://www.shepscenter.unc.edu/programs-projects/rural-health/rural-hospital-closures/, accessed September 23, 2020.
2. G. M. Holmes, R. T. Slifkin, R. K. Randolph, and S. Poley, "The Effect of Rural Hospital Closures on Community Economic Health," *Health Services Research*, 41, no. 2 (2006): 467–485.
3. Centers for Medicare & Medicaid Services, "National Health Statistics Group, Table 3 National Health Expenditures; Levels and Annual Percent Change, by Source of Funds: Selected Calendar Years 1960–2017," https://www.cms.gov/Research-Statistics-Data-and-Systems/Statistics-Trends-and-Reports/NationalHealthExpendData/NationalHealthAccountsHistorical, accessed June 4, 2021.
4. U.S. Bureau of Labor Statistics, "Occupational Employment and Wage Statistics," https://www.bls.gov/oes/tables.htm, accessed April 6, 2021.
5. U.S. Bureau of Labor Statistics, "Employment Projections," https://www.bls.gov/emp/tables/employment-by-major-industry-sector.htm, accessed April 6, 2021.
6. Centers for Disease Control and Prevention, "Data Table for Figure 18. Life Expectancy at Birth, by Sex, Race and Hispanic origin: United States, 1980–2018," http://www.cdc.gov/nchs/hus/contents2018.htm#fig18; National Vital Statistics Reports, "Table 3. Infant Mortality Rates, by Race: United States, Selected Years 1950–2017," https://www.cdc.gov/nchs/products/nvsr.htm, accessed April 6, 2021.
7. Marketing Charts, "Which Industries Are Suffering Most from Poor CX?," https://www.marketingcharts.com/customer-centric/customer-experience-111506, accessed March 9, 2021.

CHAPTER 2

Five Things the Healthcare Manager Needs to Know About Financial Management Systems

PROGRESS NOTES

After completing this chapter, you should be able to

1. Understand the four parts of a financial management system.
2. Describe an information flow for a financial transaction.
3. Describe the role and structure of the chart of accounts.
4. Explain the annual management cycle.
5. Explain the goal of responsibility center accounting.

Overview: What Does a Manager Need to Know?

Financial management is both an art and a science. You as a manager need to understand the structure and reasoning that underlie management actions. To do so, you need to be able to answer the following four questions:

1. What are the four parts of a financial management system?

2. How does financial information flow?
3. What are the functions of the **chart of accounts**, subsidiary ledgers, **general ledger, trial balance**, and financial reports in an **accounting system**?
4. What is the annual management cycle for reporting results?

This chapter provides answers to each of these four questions. It also discusses how to communicate financial information to others, a valuable if not essential skill for a successful manager.

The Financial System in Health Care

The information that you, as a manager, work with is only one part of the total financial system. To understand financial management, it is essential to recognize the overall financial system in which your organization operates. A structure exists within the system, and you must understand how the structure works to be an effective manager. The four parts that make a healthcare financial system work are (1) the **original records**, (2) the **information system**, (3) the accounting system, and (4) the **reporting system**. Generally speaking, the original records provide evidence that an economic transaction (i.e., goods or services were sold or labor, supplies, and equipment were consumed) has occurred. The information system gathers the data, and the accounting system organizes the data according to accounting principles. The reporting system summarizes and reports financial performance (i.e., revenues produced and/or expense incurred). The healthcare manager needs to know how charges for patient services, time cards, supply requests, and medical records work together to define the financial performance of an organization. The goal of managers is to ensure that their organization makes money during an accounting period, and their actions should be guided by the amount of money earned or lost.

The Information Flow

Structure of the Information System

Information systems can be simplistic or highly complex. They can be fully automated or semi-automated. Occasionally—even today—they can still be generated by hand and not by computer. Manual systems are becoming rare and continue in small and relatively isolated healthcare organizations that are not yet required to electronically submit their billings.

We will examine a particular information system and point out the basic parts a manager should understand. **Figure 2.1** shows information system components for an ambulatory care setting. The organization uses a clinical and financial data repository; in other words, both clinical and financial data are fed into the same system. An automated medical record is also linked to the system.

In addition, the financial information, both outpatient and any relevant inpatient, is fed into the data repository. Scheduling system data also enter the data repository, along with any relevant inpatient care plan and nursing information. This is the basic structure that a manager should recognize about this ambulatory care information system.

One output from the clinical and financial data repository (also shown in Figure 2.1) is insurance verification for patients through an electronic data information (EDI) link to insurance company databases. Insurance verification determines whether a patient has insurance and their coverage for planned services. Another output is decision-making information for managed care planning, including support for demand, utilization, enrollment, and eligibility, plus statistical analysis. The manager does not have to understand the specifics of all the inputs and outputs of this complex system, but he or she should recognize that these outputs occur when ambulatory services are provided.

Function of Flowsheets

Flowsheets illustrate, as in this case, the flow of activities that capture information.[1] Flowsheets are useful because they identify who is responsible for what piece of information as it enters the system. The manager needs to realize the significance of such information. We give, as an example, confirming a patient's address. The manager should know that a correct address for a patient is vital to the smooth operation of the system. An incorrect address will cause third-party billings to be rejected, patient notifications to be misdirected, and so on. Understanding this connection between deficient data such as incorrect addresses, service dates, procedure codes, and the consequences (i.e., the bill will

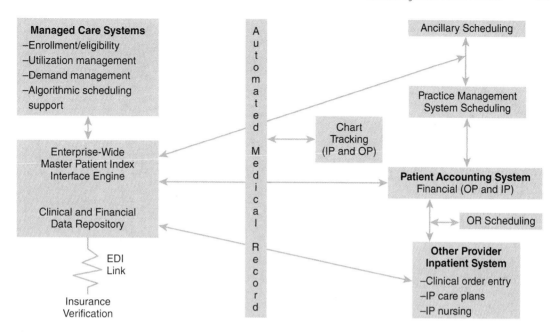

Figure 2.1 Information System Components for an Ambulatory Care Setting. OP, Outpatient; IP, Inpatient; OR, Operating Room

be rejected by the payer and thus not be paid) illustrates the essence of good financial management knowledge.

We can examine two examples of patient information flows. The first, shown in **Figure 2.2**, is a physician's office flowsheet for address confirmation. Four different personnel are involved, in addition to the patient. This physician has computed that the cost of an incorrect address is $12.30 to track down and correct each occurrence. He pays close attention to the handling of this information because he knows there is a direct financial management consequence in his operation.

The second example, shown in **Figure 2.3**, is a health system flowsheet for verification of patient information. This flowsheet illustrates the process for a home care system. In this case, the flow begins not with a receptionist, as in the physician office example, but with a central database. This central database downloads the information and generates a summary report to be reviewed the next day. Appropriate verification is then made in a series of steps, and any necessary corrections are made before the form goes to the

billing department. The object of the flow is the same in both examples—that is, the billing department must have a correct address to receive payment—but the flow is different in the two systems. A manager must understand how the system works to understand that incorrect data will delay or prevent payment for services provided and implement good financial management practices.

Basic System Elements

To understand financial management, it is essential to understand where data comes from and how it is categorized, summarized, and reported. Financial reports begin with a transaction; a good or service is sold or resources are purchased, the transaction is categorized with similar transactions, all transactions of the same type are summarized for an accounting period, and reports are produced. To comprehend financial reports, it is helpful to understand the basic system elements necessary to create the information contained in the reports.

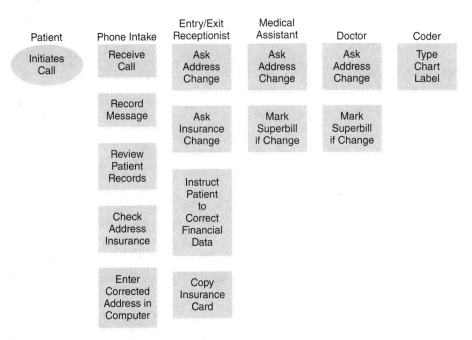

Figure 2.2 Physician's Office Flowsheet for Address Confirmation

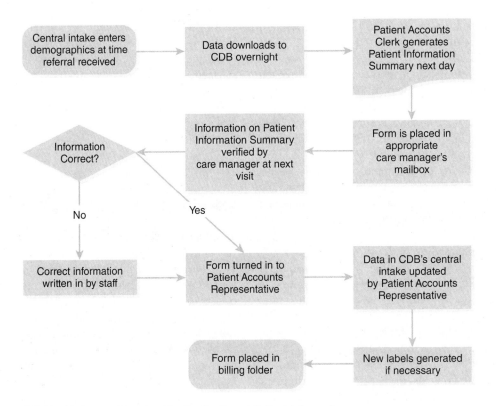

Figure 2.3 Health System Flowsheet for Verification of Patient Information

Chart of Accounts—The Map

The chart of accounts is a map that establishes numeric codes for categorizing expenses, revenues, assets, and liabilities. The goal of the chart of accounts is to compile financial data in a uniform manner that users can understand.

The accounts in the chart of accounts should match the products sold, major expenses, and authority structure of the organization. In other words, the classification on the organization chart (as discussed in Chapter 1) should be compatible with the groupings on the chart of accounts (i.e., department managers should receive reports detailing the revenues, expenses, assets, and liabilities they are responsible for). Thus, if there is a human resource department on your facility's organization chart and expenses are grouped by department, then we would expect to find a human resource grouping in the chart of accounts. Every manager working with financial data needs to understand the chart of accounts to be able to read and comprehend how the dollars are laid out and how they are gathered together, or assembled.

Basic guidance for healthcare charts of accounts is set out in publications such as Seawell's *Chart of Accounts for Hospitals*.[2] However, generic guides are just that—generic. Every organization exhibits differences in its own chart of accounts that express the unique aspects of its structure. We examine three examples to illustrate these differences. Remember, we are spending time on the chart of accounts because your comprehension of detailed financial data may well depend on whether you can decipher your organization's chart of accounts (i.e., how the information forwarded to you is mapped).

The first format, shown in **Exhibit 2.1**, is a basic use where all financial transactions are rolled up into a single responsibility center, probably a smaller organization such as a physician practice. The exhibit is in two horizontal segments, "Structure" and "Example." There are three parts to the account number. The first part is one digit and indicates the financial statement element. Thus, our example shows "1" for "Asset," "2" for "Liability," "3" for "Equity," "4" for "Revenue," and "5"

for "Expense." The second part is two digits and is the primary subclassification (i.e., the type of asset). Our example shows "10," which stands for "Current Asset," and "20" indicates a "Fixed Asset." The third and final part is also two digits and is the secondary subclassification (i.e., the type of current or fixed asset). Our example shows "11," which stands for "Petty Cash—Front Office" in this case. On a report, this account number would appear as 1.10.11, current asset, petty cash.

The second format, shown in **Exhibit 2.2**, is full use that would be used in large organizations when there is more than one responsibility center. The exhibit is again in two horizontal segments, "Structure" and "Example," and there are now two line items appearing in the Example section. The full use example has five parts to the account number. The first part is two digits and indicates the entity designator number. Thus, we conclude that there is more than one entity within this system. Our example shows "10" for "Hospital A," "20" for "Hospital B," and so on. The second part is two digits and indicates the fund designator number. Thus, we conclude that there is more than one fund within this system. In our example, "10" stands for "General Fund" and "15" for "Restricted Funds."

The third part of Exhibit 2.2 is one digit and indicates the financial statement element. Thus, the first line of our example shows "4" for "Revenue." and the second line is "5" for "Expense." The third part of this example is the first part of the example shown in Exhibit 2.1. The fourth part is four digits and is the primary subclassification, the responsibility center within the larger entity. Our example shows "3125" for "Lab—Microbiology" and "3330" for "Physical Therapy," The number 3125 appears on both lines of this example, indicating that both the revenue and the expense belong to Lab—Microbiology. The fourth part of this example is the second part of Exhibit 2.1; Exhibit 2.1 used only two digits for the primary subclassification, but the full use example uses four digits. The fifth and final part is two digits for the secondary subclassification. Our example shows "01" on the first line, the revenue line, which stands for "Payer: Medicare"

Exhibit 2.1 Chart of Accounts, Format I

Structure			
	X	XX	XX
	Financial Statement Element	Primary Subclassification	Secondary Subclassification
Example			
	1	10	11
	Asset	Current Asset	Petty Cash—Front Office
		10	12
		Current Asset	Accounts Receivable
		20	11
		Fixed Asset	Equipment
	2	10	11
	Liability	Current Liability	Accounts Payable
	3	10	11
	Equity	**	Unrestricted Equity
	4	10	11
	Revenue	Operating Revenue	Professional Services
	5	10	10
	Expense	**	Clerical salaries
	(Financial Statement Element)	(Primary Subclassification)	(Secondary Subclassification)

to indicate the source of the revenue. On the second line, the expense line, our example shows "10," which stands for "Clerical Salaries." Therefore, we understand that these are the clerical salaries belonging to Lab—Microbiology in Hospital A. On a report, these account numbers might appear as 10-10-4-3125-01 and 10-10-5-3125-10.

Every organization is unique, and the chart of accounts reflects that uniqueness. **Exhibit 2.3** illustrates a customized use of the chart of accounts adapted from a large hospital system. There are four parts to its chart of accounts number. The first part is an entity designator and designates an organization within the hospital system. The fund designator two-digit part, as traditionally used (see Exhibit 2.2), is missing here. The financial statement element

one-digit part, as traditionally used (see Exhibit 2.2), is also missing here. Instead, the second part of Exhibit 2.3 represents the primary classification, which is shown as an expense category ("Payroll") in the example line. The third part of Exhibit 2.3 is the secondary subclassification, representing a labor subaccount expense designation ("Regular per-Visit RN"). The fourth and final part of Exhibit 2.3 is another subclassification that indicates the department within the organization (e.g., "Home Health"). On a report for this organization, therefore, the account number 21-7000-2201-7151 would indicate the home care services company's payroll for regular per-visit registered nurses (RNs) in the home health department. Finally, remember that time spent understanding your organization's chart of accounts is time well spent.

Exhibit 2.2 Chart of Accounts, Format II

Structure					
	XX	XX	X	XXXX	XX
	Entity Designator	Fund Designator	Financial Statement Element	Primary Subclassification	Secondary Subclassification
Example					
	10	10	4	3125	01
	Hospital A	General Fund	Revenue	Lab—Microbiology	Payer: Medicare
	10	10	5	3125	10
	Hospital A	General Fund	Expense	Lab—Microbiology	Clerical Salaries
	10	10	4	3125	01
	Hospital A	General Fund	Revenue	Physical Therapy	Payer: Medicare
	20	10	4	3125	01
	Hospital B	General Fund	Revenue	Lab—Microbiology	Medicare
	(Entity Designator)	(Fund Designator)	(Financial Statement)	(Primary Subclassification Element)	(Secondary Subclassification Element)

Books and Records—Capture Transactions

The books and records of the financial information system for the organization serve to capture transactions. **Figure 2.4** illustrates the relationship of the books and records to each other. As a single transaction occurs, the process begins. The individual transaction is recorded in the appropriate subsidiary journal. Similar transactions are then grouped and balanced within the subsidiary journal. At periodic intervals, the groups of transactions are gathered, summarized, and entered in the general ledger. Within the general ledger, the transaction groups are reviewed and adjusted. After such review and adjustment, the transactions for the period within the general ledger are balanced. A document known as the trial balance is used for this purpose. The final step in

the process is to create statements from the trial balance to summarize financial performance for the period.

All transactions for the period reside in the general ledger. The **subsidiary journals** are so named because they are "subsidiary" to the general ledger; in other words, they serve to support the general ledger. **Figure 2.5** illustrates this concept. Another way to think of the subsidiary journals is to picture them as feeding the general ledger. The important point here is to understand the source and flow of information as it is recorded.

Reports—The Product

Reports are more fully treated in Chapter 11 of this text. Reports are designed to provide information to decision-makers and are the final product of a process that commences with an original

Exhibit 2.3 **Chart of Accounts, Format III**

Structure				
	XX	XXXX	XXXX	XXXX
	Company Category	Expense	Subaccount	Department
	(Entity Designator)	(Primary Classification)	(Secondary Subclassification)	(Additional Subclassification)
Example				
	21	7000	2200	7151
	Home Care Services	Payroll	Management salaries	Home Health
	21	7000	2201	7151
	Home Care Services	Payroll	Regular per-visit RN	Home Health
	(Company)	(Expense Category)	(Subaccount)	(Department)

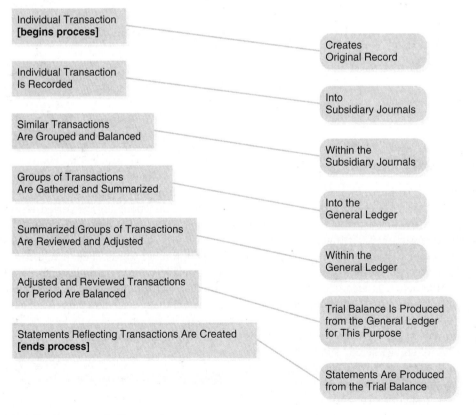

Figure 2.4 The Progress of a Transaction

THE BOOKS

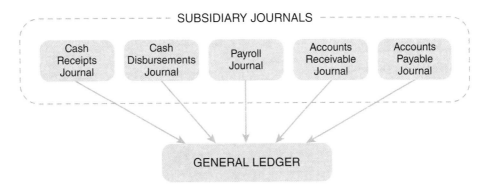

Figure 2.5 Recording Information: Relationship of Subsidiary Journals to the General Ledger

Courtesy of Resource Group, Ltd., Dallas, Texas.

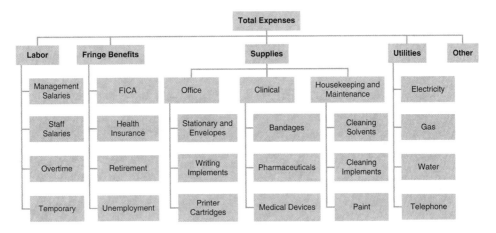

Figure 2.6 Another View of the Chart of Accounts

transaction. The goal of the chart of accounts is to categorize similar transactions so decision-makers understand the revenues, expenses, assets, and liabilities of an organization or department. **Figure 2.6** focuses on expenses to highlight how the chart of accounts can be used to understand organizational and department performance.

A report of simply total expenses would not illuminate how expenses are used, so the chart of accounts divides expenses into salaries, fringe benefits, supplies, utilities, and other expenses. Managers can then determine whether one or more categories of expenses are excessive. If salaries are higher than similar providers, the manager

can then determine why salaries are high. Is the difference due to excessive management or staff salaries, overuse of overtime or temporary staff, or a combination of factors?

The Annual Management Cycle

The annual management cycle affects the type and status of information that the manager is expected to use. Some operating information is "raw"—that is, unadjusted. When the same information has passed further through the accounting system and has been verified, adjusted, and balanced, it will usually vary from the initial raw data. These differences are a part of the process just described.

Daily and Weekly Operating Reports

The daily and weekly operating reports generally contain raw data, as discussed in the preceding paragraph. The purpose of such daily and weekly reports is to provide immediate operating information on output, revenues, and expenses to use for day-to-day management purposes (e.g., are revenues too low or expenses too high and should actions be taken to increase revenue or decrease expenses?).

Monthly and Quarterly Reports and Statistics

The quarterly reports and statistics generally have been verified, adjusted, and balanced. They are called interim reports because they have been generated some time during the reporting period of the organization and not at the end of that period. Managers often use quarterly reports as milestones. A common milestone is the quarterly budget review that compares actual and budgeted revenues and expenses over three months to determine if corrective action is needed before the end of the fiscal year.

Annual Year-End Reports

Most organizations have a 12-month reporting period known as a fiscal year. A fiscal year, therefore, covers a period from the first day of a particular month (e.g., January 1) through the last day of a month that is one year, or 12 months, in the future (e.g., December 31). If we see a heading that reads, "For the year ended June 30," we know that the fiscal year began on July 1 of the previous year. Anything less than a 12-month year is called a "stub period" and is fully spelled out in the heading. If, therefore, an organization is reporting for a three-month stub period ending on December 31, the heading on the report will read, "For the three-month period ended December 31" or "For the period October 1 to December 31."

Annual year-end reports cover the full 12-month reporting period or the fiscal year. Such annual year-end reports are not primarily intended for managers' use. Their primary purpose is reporting the operations of the organization for the year to outsiders or third parties. Annual year-end reports represent the closing out of the information system for a specific reporting period and are used to assess managerial performance; in other words, did the manager meet their financial goals? The recording and reporting of operations will now begin a new cycle with a new year.

Communicating Financial Information to Others

The ability to communicate financial information effectively to others is a valuable skill. It is important to

- Create a report as your method of communication.
- Use accepted terminology.
- Use standard formats that are accepted in the accounting profession.
- Begin with an executive summary.
- Organize the body of the report in a logical flow.
- Place extensive detail into an appendix.

The rest of this book will help you learn how to create such a report. This book will sharpen your communication skills by helping you understand how healthcare finance works.

Responsibility Center Accounting

Effective financial management requires managers be supplied with timely and accurate information on their area(s) of responsibility and have the authority to make decisions. Managers at different levels of an organization have different duties, and those at the highest levels have the greatest responsibilities and authority. Responsibility center accounting clarifies managerial roles. Authority ranges from control over how work is performed at the lowest level to control over what products are produced and where investments will be made at the top of the organization. Responsibility centers include cost, expense, revenue, profit, and **investment centers** and each highlight that managers should only be held accountable for financial performance that is within their control.[3]

Cost Centers

A manager of a **cost center** is responsible for producing an easily measured good or service at the lowest cost (i.e., the number of units produced can be counted). A head nurse or clinical lab manager is responsible for efficiency, minimizing the cost per patient day or lab test while meeting expected quality standards. Their authority extends to determining how work is performed and the mix of inputs (i.e., the amount of labor, supplies, and equipment used). Cost center managers should not be evaluated on volume or profit as they have no control over product mix or selling prices.

Expense Centers

Expense centers, unlike cost centers, do not produce an easily measured good or service; the output of expense centers is more subjective. Examples of expense centers include accounting, human resources, public relations, and research and development. The output of these departments is subjective; the role of these departments is clear, but the quality of the service delivered is not easily measured (i.e., what is the quality of hires, accounting reports, or research?). The manager of an expense center should be responsible for minimizing the cost per service where the appropriateness of cost should be measured against departments in similar size organizations (e.g., is the accounting department staff and budget comparable to similar size organizations?). The authority of expense center managers extends to determining how work is performed and the mix of inputs, labor, supplies, and equipment used, and these managers should not be evaluated

on volume or profit as they have no control over product mix or selling prices.

Revenue Centers

Revenue centers are responsible for selling activities; they should maximize revenue based on a given price for goods and services and a fixed budget for inputs, labor, supplies, and equipment. Revenue center managers' authority extends to determining how work is performed and the mix of inputs, labor, supplies, and equipment used; like cost and expense center managers, they should not be evaluated on profit as they have no control over product mix or selling prices.

Profit Centers

Profit center managers have the authority to set prices and decide the type of products to sell in addition to making input mix decisions. Given their broader authority and responsibilities, profit center managers should be assessed on the difference between budgeted and actual profits (i.e., superior performance would result in higher than budgeted profits). The accounting system should thus provide the information needed to determine if profit center managers have made optimal decisions on input mix, product mix, and pricing.

Investment Centers

Investment center managers, typically the chief executives, should be assessed on return on investment. A profit center manager should maximize profit given a fixed set of resources; the investment center manager has additional authority to determine where future investments should be made (i.e., identify and invest in the areas that will provide the highest returns in the future). These managers determine not only where future investments should be made but also the level of investment. Their performance should be measured against similar organizations (i.e., superior investment center managers should earn higher profits than their peer group).

Accounting systems should define managers' goals and provide them with the information and incentives they need to meet these goals.

WRAP-UP

Summary

Understanding healthcare finance begins with knowing how data enters the system, is collected and organized, and finally is reported. Managers should understand (1) the original records (initiating event), (2) the information system (data collection), (3) the accounting system (how it is organized), and (4) the reporting system (what is distributed). Effective management requires managers know where information comes from, how it flows and is grouped, what it is needed for, and the consequences of bad information.

Managers should understand the role and structure of the chart of accounts, subsidiary ledgers, general ledger, trial balance, and reports to gain the maximum information from the financial system and take effective action when needed. The goal of responsibility center accounting is to highlight a manager's areas of responsibility and supply information to allow them to assess their performance.

Key Terms

Accounting System

Chart of Accounts

Cost Center

Expense Center

General Ledger

Information System

Investment Center

Original Records

Profit Center

Reporting System

Revenue Center

Subsidiary Journals

Trial Balance

Discussion Questions

1. Describe the four parts of a financial management system.
2. Describe the information flow needed to record and bill patient services. What are the potential consequences of poor information?
3. Describe the role of the chart of accounts, subsidiary ledgers, general ledger, trial balance, and financial reports.
4. Explain the role of weekly, monthly or quarterly, and annual reports in the annual management cycle.
5. Explain the goal of responsibility center accounting.

Notes

1. J. J. Baker, *Activity-Based Costing and Activity-Based Management for Health Care* (Gaithersburg, MD: Aspen Publishers, Inc., 1998).
2. L. V. Seawell, *Chart of Accounts for Hospitals* (Chicago: Probus Publishing Company, 1994).
3. J. A. Brickley, C. W. Smith, and J. L. Zimmerman, *Managerial Economics and Organizational Architecture,* 2nd ed (Boston, MA: McGraw-Hill Irwin, 2001).

CHAPTER 3

Using Excel

PROGRESS NOTES

After you complete this chapter, you should be able to

1. Create an Excel worksheet, enter data, sort the table, and save the file.
2. Add, subtract, multiply, and divide using mathematical operators and understand fixed cell references and order of operation.
3. Use and interpret formulas.
4. Create and interpret graphs.

Overview: Excel

Excel is an essential tool for gaining insight into financial information and operating performance. Excel is used for data storage, data analysis using mathematical operators and formulas, and information reporting using tables and graphs. Excel links finance to data analysis and facilitates identifying where improvements should be made to increase value for patients, employees, and/or organization owners. Financial data is an unintelligible mass of numbers to most people; transforming data into information, information into knowledge, and knowledge to effective action requires understanding where the data came from, determining if data are valid, and converting them into meaningful information that people can understand and use to make decisions and take action.

Plans generally fail when the supporting data are wrong or the information gained from the data is inappropriately used. Managers should recognize that the data collected and/or reported on system performance may not be accurate and should not be used for decision-making until they are critically assessed. Data often do not reflect how systems perform; this may be due to poor data collection or attempts by those working in the system to make themselves look good. Avoiding the garbage in, garbage out problem requires the ability to assess and correct data when needed—the launch point for effective action. Second, after validating the data, we must have the skills to transform it into the information needed for a particular situation at a particular point of time. Applying a proven action to an inappropriate situation or at the wrong time may be useless if not detrimental. Excel is a tool that enables us to assess the validity of data and obtain the information needed for effective decision-making and action.

Navigating the Ribbon

Excel is a spreadsheet program that stores and manipulates data, numbers and words, in tables and creating useful information requires

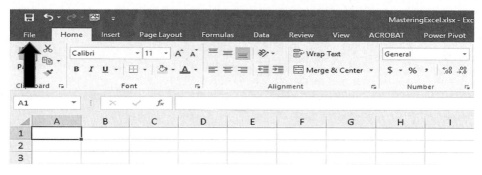

Figure 3.1 The Excel Ribbon

mastering its capabilities. Excel proficiency begins with the Ribbon. First-time Excel users can be overwhelmed by the 10 tabs on the Ribbon (**Figure 3.1**) and the hundreds of underlying functions. The journey to better financial skills begins with the **File** tab. **File** provides the ability to create worksheets, access existing worksheets, save updates, and print a worksheet or portion of a worksheet.

The first step is creating a worksheet or accessing a previously created worksheet. When creating a worksheet, the manager must select **File <tab>** and **New <function>** on the next screen. Excel provides a multitude of formats, such as a blank workbook, calendars, budgets, and invoices, geared for different tasks. Selecting **Blank workbook** provides a blank series of rows (indicated by numbers) and columns (indicated by letters). When a user wants to update an existing worksheet, the user selects **File** and **Open <function>.** Recently updated files are shown in the third column, and the user can right-click on the desired file. When the file has not been recently updated, the user must use 🗁 **Browse** to access other files. Once a file has been created, data must be entered into its cells; once entered, the data can be summarized or manipulated using Excel's mathematical operators and functions (discussed later).

After data are entered or existing data have been summarized or otherwise manipulated, the file must be saved to retain the changes. The user selects **File** and **Save/Save As** to save changes. **Save** requires the user to enter a file name and

specify where the file will be saved (e.g., 🌐 One-Drive, 🖥 This PC, or ➕ Add a Place for a new file). Saving changes to an existing file overwrites the original file (i.e., modifies, supplements, and/or deletes existing data). The file will remain open until the user selects **File** and **Close** to exit the worksheet. If you select **Close** without saving your updates, Excel will prompt, "Want to save your changes to 'Your File Name.xlsx'"? and you must select Save, Don't Save, or Cancel to save the file, exit without updating, or continuing working, respectively. When you want to save recent work without overwriting the existing file, select **Save As** and enter a new file name to retain the original file.

The third critical function on the **File** tab is **Print**, which allows the user to print all or portions of a worksheet. Print allows the user to specify the printer where the document will be printed and the range of rows and columns to print and to review what the printout will look like before it is printed. The Print Area and Preview functions are essential when working with large data sets when you do not want to print every row and column in a spreadsheet and you want to see what the output will look like before it is printed. We will return to tailoring print outputs in **Page Layout, Page Setup**.

The second tab, **Home**, provides the ability to cut and paste data, set fonts, format numbers, and insert and delete rows and columns. The **Clipboard** function provides the ability to move or copy data from one cell to another. Users highlight the cells to be moved and select **Cut** to move the data to a new location or **Copy** to copy the highlighted data to new cells and leave the numbers or formulas in the original location. After Cut or Copy is chosen, the user moves to the destination cell and selects **Paste** to move or copy the highlighted data to the new location. **Paste** provides six options: **Paste (P)** retains the content of the originating cell (numbers or formulas) and increments the rows and columns to the new location, **Value (V)** enters the number only (i.e., formulas are converted to their sum, difference, product, or quotient), **Formula (F)** retains the formulas in the originating cell, **Transpose (T)** shifts the rows to columns and columns to rows in the destination cells, **Formatting (R)** does not transfer the numbers or formulas in the originating cells but only the format (i.e., font, font size, bold, italic, underline,…), and **Paste Link (N)** is for copying hypertext links. **Cut** can also be used to remove unwanted data.

Proper formatting of numbers is essential to convey information. **Home** and **Number** provide 12 formatting options. Entering 200000 results in 200000 appearing in a cell, which is difficult to interpret; selecting **Currency ($)** translates this value into dollars with commas separating every three numbers and two decimal places (i.e., $200,000.00). **Percentage (%)** converts the value to 200000.00%, and **Number (,)** results in 200,000.00. Users can increase the number of decimal points by selecting ←0.0 or reduce the number of decimal points by selecting →0.0. Other formatting options include **Date**, **Time**, and **Scientific**. Right-clicking while in a cell also allows formatting to be changed. **Format Cells…** is the fourth to last option on the pop-up menu.

The **Insert <third tab>**, **Tables** function allows users to create PivotTables and Tables. **PivotTable** allows users to summarize data and highlight relationships between two or more variables in a data set; PivotTables are a powerful yet complex function and cannot be given their due in a short review. **Table** requires the user to identify variables to include in the rows and columns of a table. **Table** transforms the data entered into rows and columns into eye-appealing and dynamic

tables. First, it applies different color background for titles and alternating colors for rows. Second, it facilitates data sorting by column and gives a manager the ability to determine what is presented in a table, all data or simply the observations that meet a user-defined criteria (e.g., **Number Filters** allow a user to display only patients over or under a defined age or males or females).

One of Excel's strongest features is the ability to create **Charts**; a picture is worth a thousand words, and a single chart can convey more information than a data table, especially tables with numerous rows and columns. Selecting **Insert** and **Charts** allows a user to produce pie, column, run, scatter, and other charts. This feature will be explored further in **Graphing**.

The **Page Layout <fourth tab>**, **Page Setup** function allows a user to specify the parts of a worksheet to print. Simply selecting **Print** (on the File tab) and **Print** prints the entire spreadsheet; multiple pages of output will be printed when there are more than 26 rows and/or 7 columns of data. Selecting **Margins** from **Page Setup** allows a user to increase or decrease the top, bottom, left, and right margins. **Scale to Fit** allows a user to specify the paper orientation and size of print. Under **Orientation**, selecting ⭕ **Portrait** prints the specified print range on 8.5-inch-wide-by-11-inch-tall paper; Portrait is the default and should be used when the print area has more rows than columns. Selecting ⭕ **Landscape** prints the output on 11-inch-wide-by-8.5-inch-tall paper and should be used when the print area has more columns than rows. Under **Scaling**, selecting ⭕ **Adjust to:** allows the user to increase or decrease the size of the printing. More useful is the ⭕ **Fit to:** feature, which automatically calculates the font size required to print the specified print area on the desired number of pages; the default is 1 page wide by 1 page tall. **Size** allows the user to specify the paper to be printed on. The default is standard letter size (8.5-by-11-inch); other sizes can be selected including legal (8.5-by-14-inch). Assume you have a file with 1,000 rows of data; Print will produce 22 pages of output. Few people want to see all your data, so the user should select **Print Area** to limit printing to a user-defined range of rows and columns (i.e., a summary versus every row and column).

After **Print…** is selected, Excel displays on the screen what the printout will look like when it is printed. If the printout is satisfactory, the user should click on **Print** to create the hard-copy output. When the printout is unsatisfactory, the user should move to Setting and Print Active Sheets or specify a page range, Portrait Orientation, Letter (size of paper), Normal Margins, and/or No Scaling to respecify what should be printed and how it should be printed. These options are also available on the **Print** function on the **File** tab.

Formulas <fifth tab> is another Excel strongpoint as worksheets are designed to process numeric data. Formulas can be typed into a cell or inserted using **Insert Function** or the **Function Library**. There are more than 400 functions listed alphabetically or by category such as Financial, Logical, and so on. After a function is used, it is stored in the Recently Used ▼ category for ease of reuse. Formulas will be explored in the **Mathematical Operations** section.

Under **Data <sixth tab>**, **Sort & Filter** is an essential function as it allows a manager to assess the accuracy of and understand the data they are working with. Sort requires the manager to specify the column to sort on (**Sort by**) and what to sort

(**Sort On**) with options of **Values, Cell Color, Font Color,** or **Cell Icon** and **Order** with the options of **Smallest to Largest, Largest to Smallest, A to Z, Z to A,** or **Custom List**. A simple ascending or descending sort of cell value can highlight potential data problems. Are the minimum and maximum values reasonable or possible?

Assume the chief medical officer (CMO) wants to assess the productivity of hospitalists during the first six months of the year and received the following data table listing the number of patients seen and total charges by physician number from lowest to highest (**Table 3.1**). Create a new Excel file (i.e., Blank workbook) and enter these values into the spreadsheet as subsequent work will utilize this data. The table requires effort to determine which physician is seeing the most and fewest patients and generating the highest and lowest charges.

A more useful presentation given the goal is to understand productivity would rank hospitalists based on the number of patients seen and format charges as currency with no decimals. Resorting Table 3.1 from the most to fewest admissions requires highlighting cells starting with "Hospitalist" and ending with "4466406.62" (three columns and eleven rows), clicking on **Data**, clicking on **Sort**, moving to **Sort by** and selecting

Table 3.1 Patients Seen by Hospitalists

Physician #	Total Admissions	Total Charges
156	407	2926400.49
175	329	2252902.74
188	573	3214040.14
206	525	2800595.38
207	757	4549200.79
217	489	2853997.96
230	448	2086428.57
251	425	2595588.24
263	349	2318065.90
311	846	4466406.62

Table 3.2 Hospitalists Ranked from Most to Fewest Patients Seen

Physician #	Total Admissions	Total Charges	
311	846	$4,466,407	Maximum
207	757	$4,549,201	
188	573	$3,214,040	
206	525	$2,800,595	
217	489	$2,853,998	Midpoint
230	448	$2,086,429	
251	425	$2,595,588	
156	407	$2,926,400	
263	349	$2,318,066	
175	329	$2,252,903	Minimum

Total Admissions, moving to **Order** and selecting **Largest to Smallest**, and hitting **OK**, converts Table 3.1 to **Table 3.2**.

Table 3.2 is easier to interpret than Table 3.1; hospitalist #311 treats the most patients, 846, and #175 the fewest, 329. The CMO can quickly identify physicians seeing the most and fewest patients and generating the highest charges during the period. The CMO can also get a feel for the average number of patients seen by a hospitalist by looking at the midpoint of the table. These hospitalists on average see between 448 and 489 patients every six months.

Table 3.3 supplies a quick reference guide to the most common Excel functions residing under the eight primary Excel tabs; **Review** and **View** <seventh and eighth tabs> were not discussed as the authors do not believe either supplies essential functions. Mastering the highlighted essential functions will make your tasks easier and improve the quality of your analyses.

After familiarizing yourself with the tabs and their underlying functions, you are ready for more advanced features. Mathematical operators allow you to add, subtract, multiply, and divide numbers in a cell by the values in other cells or constants.

Mathematical Operators

Data must be processed to create information and understand the system from which the data were drawn. Data processing often requires adding, subtracting, multiplying, and dividing values. For example, effective management of healthcare resources and operations requires knowing mortality rates (versus the number of deaths), average length of stay (versus total patient days), and average reimbursement and cost (versus total revenue and expense) to determine if outcomes, admitting and discharge decisions, prices, and/or use of staff, supplies, and equipment are appropriate.

Excel is designed to perform mathematical operations on the data entered into its cells—adding (+), subtracting (-), multiplying (*), and dividing (/) cells or raising a cell by an exponent (^). A data file (**Table 3.4**) has been compiled with the results of 50 normal deliveries at a hospital from October through December, available in the accompanying Excel files. The 50 individual entries provide little information, so we will use mathematical operators and formulas to gain insight into financial performance. The data file contains patient number, the month of admission, admitting physician number, reimbursement, cost, and length of stay (LOS) by

Table 3.3 Excel Function Quick Reference

Tab: File	Home	Insert	Page Layout	Formulas	Data	Review	View
Info	Clipboard (Copy/Paste)	Tables	Themes	Insert Function	Get External Data	Proofing	Workbook Views
New	Font	Illustrations	Page Setup	Function Library	Get & Transform	Insight	Show
Open	Alignment	Add-ins	Scale to Fit	Defined Names	Connections	Languages	Zoom
Save	Numbers	Charts	Sheet Options	Formula Auditing	Sort & Filter	Comments	Windows
Save As	Styles	Sparklines	Arrange	Calculation	Data Tools	Changes	Macros
Save as Adobe PDF	Cells (Insert, Delete & Format)	Filters			Forecast		
Print	Editing	Links			Outline		
…		Text			Analyze (add-in)		
Options		Symbols					

Table 3.4 Inpatient Admissions

	A	B	C	D	E	F
5	Patient #	Reimbursement	Cost	LOS	MD	Month
6	1	$6,966	$6,769	3	114	October
7	2	$8,537	$6,689	2	114	October
8	3	$6,498	$6,871	2	232	October
9	4	$6,768	$6,163	2	295	October
10	5	$6,715	$6,529	2	114	October
⋮	⋮	⋮	⋮	⋮	⋮	⋮
55	50	$4,846	$6,551	2	295	December

patient; Table 3.4 displays the first five admissions and the 50th admission.

This data file provides a lot of data but little information, so a first step is calculating the profit per admission, reimbursement minus cost; in Excel, the user would type =B6-C6 into cell G6. When the first entry in a cell is "=", "+", or "−," it informs Excel that a mathematical operation will occur. Typing B6-C6 into G6 would produce the label "B6-C6" rather than a number. For the first admission, patient #1 generated $197 in profit for the hospital, $6,966 – $6,769. The amount of profit (or loss) should vary by how long a patient is hospitalized, so we will calculate the profit margin, profit divided by reimbursement. Typing =G6/B6 in cell H6 shows that patient #1 generated a 2.8% profit on reimbursement.

Similarly, we may want to examine the cost per day to determine if cost is high due to length of stay or high resource use per day. Cost per day is calculated as =C6/E6. Similar work is required to multiply (=B6*G6 = profit), add (=C6+G6 = reimbursement), or raise a number by an exponent (=A6^2 would square the patient number $1^2 = 1$; a better example is A7, as A7^2 produces 4, $2^2 = 4$). The next step is to copy the formulas from G6 and I6 to the end of the file (line 55). Highlight cells G6 through I6, select **Copy**, simultaneously depress **Crtl**, **Shift**, and (down arrow) to move to the last row (the equations can also be dragged down the worksheet using the square in the bottom, right hand corner of cell F6), and hit

Enter ↵; profit, profit margin, and cost per day are calculated for every patient. **Table 3.5** shows the results of the mathematical calculations.

A review of the first five patients in Table 3.5 suggests that routine deliveries are a profitable service; four out of five patients produced a profit, with a cost of approximately $3,000 per day. Formulas provide the ability to quickly determine the actual profit, profit margin, and average cost per day for all 50 patients.

Fixed Cell References

When copying an equation with cell references from one cell down the worksheet, Excel increments the row number (1 to 2 to 3…), and when cells are copied across a worksheet, the column is incremented (A to B to C…). There are times when a manager wants to add, subtract, multiply, or divide a cell by a constant (e.g., divide the profit margin for patients by the average profit margin for all patients to identify patients with significantly higher or lower margins). In the data files supporting Chapter 3, you may have noticed the use of "$" before column letters or cells; the author used the dollar sign to ensure that rows or columns were not incremented when copying cells to other cells.

Fixed cell references are created by placing a $ in front of the column letter and/or row number. The manager may also use the F4 function key while on an equation; hitting F4 once fixes the column and row, $Column$Row (i.e.,

Table 3.5 Inpatient Admissions with Mathematical Operations

Patient #	Reimbursement	Cost	LOS	MD	Month	Profit	Profit Margin	Cost per Day
1	$6,966	$6,769	3	A	October	$197	2.8%	$2,256
2	$8,537	$6,689	2	A	October	$1,848	21.6%	$3,345
3	$6,498	$6,871	2	B	October	-$373	-5.7%	$3,436
4	$6,768	$6,163	2	C	October	$605	8.9%	$3,082
5	$6,715	$6,529	2	A	October	$186	2.8%	$3,265
...	...	...	...	...	...	...	...	...

Excel always references the same cell). Hitting F4 a second time fixes the row and allows the column to increment, Column$Row. Hitting F4 a third time fixes the column but allows the row to increment, $ColumnRow. If F4 is hit again, a fourth time, the columns and rows return to their original form; columns and rows are incremented as cells and are copied down or across the worksheet. For example, the variation in total cost for a patient could be calculated as =C6/C57, where the C57 is the calculated average cost for all 50 patients (e.g., patient #1's cost is 1.024 or 2.4% higher than average).

Order of Operation

The order in which mathematical operations are performed has a substantial impact on the result; for example, what is the result of 2 multiplied by 3 plus 4? The answer could be 10 ([2 × 3] + 4) or 14 (2 × [3 + 4]). When =2*3+4 is entered into a cell, Excel calculates 10; when 14 is the desired result, the user must enter =2*(3+4). Excel calculations use the following rule: Data enclosed in <u>P</u>arentheses are calculated first, followed by <u>E</u>xponents, <u>D</u>ivision and <u>M</u>ultiplication, and finally <u>A</u>ddition and <u>S</u>ubtraction (**PEDMAS**). You should review all complicated calculations to ensure that the equations are properly structured so the results are correct.

Formulas

If we wanted to know total cost for all 50 patients in Table 3.4, we could type =C6+C7+C8...C55, but specifying 50 cells in the calculation would be time-consuming. Calculating the profit and profit margin per patient was easy, but calculating total profit, average profit per patient, and average profit margin requires the use of formulas (**Figure 3.2**). Excel supplies numerous formulas to facilitate mathematical operations; these functions can be inserted into a cell by selecting the **Formulas** tab and **Insert Function** or **Function Library** or by typing the formula directly into a cell.

When **Insert Function** is selected, the user receives the following screen (**Figure 3.3**).

To determine the total reimbursement for the 50 patients, type =SUM(B6:B55) (or select =SUM from the Insert Function menu, enter B6:B55 in the **Number1** range, and hit **OK**) into cell B56 and hit **Enter↵**. Likewise typing =SUM(C6:C55) into cell C56 calculates total cost, and subtracting total cost from total reimbursement provides total profit, $336,272 – $330,463 = $5,809. To calculate the average profit margin, 1.7%, type =G56/B56 in cell H56 and hit Enter.

To calculate the average reimbursement, type =AVERAGE(B6:B55) in cell B57, $6,725; copying the formula to columns C and G shows that average cost is $6,609 and average profit is $116. Note in column G that when the average profit margin formula was copied to all patients, it produced #DIV/0! because two patients had zero reimbursement and a number cannot be divided by zero. Other measures of central tendency that can be calculated include the median, which is the number that separates the highest 50% from the lowest 50%, =MEDIAN(range); and the mode, the most frequently occurring value, =MODE(range).

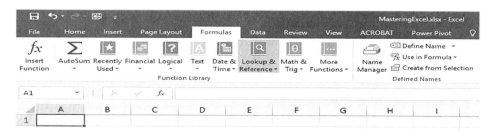

Figure 3.2 The Formulas Tab

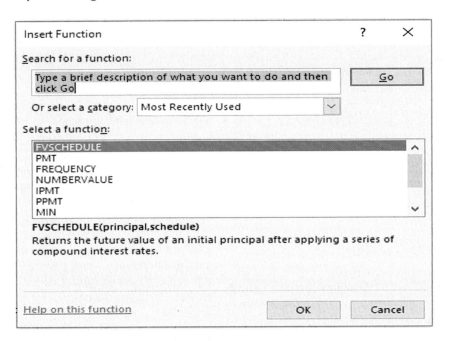

Figure 3.3 Insert Function Screen

Table 3.6 highlights 10 of the most frequently used formulas plus two closely related formulas.

After assessing profitability, we can assess the variation in patient reimbursement and cost (i.e., the maximum and minimum reimbursement and cost per patient). The MAX(range) formula reports the highest value in the group, =MAX(B6:B55) reports the highest reimbursement was $9,551, and =MIN(B6:B55) reports $0.00 (no pay), a range of $9,551. **Table 3.7** reports the average, minimum, maximum, range, and standard deviation for reimbursement and cost for the 50 patients.

Table 3.6 Commonly Used Excel Formulas

1. =SUM(number1, [number2], ...): sums the total in a defined range (e.g., cost).
2. =SUMIF(range, criteria, [sum_range]): sums the total for all cells in a range meeting a defined criteria (e.g., total cost for MD 114, =SUMIF(E6:E55,"114",C6:C55)).
3. =AVERAGE(number1, [number2], ...): calculates the mean for a defined range (e.g., mean cost or LOS). Closely related functions: =MEDIAN and =MODE.
4. =AVERAGEIF(range, criteria, [average_range]): calculates the mean for all cells in a range meeting a defined criteria (e.g., average cost for MD 114, =AVERAGEIF(E6:E55,"114",C6:C55)).
5. =MAX(number1, [number2], ...): reports the largest value in a range (e.g., cost).
6. =MIN(number1, [number2], ...): reports the smallest value in a range (e.g., cost).
7. =STDEV(number1, [number2], ...): reports the standard deviation for values in a defined range (e.g., cost).
8. =COUNT(value1, [value2], ...): counts the number of cells in a defined range with numbers (e.g., total patients by counting patient number, cost, or LOS).
9. =COUNTA(value1, [value2], ...): counts the number of cells in a range that are not blank (e.g., total patients by counting MD or month).
10. =COUNTIF(range, criteria): counts the number of cells in a range with a defined value (e.g., total patients for MD A, =COUNTIF(E6:E55,"114")).

Table 3.7 Variability of Reimbursement and Cost

	Reimbursement	Cost
Mean	$6,725	$6,609
Maximum	9,551	7,759
Minimum	0	5,705
Range	9,551	2,054
Standard deviation	1,872	465

Range reports variability using only the two extreme values; standard deviation incorporates every case to calculate a value that specifies the percent of observations that should fall within a specified range from the mean assuming the variable follows a normal or bell curve distribution. Entering =STDEV(C6:C55) and hitting **Enter↵** produces a standard deviation for average cost per admission of $465. Assuming the cost per patient is normally distributed, 68% of cases should fall between $6,144 and $7,074, $6,609 ± $465 (one standard deviation), and 95% should cost between $5,679 and $7,540, $6,609 ± 2 × $465 (two standard deviations). Knowing how many observations *should* fall within a defined range allows managers to determine whether their population is normal or if there is an excessive number of high and/or low values. When more than 2.5% (5% ÷ 2) of patients have a cost greater than $7,540, managers may want to investigate the cause for the large number of high-cost cases and whether corrective action is necessary.

Data users often need to know the number of people or events in a data set to determine if information gathered is valid (i.e., is the information based on all members of the population or a subset?). When the count does not match the population total, a user should consider if the information gathered should be used to draw conclusions about or institute action for other groups. The =COUNT formula reports the number of cells with numbers (i.e., =COUNT(B6:B55) = 50). When a cell contains alphabetic characters, =COUNTA(range) will report the number of

cells with nonnumeric data; this formula can be used to count the number of patients by physician (i.e., =COUNTA(E6:E55) = 50). A third useful count formula is =COUNTIF(range, criteria, [average_range]), which only reports the number of cells meeting a user-defined criteria (e.g., how many patients did physician A treat?). Entering =COUNTIF(E6:E55,"A") reports 23 patients; 46% of all patients were treated by physician A.

Formulas supply insight into data. We now know total and average reimbursement, cost, and profit and have the ability to extract the same values for specific physicians using =AVERAGEIF(range, criteria) so interventions can be targeted to areas where they can produce the greatest improvement. Improvement often requires convincing others that change is needed, and graphs are often the best way to present information.

Graphing

Excel's graphing capabilities are another of its strongpoints. Graphs allow vast amounts of data to be understood using pictures. Users can contrast size across groups, see trends over time, and highlight the relationship between two variables. More sophisticated graphing allows users to determine whether a variable is normally distributed (i.e., are there few or many extreme cases in a data set?).

Insert Pie or Doughnut Chart

The different forms of hospital ownership were discussed in Chapter 1, but that discussion did not demonstrate the composition of the industry. **Table 3.8** shows the distribution of hospitals by ownership in 2018, available in the accompanying Excel files. Careful review of the table shows that nonprofits make up more than half of all hospitals, one-quarter are for-profits, and fewer than 20% are public, federal, state, or local organizations.

The benefit of charts over data tables is charts can quickly convey information while data tables require examination. Creating a pie chart for hospital ownership requires highlighting the % of Total column, 18.6% through 24.9%; selecting **Insert** and **Insert Pie or**

Table 3.8 Hospitals by Ownership

Ownership	% of Total
Public	18.6%
Nonprofit	56.5%
For-profit	24.9%
Total	100.0%

Doughnut Chart (in Charts); and choosing **2-D Pie** (or 3-D Pie). You should not include the Total, 100.0%, in the range as the Pie chart will then calculate shares based on 200% rather than 100%. When the column highlighted includes a heading, % of Total, the heading will be the title of the chart. Otherwise "Chart Title" will be displayed (which can be clicked on and edited). Similarly, if the Ownership column is highlighted, the data labels will be included in the chart. When the labels are not highlighted, they can be inserted by right-clicking while within a chart, selecting **Select Data**, clicking on **Edit** under **Horizontal (Category) Axis Labels**, entering the range for Ownership in the **Axis label range:** input box, and hitting **OK**.

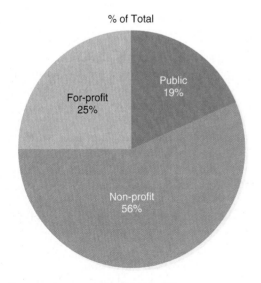

% of Total

Figure 3.4 Hospitals by Ownership

Figure 3.4 immediately conveys the composition of the hospital industry; nonprofits dominate, and the number of for-profit hospitals is considerably larger than public hospitals.

Insert Column or Bar Chart

Column and bar charts are used to display the numeric differences between groups. Column charts place the variables of interest on the x-axis and the magnitude of the variable on the y-axis; bar charts place the variables on the y-axis and their numeric values on the x-axis. **Table 3.9** shows the difference in life expectancy across educational groups, available in the accompanying Excel files.

Creating a column chart for the difference in life expectancy across educational groups requires highlighting the Education and Life expectancy columns, selecting **Insert** and **Insert Column or Bar Chart** (in Charts), and choosing **2-D Column** (or 3-D Column). The vertical axis label "Life expectancy (years)" was inserted by accessing **Chart Tools** (a new tab), **Design**, **Add Chart Element ▼**, **Axis Titles**, and **Primary Vertical**.

Figure 3.5 is a vast improvement over Table 3.9 and highlights life expectancy increases with the amount of education a person has completed. The leap in life expectancy corresponds with going to college; those with a high school education or less have a life expectancy of 70.8 to 72.8 years, and obtaining an associate's degree increases life expectancy by 5.9 years. Additional education, completing

Table 3.9 Education and Life Expectancy

Education	Life Expectancy (years)
Less than high school	70.8
High school	72.8
Associate	78.7
Bachelor	81.5
Master+	82.2

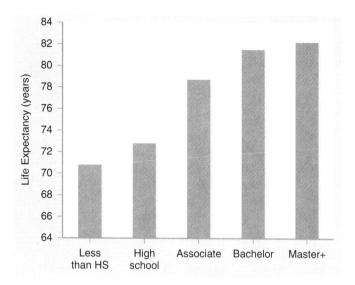

Figure 3.5 Column Chart of Life Expectancy by Education

a four-year or master's degree, increases life expectancy by 2.8 and 3.5 years over an associate's degree.

Insert Line or Area Chart

Assume you want to know how operating margins have changed over time. Is financial performance improving, stable, or deteriorating? **Table 3.10** shows average hospital operating margins from 2011 through 2015.[1] (These data are available in the accompanying Excel files.) As a manager, you should ask whether your organization is above or below the average and whether its performance is moving in the same direction as the industry. Line or Run charts visually display the change in a variable over time.

Examining Table 3.10 does not reveal much information. Operating margins vary from 3.0% to 3.8%, so the next step is to create a run chart with the variable of interest on the y-axis and time on the x-axis. The manager should highlight the operating margin column, select **Insert, Insert Run or Area Chart** (in Charts), and choose **2-D Line**. The run chart (**Figure 3.6**) shows the variability of operating margins over time, and it lacks a clear trend. The operating margin in 2015 exceeds 2011,

Table 3.10 Hospital Operating Margins

Year	Operating Margin
2011	3.0%
2012	3.4%
2013	3.2%
2014	3.2%
2015	3.8%

but additional insight can be obtained by inserting a **trend line** into the run chart; right-click on any data point, select **Add Trendline, Linear,** and press **Enter**.

The trend line shows an upward trend from 2011 to 2015; the best-fitting line begins at slightly over 3% in 2011 and ends at slightly more than 3.5% in 2015. Managers may believe and act on the assumption that the trend will continue but should recognize the reduction between 2012 and 2013 (i.e., operating margin may decrease from year to year).

Add Trendline provides multiple options for inserting the best-fitting line for the data, **Trendline Options** include exponential, linear, logarithmic, and polynomial lines. **Exponential** should be used when a variable increases

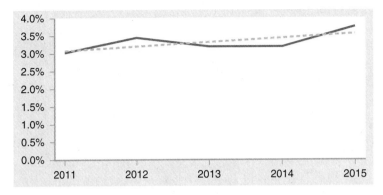

Figure 3.6 Operating Margins, 2011–2015

or decreases at an increasing rate (e.g., compounding of interest on an investments). **Linear** should be used when a variable increases at a constant rate (i.e., a straight line). **Logarithmic** should be used for variables that increase or decrease at a decreasing rate (i.e., diminishing returns); increases in one variable have a decreasing effect on another. For example, public health expenditures initially target the most at-risk populations and produce large health gains; expanding screening or vaccination to lower-risk groups produces lower health improvements. **Polynomial** should be used when a DV increases <u>and</u> decreases over time. An order 2 polynomial function has a single turning point, a peak or trough, an order 3 function has two turning points.

Insert Scatter (X, Y) or Bubble Chart

Scatter or XY diagrams plot a set of coordinates in a two-dimensional space to determine if a change in one variable is correlated with changes in another variable (i.e., are increases or decreases in one variable associated with changes in another variable?). The variable plotted on the x-axis is the variable expected to predict or cause a change in another variable—that is, the independent variable (IV). The variable plotted on the y-axis is the variable expected to be changed by increases or decreases in the independent variable, the dependent variable (DV). For example, does the

number of hospital beds (IV) predict operating margin (DV) (**Table 3.11**, available in the accompanying Excel files)?[2]

Scatter diagrams reveal four types of relationships between two variables: positive, negative, nonlinear, or no relationship. A positive or direct relationship exists when an increase (decrease) in the IV is accompanied by an increase (decrease) in the DV; in this example, are operating margins higher in hospitals with more beds? A negative or inverse relationship exists when an increase in the IV is accompanied by a decrease in the DV or vice versa; that is, does operating margin fall as bed size increases? A nonlinear relationship exists when the DV increases with increases in the IV up to a point and thereafter decreases or vice versa; that is, are operating margins low for small and large hospitals and higher for hospitals with 100 to 299 beds or vice versa? No relationship

Table 3.11 Beds and Operating Margin

	(X or IV)	(Y or DV)
Beds	Bed size	Operating Margin
<25	12	2.97%
25–99	50	3.30%
100–199	150	3.85%
200–299	250	4.88%
300–399	350	4.69%
>400	450	5.38%

exists when the DV shows no definite changes with changes in the IV; that is, operating margin does not change with increases or decreases in the number of beds.

Figure 3.7 plots the relationship between operating margin (Y) and bed size (X). Note that an average bed size was calculated to provide a single *x*-coordinate for each range, column 2 [e.g., (100 + 199) ÷ 2]. The scatter diagram shows that operating margins increase with bed size. The strength of the relationship between the IV and DV can be assessed by the distance between the points and the trend line. When points lie on or close to the trend line, it shows that changes in the DV closely track changes in the IV. Managers should be less confident that the DV moves with changes in the IV when points are far from the trend line (i.e., changing the DV will be less likely to produce the desired effect). In this case, the points lie close to the line; the minor exceptions are a higher than expected operating margin for hospitals with 200 to 299 beds and lower than expected margin for hospitals with 300 to 399 beds.

Scatter diagrams speak to the level of confidence we have in the relationship between our identified causes (X) and our objective (Y). The tighter the fit around a trend line, whether positive or negative, the more confidence we should have that changing the identified cause will produce the desired result. On the other hand, when there is no relationship between X and Y, a horizontal trend line, we should not expect that changing X will have any impact on Y. Finally, when a nonlinear relationship exists between X and Y, the variable of interest may improve up to a point and decrease thereafter or show no additional improvement or diminishing marginal returns (e.g., additional physical or occupational therapy sessions beyond 10 visits may be unable to improve patient mobility or the patient's ability to complete activities of daily living).

Insert Statistics Chart (Histogram, Box, and Whisker)

Histograms examine the distribution of variables measured on a continuous scale such as dollars, pounds or kilograms, and temperature to identify excessive variation or outliers (i.e., disproportionate occurrences of high or low values). Many natural phenomena such as height, weight, and IQ follow a normal or bell curve distribution. In a normal distribution, approximately 68% of all observations fall within one standard deviation of the mean, 95% fall within two standard deviations, and 5% fall outside two standard deviations. Histograms are used to identify extreme values, typically more than two standard deviations from

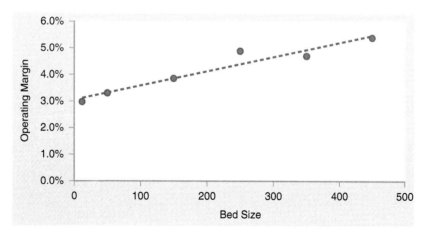

Figure 3.7 Operating Margin and Bed Size

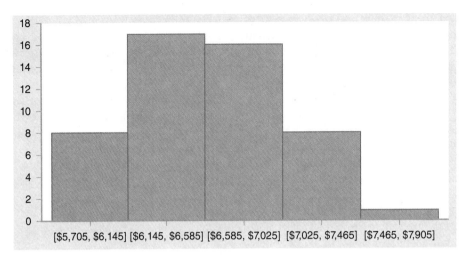

Figure 3.8 Insert Statistics Chart

the mean, and assess whether extreme values are occurring more or less frequently than we would expect. Using the data from Table 3.4, we can assess whether the average cost for the 50 patients is approximately normal by highlighting C5 through C55, selecting **Insert, Statistics Chart, Histogram,** and hitting **Enter.**

The histogram in **Figure 3.8** shows that 33 patients, 17 + 16, or 66%, have a cost between $6,145 and $7,025 and the distribution is approximately normal. **Insert Statistics Chart** determines how many columns to create, and Excel's determination may poorly present data. The common rule for presenting data recommends five to eight columns. In lieu of Insert Statistics Chart, the author recommends that the manager determine how to group the data (i.e., define the ranges and the number of columns the chart should report).

Using the **Histogram** function in **Data, Data Analysis** (must be added into the standard Excel package) creates the frequency table in **Table 3.12**, dividing cases into nine groups. The table should be interpreted as one case

with a cost of $5,705 or less, five cases under $5,998 but greater than $5,705, and so on. The manager would then need to highlight the Frequency column and select **Insert** and **Insert Column or Bar Chart** to create the histogram in **Figure 3.9**.

Cost per CMI/WI Adjusted Discharge

The distribution in Figure 3.9 provides greater detail and appears more bell-shaped; six cases cost less than $5,998 and five cases more $7,466 or more—that is, there are few low- and high-cost cases. The usefulness of the histogram is demonstrated by contrasting Figures 3.9 and 3.10.

The distribution of **Figure 3.10** is similar to Figure 3.9 except for the high number of cases over $7,466. The greater-than-expected number of high-cost cases should spur investigation. What were the cause(s) of the high cost, are the cause(s) controllable, and, if so, what actions can be taken to lower cost?

Table 3.12 Bins and Discharges

Bins	Frequency	%
$5,705	1	2.0%
$5,998	5	10.0%
$6,292	6	12.0%
$6,585	13	26.0%
$6,879	13	26.0%
$7,172	7	14.0%
$7,466	4	8.0%
More	1	2.0%
	50	100.0%

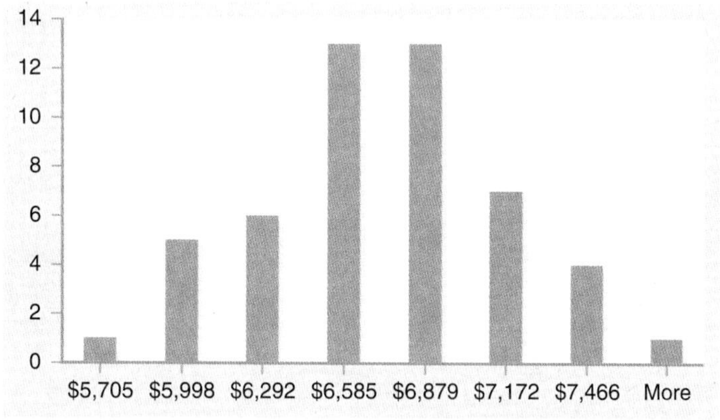

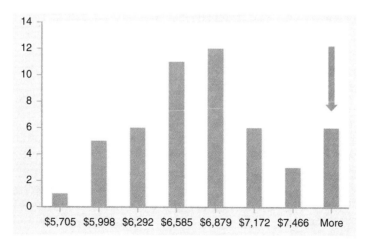

Figure 3.9 Distribution of Average Discharge Cost: Expected Number of Cases

Figure 3.10 Distribution of Average Discharge Cost: Actual, Unexpected Number of High-Cost Cases

WRAP-UP

Summary

After reading this chapter and working through the examples and problems, you should have a greater understanding of how Excel can be used to organize and present financial data. The first step in achieving Excel proficiency is navigating the Ribbon to access Excel functions. One of Excel's most useful functions is Sort; it allows a user to rank data in ascending or descending order by any variable in the data set to assess and understand collected data. Excel allows a manager to quickly perform mathematical calculations such as addition, subtraction, multiplication, and division on hundreds or thousands of data points. It is often necessary to process a data set for information to assess performance and determine if and what type of action is needed. Means, standard deviations, and other more complex calculations are easily performed using formulas, and you are now familiar with the use of 10 of the most common formulas used in finance.

Mathematical operations and formulas allow managers to create information, but numbers and data tables should be used cautiously. One number, such as an average, provides a single piece of information such as average cost, but averages do not reveal the number of cases or variation in cost. A data table may provide the number of cases and cost ranges, but the magnitude of the information conveyed is often difficult to interpret, especially by users who are not numerically confident. Graphs can quickly convey large amounts of information and are easy to understand. Pie charts show the composition of a variable (i.e., the proportion of events that fall into distinct classes). Column charts show the number of events by group and highlight differences between groups. Run charts demonstrate change over time, scatter or XY diagrams highlight the relationship between two variables, and histograms show the distribution of events. Graphing is often the most effective means to convey information, so managers should master Excel charts to ensure that the intended audience understands their message.

Key Terms

Column or Bar Chart	Line (Run) or Area Chart	Scatter or XY Diagram
Fixed Cell Reference	Pie or Doughnut Chart	Trend Line
Histogram	PEDMAS	

Discussion Questions

1. When dealing with a large data set containing hundreds of rows and/or columns that would take multiple pages to print, how can a user customize the printout to one or two pages?
2. Explain how Excel copies formulas containing cell references down a worksheet and how a user can establish a fixed cell reference.
3. Explain PEDMAS and how the order of operations can affect calculations.
4. Explain the difference between the =AVERAGE and =AVERAGEIF functions. Why is the =AVERAGE function necessary?
5. Explain the purpose of pie charts, column charts, run charts, scatter diagrams, and histograms.

Problems

1. Using the problem 3–1 tab in the Chapter 3 Excel files (provided in the online resources), sort the 44 countries by life expectancy and infant mortality rate. What countries have the highest and lowest life expectancy and infant mortality rate, and where does the United States rank on life expectancy and infant mortality rate?

2. Given the following table, calculate profit margin for each medical service, total revenue and profit for all services, the average revenue and profit, and maximum and minimum revenue, profit, and profit margin.

Service	Revenue (millions)	Profit (000)
Cardiovascular surgery	$11.4	$625
Invasive cardiology	8.0	690
Neurosurgery	7.5	687
Orthopedic surgery	5.6	533
Gastroenterology	5.0	487
Oncology	4.8	425
General surgery	4.4	350
Internal medicine	3.4	161
Pulmonology	3.0	278
Cardiology-noninvasive	2.8	227

3. Using the table in problem 3–2, create a pie chart showing the percent of revenue generated by each medical service. What percent of total inpatient revenue is generated by the three largest services?

4. Using the table in problem 3–2, create a column chart displaying profit margin by medical service ordered from highest to lowest margin. What services have the highest and lowest profit margins?

5. Given the following table, create a line (combo) chart for pulmonary revenue and profit margin by year. How are revenue and profit margin changing over time?

Year	Revenue	Profit margin
2012	$1.5	5.6%
2013	$1.3	4.1%
2014	$1.4	3.9%
2015	$1.3	4.0%
2016	$1.6	4.2%
2017	$2.0	5.1%
2018	$2.0	5.3%
2019	$2.1	5.1%
2020	$2.3	5.9%
2021	$2.6	7.5%
2022	$3.0	9.3%

6. Using the table in problem 3–5, create a scatter graph plotting pulmonary revenue on the x-axis and profit margin on the y-axis. Explain the relationship between revenue and profit margin.

7. Given the following table (also available in the online resources) reporting the LOS for 60 pulmonary patients, create a statistics graph (histogram) of the number of pulmonary patients by their LOS and complete the table. What is the most frequent LOS for pulmonary patients, and how often are patients hospitalized for three or seven days?

Patient #	LOS	Patient #	LOS	Patient #	LOS
1	4	21	7	41	3
2	7	22	4	42	5
3	4	23	4	43	5
4	3	24	5	44	3
5	5	25	4	45	5
6	5	26	5	46	4
7	3	27	6	47	4
8	3	28	5	48	6
9	4	29	5	49	5
10	4	30	3	50	5
11	3	31	4	51	6
12	5	32	6	52	6
13	4	33	4	53	3
14	7	34	4	54	5
15	5	35	4	55	6
16	4	36	6	56	6
17	6	37	7	57	5
18	3	38	5	58	6
19	4	39	6	59	6
20	4	40	5	60	4

LOS	Count
3	_____
4	_____
5	_____
6	_____
7	_____

Note

1. Optum360°, *2017 Almanac of Hospital Financial and Operating Indicators* (Salt Lake City, UT: Author, 2016).

Assets, Liabilities, Revenues, and Expenses

CHAPTER 4

Assets, Liabilities, and Net Worth

PROGRESS NOTES

After completing this chapter, you should be able to

1. Describe typical assets and explain the difference between current and long-term assets.
2. Describe typical liabilities and explain the difference between current and long-term liabilities.
3. Describe the different terms for net worth and their use across organizations.
4. Explain how assets, liabilities, and net worth fit together.

Overview: Assets, Liabilities, and Net Worth

Assets, **liabilities**, and **net worth** are part of the language of finance. As such, it is important to understand both their composition and how they fit together. Assets are the tools employees have to complete work, and due to their high cost, it is essential to track them and how they are used. Liabilities identify the amount of assets acquired by debt (i.e., how much the organization owes to others). Net worth is the difference between total assets and liabilities (i.e., the value of the organization). The chart of accounts as discussed in Chapter 2 establishes how assets, liabilities, and net worth are summarized and reported on financial statements.

Assets

Assets are economic resources such as supplies, equipment, and buildings that are expected to produce future benefits for an organization. In other words, assets are what the organization owns and/or controls. Opening a physician practice may require assets of $100,000 or more, a small hospital requires assets of $50 million or more, and health systems routinely have billions in assets. One of the primary duties of managers is to ensure that the organization has the appropriate level of assets; purchasing more or less assets than needed to deliver care imposes unnecessary costs on the organization. Overinvestment in assets results in underutilized resources and higher costs, and having less assets than needed to delivered care reduces the number of patients that can be treated, quality of care, and revenue.

© dinn/E+/Getty Images.

47

Liabilities

The cost of assets needed to run an organization must be paid by its owners or others; liabilities are "outsider claims" consisting of economic obligations, or debts, owed to outsiders. Liabilities are what the organization owes, and the outsiders to whom the debts are due are creditors of the business. Interest must often be paid on borrowed money, so managers should carefully consider whether the organization will be able to meet the interest expense when debt is used to acquire assets. Interest expense varies based on the type of debt used; short-term debt often carries no explicit interest expense, while interest rates generally increase with the length of a loan. Managers should consider the type of debt as well as the amount of debt used.

Net Worth

Net worth or "insider claims" are also known as owner's **equity** or **fund balance**. Organization owners have the residual claim to the entity's assets—that is, they own any assets remaining after debts are paid. No matter what term is used, the difference between total assets and liabilities is the business's "net worth."

The Three-Part Equation

The relationship among assets, liabilities, and net worth is reflected in the accounting equation: assets equal liabilities plus net worth.

$$\text{Assets} = \text{Liabilities} + \text{Net Worth}$$

The three parts always balance among themselves because net worth is the residual claim. For example, when an organization has $100 million in assets and $45 million in liabilities, its net worth (or book value) is $55 million. If the value of its assets falls to $90 million due to a decline in customer demand, increase in operating costs, technological obsolescence… and liabilities do not change, its net worth falls to $45 million. Likewise, if the value of assets grows to $110 million, net worth increases to $65 million, and owners gain $10 million.

Assets

Cash, accounts receivable, notes receivable, and inventory are all assets. For example, the Nightingale Home Health Agency has cash in its bank account; it is an economic resource—an asset. Accounts receivable reports the amount of money Nightingale is owed for services rendered to patients; this is an economic resource—an asset. When patients sign a formal agreement to pay Nightingale for the services they receive, the notes receivable are economic resources—assets. Nightingale also has an inventory of medical supplies, such as dressings, syringes, IV tubing, and so on, that are used in its day-to-day operations. Inventory on hand is an economic resource—an asset. More expensive assets needed to run a business include equipment, buildings, and land. **Exhibit 4.1** summarizes asset examples. It is important to understand that these categories contain multiple, if not thousands of, distinct items.

Figure 4.1 show the distribution of assets for a hypothetical hospital and physician practice. Actual assets may differ based on the type and location of the hospital or practice; however, these charts provide insight into the investment needed to run these organizations.

The average hospital was estimated to have $675,484,000 in assets in 2020, with the majority of assets being equipment, buildings, and land.[1] Putting $675,484,000 in perspective, this is the cost of 1,827 homes at the 2021 U.S. average price of $369,800[2] or 15,985 vehicles at an

---

Exhibit 4.1 Assets

Cash
Accounts receivable
Notes receivable
Inventory
Equipment
Buildings
Land

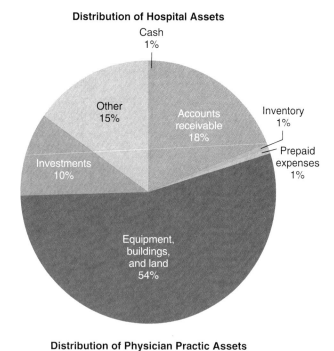

Distribution of Hospital Assets

Cash
1%

Other
15%

Accounts
receivable
18%

Inventory
1%

Prepaid
expenses
1%

Investments
10%

Equipment,
buildings,
and land
54%

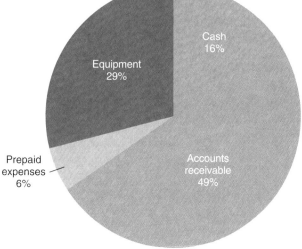

Distribution of Physician Practic Assets

Equipment
29%

Cash
16%

Prepaid
expenses
6%

Accounts
receivable
49%

Figure 4.1 Hospital and Physician Practice Assets

average price of $42,258.[3] The cost of providing one hospital bed (including the building and equipment) has been estimated to run between $1 million and $2 million or $400 to $700 per square foot.[4]

Starting a physician practice is estimated to cost up to $100,000 with the majority devoted to accounts receivable (i.e., waiting for patients or insurance to pay for services provided).[5] Cash to pay staff wages, insurance, and monthly rent also accounts for a large percentage of assets. Unlike hospitals, physicians do not require large investments in equipment and facilities as they often lease equipment and rent office space.

Short-Term Versus Long-Term Assets

Assets are divided between either "current" or "short-term" and "long-term" assets. When an asset can be turned into cash within a 12-month period, it is categorized as a current asset. When an asset cannot be converted into cash within a 12-month period, it is considered long-term. In our Nightingale example, accounts receivable should be collected within one year and is a current asset. Likewise, inventory should be used to provide patient care, billed, and collected within one year; thus, it too is considered a short-term asset.

Classification of the note receivable depends on the length of time that payment is promised. If the entire note receivable should be paid within one year, it is a short-term asset. However, if the note is to be paid over three years, a portion of the note—the amount to be received in the coming 12 months—will be classified as a current asset. The portion of the note to be paid in the second and third years will be classified as long-term asset.

Equipment, buildings, and land are generally classified as long term because these assets will not be converted into cash in 12 months. Equipment, buildings, and land should provide an organization with the tools to generate revenue for many years into the future. Equipment and buildings are also generally stated at a net figure called book value, which reduces their historical cost, their purchase price, by any accumulated depreciation. Depreciation recognizes the wear and tear on equipment and buildings (i.e., the loss in value) due to use and/or age. The concept of depreciation is discussed in Chapter 10, and reporting the value of total assets is covered in Chapter 11.

Liabilities

Accounts payable, payroll taxes due, notes payable, and mortgages payable are all liabilities. Nightingale owes vendors for the medical supplies it has purchased on credit. The amount owed to the vendors is recognized as accounts payable. When Nightingale pays its employees, it withholds income and payroll taxes, as required by the government. The income and payroll taxes withheld are to be paid to the government in the future and thus are also a liability. Nightingale has borrowed money to acquire needed assets and signed a formal agreement; thus, the note payable is a liability. Nightingale also has a mortgage on its building, a liability. Large healthcare organizations may issue bonds to raise large amounts of money when notes or mortgages are not appropriate. Bonds are sold to multiple investors, so they offer lower interest rates than mortgages that are often held by a single institution. **Exhibit 4.2** summarizes liability examples.

Short-Term Versus Long-Term Liabilities

Liabilities are also categorized as "current" or "short-term" and "long-term" liabilities. When a liability is expected to be paid within a 12-month period, it is a current liability. When a liability cannot reasonably be expected to be paid within a 12-month period, it is a long-term liability. In our Nightingale example, accounts payable and payroll taxes due should be paid within one year and thus should be labeled as current liabilities. Current liabilities generally do not require the payment of interest for the use of funds.

Exhibit 4.2 Liabilities

Accounts payable
Payroll taxes due
Notes payable
Mortgage payable
Bonds payable

Classification of the note payable depends on the length of time that payment is promised. If Nightingale is planning to pay the entire note payable within one year, it is a short-term liability. If the note is to be paid over three years, the amount to be paid in the coming 12 months will be classified as a current liability, and the rest of the note—that amount to be paid further in the future—will be classified as a long-term liability. Mortgages are treated slightly differently; the portion to be paid within the coming 12 months may be classified as a short-term liability, while the remaining mortgage balance will be labeled as a long-term liability. Notes payables and long-term liabilities typically require the organization to pay interest for the use of the funds.

Net Worth

Net worth—the third part of the accounting equation—is labeled differently depending on the type of organization. For-profit organizations report their net worth as equity. Equity is the ownership right in property or the money value of property. For example, a sole proprietorship or a partnership's net worth may simply be labeled as "Owners' Equity." A corporation will generally report two types of equity accounts: "Capital Stock" and "Retained Earnings." Capital Stock represents the owners' investment in the company, indicated by their purchase of stock. Retained Earnings, as the name implies, represents undistributed profits that have been left in the business. Net worth can be understood by rearranging the three-part equation:

Net Worth = Assets − Liabilities

Nonprofit organizations generally use a different term such as "Fund Balance" to report the difference between assets and liabilities in their report. This is because nonprofits should not, by definition, have equity. Governmental entities in the United States may also use the term "Fund Balance" in their reports. Equity in for-profit organization is based on owners' investment and retained earnings, while in not-for-profits the fund balance consists of

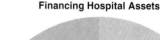

Exhibit 4.3 **Net Worth Terminology**

For-profit sole proprietors or partnerships:
   Owners' Equity
For-profit corporations:
   Capital Stock
   Retained Earnings
Nonprofit entities:
   Fund Balance

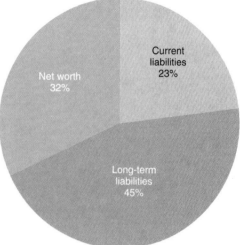

Financing Hospital Assets

Current liabilities 23%
Net worth 32%
Long-term liabilities 45%

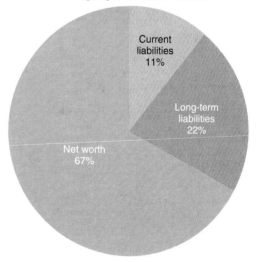

Financing Physician Practice Assets

Current liabilities 11%
Long-term liabilities 22%
Net worth 67%

Figure 4.2 Financing of Hospital and Physician Practice Assets

donor contributions, government grants, and retained earnings. **Exhibit 4.3** summarizes terminology examples for net worth as just discussed.

Figure 4.2 showing a hypothetical breakdown of how assets are financed by hospitals and physician practices. Again, different hospitals and physicians will choose a different mix of liabilities and net worth to acquire assets. Owners and managers adverse to risk choose to rely more on net worth, while those who believe their organization can handle the

interest expense that accompanies debt use more liabilities to finance assets.

As the pie charts show, hospitals rely heavily on long-term debt to finance their assets due to the high cost of hospital facilities and equipment. On the other hand, physicians rely heavily on net worth, their personal investment in their practice. Physicians just out of residency and entering practice may be forced to use debt due to their limited funds, while established doctors often use the proceeds of their practice to purchase their office space and equipment to reduce rental costs.

WRAP-UP

Summary

Healthcare organizations require substantial investments in supplies, equipment, facilities, and other assets to provide patient care. This chapter described how assets are categorized for financial reporting. Understanding the assets needed to provide care is the first step to ensuring that an efficient amount of resources is employed.

The second step to minimizing costs is using the least costly method to acquire assets.

Assets can be purchased using debt, external funds, or owners' funds. The cost of financing assets ranges from zero for short-term debt to high rates based on the borrower's credit history and type of debt sought. The difference between assets and liabilities is net worth, the owners' interest in the organization. Financial statements in Chapter 11 will explore how assets, liabilities, and net worth report the financial performance and status of an organization.

Key Terms

Assets

Equity

Fund Balance

Liabilities

Net Worth

Discussion Questions

1. Describe the different types of assets needed to operate a business and explain the difference between current and long-term assets.

2. Describe the different types of liabilities.

3. Describe the different terms for net worth and their use in for-profit, nonprofit, and public organizations.

4. Explain the relationship between assets, liabilities, and net worth.

Notes

1. Merritt Research Services, "Hospital Medians," https://www.merrittresearch.com, accessed September 29, 2021.

2. St. Louis Federal Reserve Bank, "Median Sales Price of Houses Sold in the United States," https://fred.stlouisfed.org, accessed September 29, 2021.

3. Kelley Blue Book, "Average New-Vehicle Prices Hit All-Time High, According to Kelley Blue Book," https://mediaroom.kbb.com, accessed September 29, 2021.

4. AssetsAmerica, "How Much Does It Cost to Build a Hospital?," https://assetsamerica.com, accessed September 29, 2021.

5. W. J. Palmer, "What Is the Cost of Starting a Medical Practice?," https://www.wolterskluwer.com/en/expert-insights/what-is-the-cost-of-starting-a-medical-practice?.html, accessed March 28, 2021.

CHAPTER 5

Revenues

PROGRESS NOTES

After completing this chapter, you should be able to

1. Explain the difference between operating and nonoperating revenue.
2. Define contractual allowances and discounts and explain their impact on revenue.
3. Describe the different sources of healthcare revenue.
4. Explain how to group revenue for planning and control.

Overview: Revenue

Managers should ensure that the organization's revenues exceed its expenses and provide enough additional funds to replace and improve assets and increase capacity. Revenue represents the amount earned by an organization—that is, actual or expected cash inflows due to the organization's major business. In the case of health care, revenue is mostly earned by rendering services to patients; however, some organizations earn substantial income from donations, investments, and other sources. Revenue flows into the organization and is sometimes referred to as the revenue stream. Maximizing revenue by producing the maximum amount of services from the resources employed and obtaining the highest possible payment for these services is one means of ensuring the financial health of an organization.

Revenue is generally defined as the value of services rendered, expressed at the facility's full established rates. For example, Codman Medical Center's full established rate for a chest X-ray is $100, but Giant Health Plan has negotiated a **managed care** contract whereby the plan pays only $90 for the procedure. The revenue figure—the full established rate—is $100. Revenues can be received in the form of cash or credit. Most, but not all, healthcare revenues are received in the form of credit.

Operating and Nonoperating Revenues

The major source of revenue for most healthcare providers is received for services provided to patients. Payment for services may be received before or after the services are delivered. The other source of revenue is nonoperating; this is income or payments received for goods or services that are tangentially related to an organization's main business.

Payment After Service Is Delivered

The traditional payment method in health care is that of payment after service is delivered. Two basic types of payment after service is delivered are discussed in this section: **fee for service** and **discounted fee for service**.

1. *Fee for service.* The traditional method of receiving revenue for services in the United States was fee for service. The provider of services is paid according to the price charged for the services performed (i.e., if $100 is charged for a physician visit, $100 was collected unless the patient did not pay (bad debt) or all or a portion was written off as charity). Before the 1960s, with very few exceptions, fee for service was the dominant method of payment for health services in the United States.[1]

2. *Discounted fee for service.* In this variation on the original fee for service, a contracted discount is agreed upon by the provider and third-party payer. The provider of services receives a payment that is discounted in accordance with the contract (i.e., if a 20% discount is agreed upon, the provider receives $80 for a $100 billed service and $20 is written off as a contractual discount). After **Medicare** was established, hospitals were paid on the basis of the cost of services performed— **cost reimbursement**—rather than charges, while physicians were paid on the basis of reasonable and customary charges. Discounted fee for service now includes fee schedules that are unrelated to either charges or costs. **Per case reimbursement** is now used by Medicare and other payers to pay hospitals a flat rate based on the type of inpatient service provided, called diagnostic related groups (DRG). A third method pays a flat fee per service; in the case of hospitals, this is a **per diem reimbursement** based on the number of days hospitalized. A large healthcare provider often has many different contracts with third-party payers with different payment arrangements and rates for the same services.

Payment Before Service Is Delivered

Traditional payment methods in the United States have begun to give way to payment before service is delivered. There are multiple names and definitions for such payment. We have chosen to use the term *predetermined per-person payment* when payment is received for services before they are delivered. The payment methods and rate-setting variations are discussed in this section.

1. *Predetermined per-person payment.* Payment received before service is delivered is generally at an agreed-upon predetermined rate. Payment therefore consists of the predetermined rate for each person covered under the agreement: **capitation reimbursement**. Thus, the provider receives a per-person, per-month (PMPM) payment based on the number of patients they are obligated to provide care for.

2. *Rate-setting differences.* Different agreements can use varying assumptions about the group to be served, and these variations will affect the rate-setting process. We know older people tend to use more services than younger people, so a contract may specify a rate of $4,000 per year to cover enrollees between the ages of 19 and 64 and $12,000 for people 65 years of age and older. Numerous variations are therefore possible.

Nonoperating Revenues

In addition to revenues generated from patient services, hospitals often supplement their revenues from other sources. The three main sources are related income from parking, cafeteria, and gift shops; investment income; and charitable contributions. Many hospitals do not generate sufficient operating revenues to cover their expenses, so these other sources of revenue may be vital to their ability to continue operations.

In 2015, average nonoperating income, investment income, charitable contributions, and grants for hospitals was 0.02% of total revenue.[2] Over half of hospitals reported no nonoperating revenues, and hospitals with more than 400 beds reported an average of 0.09%. While nonoperating revenues are negligible in most hospitals, Mayo Clinic is a notable exception. In 2018, Mayo reported $323 million in investment income and $1.975 billion in contributions and grants.[3] Obviously, few healthcare organizations are as capable of generating nonservices revenues as Mayo.

Contractual Allowances and Other Deductions from Revenue

Revenues are recorded at the organization's full established rates, as previously discussed. The amounts estimated to be uncollectible are considered to be deductions from revenues and are recorded as such on the books of the organization. For purposes of the external financial statements released for third-party use, reported revenue must represent the amounts that payers or patients are obligated to pay. Therefore, the terms *gross revenue* and *deductions from revenue* will not be seen on external financial statements. The discussion that follows, however, pertains to the books and records that are used for internal management, where these classifications will be used.

Contractual allowances are the difference between the full established rate and the agreed-upon contractual rate that will be paid. Contractual allowances are often for composite services. Take the case of Codman Medical Center as an example. As discussed in the introduction to this chapter, Codman's full established rate for a certain procedure is $100, but Giant Health Plan has negotiated a contract whereby the plan pays $90 for the procedure. The $10 difference between the $100 charge and the contracted amount that the plan pays, $90, represents the contractual allowance and is written off. Contractual discounts reduce provider's revenue. The average hospital collected less than 31 cents for every $1.00 charged in 2015, demonstrating the impact of contractual discounts on revenue.[4]

It is common for different third-party payers to pay different contractual rates for the same service. This practice is illustrated in **Table 5.1**, which shows contractual rates to be paid for brief physician visits, CPT code 99211, and comprehensive visits, CPT code 99215, for different third-party payers.

The second major deduction from revenue is the allowance for bad debts, also known as

Table 5.1 Payment Rates for Physician Office Visits

	CPT Visit Codes	
Payer	**99211**	**99215**
Charge/Self-pay	$60.00	$100.00
Medicare	39.50	54.90
Medicaid	29.90	35.40
Blue Cross	48.00	80.00
Managed Care—Giant	55.00	85.00
Managed Care—Sigma	42.00	70.00
Managed Care—Unity	52.00	65.00
Charity/No-pay	0.00	0.00

Table 5.2 Calculating Average Reimbursement

Payer	CPT 99211	Payer Mix	Average Reimbursement
Charge/Self Pay	$60.00	8%	$4.80
Medicare	39.50	45%	17.78
Medicaid	29.90	5%	1.50
Blue Cross	48.00	15%	7.20
Managed Care—Giant	55.00	10%	5.50
Managed Care—Sigma	42.00	8%	3.36
Managed Care—Unity	52.00	7%	3.64
Charity/No-pay	0.00	2%	0.00
Average reimbursement	$40.80	100%	$43.77

a provision for doubtful accounts. The allowance for bad debt represents amounts owed by patients or their third-party payer that are not expected to be paid. Again, for purposes of the external financial statements released for third-party use, the provision for doubtful reports must be reported separately as an expense item. The discussion that follows, however, still pertains to the books and records that are used for internal management, where the classification of deductions from revenue will be used. The allowance for bad debts is charged with the amount of services received on credit (recorded as accounts receivable) that are expected to not be paid by patients or third-party payers.

Beyond contractual allowances and a provision for bad debts, the third major deduction from revenue classification is charity service. Charity service is generally defined as services provided to financially indigent patients. The Centers for Disease Control and Prevention estimated the number of uninsured under the age of 65 as 32.8 million people in 2019,[5] and EMTALA requires all Medicare-participating hospitals to provide emergency care to all regardless of insurance status. Thus, providers deliver many charity services or services that go unpaid (bad debt).

Determining how much revenue will be earned from a typical patient is complicated by the **payer** mix (i.e., how many patients are reimbursed at each rate). **Table 5.2** shows how average reimbursement should be calculated for CPT 99211.

Table 5.2 shows calculating a simple average that assumes an equal number of patients are paid at each rate will underestimate actual reimbursement (i.e., $40.80, the average of column 2). When payer mix is considered, multiplying the reimbursement rate (column 2) by payer mix (column 3) and adding the products in column 4, the weighted average reimbursement is $43.77. Fortunately for most providers, the percent of charity or no-pay patients is small. Table 5.2 demonstrates that a simple average underestimates reimbursement by $2.97 per patient; considering many physician practices see 5,000 or more patients per year, this error can result in substantial under- or overestimation of total revenue.

Sources of Healthcare Revenue

Healthcare revenue in the United States comes from a variety of public programs and private payers. The sources of healthcare revenue are generally termed *payers*. Payer mix—the proportion of revenues realized from the different types of payers—is a measure that is often included in the profile of a healthcare organization. For example, Codman Medical Center has a patient or payer mix that is 45% Medicare, 30% managed care, 15% traditional insurance, 8% **Medicaid**, and 2% self-pay.

Public Programs

The Medicare Program

Title XVIII of the Social Security Act, "Health Insurance for the Aged and Disabled," is commonly known as Medicare. Medicare established a health insurance program for the aged in 1965 and was intended to complement other benefits (such as retirement, survivors', and disability insurance benefits) under other titles within the Social Security Act.

The Medicare program currently has four parts. The first part, known as Part A, is hospital insurance (HI) and is funded primarily by a 1.9% payroll tax on workers and employers. Part A expenditures in 2019 were $318.4 billion; payroll taxes covered $281.4 billion, and taxation and interest covered $33.3 billion. The HI trust fund loses billions per year and is expected to be depleted in 2026.[6]

The second part, known as Part B, is called supplementary medical insurance (SMI) and covers outpatient and professional fees. SMI is voluntary and is funded primarily by insurance premiums (usually deducted from monthly Social Security benefit checks of those enrolled) and federal general revenue funds. In 2019, expenditures were $435.5 billion with premiums covering $113.5 billion and general revenue covering $331.8 billion. Guidelines determine both the services to be covered and the eligibility of the individual to receive the services under the Medicare program. Medicare claims (billings) are processed by fiscal agents who act on behalf of the federal government.

Medicare's third part, Part C, is known as "Medicare Advantage." Medicare Advantage consists of managed care plans, private fee-for-service plans, preferred provider organization plans, and specialty plans. Although Medicare Advantage is offered as an alternative to traditional Medicare, coverage cannot be less than what Parts A and B (traditional Medicare) would offer the beneficiary.

Medicare's fourth part, Part D, is the prescription drug benefit, implemented on January 1, 2006. It is a voluntary program that requires payment of a separate premium and contains cost-sharing provisions. Part D expenditures in 2019 were $95.3 billion, premiums covered $15.8 billion, and transfers from federal and state revenues covered $80.1 billion.

The Medicare program covers approximately 95% of the aged population in the United States along with eligible individuals receiving Social Security disability benefits.[7] Medicare is an important source of healthcare revenue to most healthcare organizations.

The Medicaid Program

Title XIX of the Social Security Act is commonly known as Medicaid. Medicaid legislation established a federal and state matching entitlement program in 1965 to provide medical assistance to eligible needy individuals and families.

The Medicaid program is state specific, although the federal government has established minimum national guidelines. Each state has the power to set eligibility, service restrictions, and payment rates for services within their state. In doing so, each state is bound only by the broad national guidelines. Medicaid policies are complex, and considerable variation exists among states. The federal government is responsible for a certain percentage of each state's Medicaid expenditures; the specific amount due is calculated by an annual formula. Providers of Medicaid services are paid directly by the states.

The Medicaid program is the largest U.S. government program providing funds for medical and health-related services for the poor.[8] Therefore, although the proportion of Medicaid services within the payer mix may vary, Medicaid is a major source of healthcare revenue in almost every healthcare organization.

Other Programs

There are numerous other sources of federal, state, and local revenues for healthcare organizations. Generally speaking, for most organizations, none of the other revenue sources exceed the Medicare and Medicaid programs just discussed. Other programs include the Children's Health Insurance Plan (CHIP), Department of Defense and Veterans' Affairs health programs, workers' compensation programs, and state-only general assistance programs. Other public programs include school health programs, public health clinics, maternal and child health services, migrant healthcare services, mental health and drug and alcohol services, and special programs such as Native American healthcare services.

Managed Care

In the 1970s, managed care began to appear in healthcare systems in the United States although they did not become large sources of revenue until the 1980s. An all-purpose definition of managed care is managed care is a means of providing healthcare services within a network of healthcare providers. The responsibility to manage and provide high-quality and cost-effective health care is delegated to this defined network of providers.[9] A central concept of managed care is the coordination of all healthcare services for an individual. In general, managed care plans receive a predetermined amount per member in premiums.

Types of Plans

One type of managed care is the health maintenance organization (HMO). Members enroll in the HMO. They prepay a fixed monthly amount; in return, they receive comprehensive health services. The members must use the providers who are designated by the HMO; if they go outside the designated providers, they must pay all or a large part of the cost themselves. The designated providers of services in turn contract with the HMO to provide services at agreed-upon rates. Several different forms of HMOs have evolved over time.

The most prevalent type of managed care plan today in the United States is the preferred provider organization (PPO) that consist of a group of providers called a panel. The panel members are an approved group of various types of providers, including hospitals and physicians. The panel is limited in size and generally has utilization review powers. When patients in a PPO use providers who are not in the PPO, they must pay

a higher amount in deductibles and coinsurance. As of 2018, 94.8 million people were enrolled in HMO plans and 165.8 million in PPOs.[10]

Types of Contracts

In the case of an HMO, the designated providers of health services contract with the HMO to provide services at agreed-upon rates. The different types of HMOs—including the staff model, the group model, the network model, the point-of-service model, and the individual practice association (IPA) model—have various methods of arriving at these rates. A PPO contracts with its selected group, who are all participating payers, to buy services for its eligible beneficiaries on the basis of discounted fee for service. A large healthcare facility will have one or more individuals responsible for managed care contracting.[11]

Other Revenue Sources

A considerable amount of healthcare revenue is still realized from sources other than Medicare, Medicaid, and managed care:

- *Commercial insurers.* Generally speaking, conventional indemnity insurers, or commercial insurers, simply pay for the eligible health services used by those individuals who pay premiums for healthcare insurance. They do not tend to have a say in how those health services are administered.
- *Private (or self) pay.* This is payment by patients themselves or by the families of patients. Private pay is more prevalent in nursing facilities and in assisted-living facilities than in hospital settings. Physicians' offices also receive a certain amount of private pay revenue.
- *Other.* Additional sources of revenue for healthcare facilities include donations received by voluntary nonprofit organization, tax revenues levied by governmental nonprofit organizations, and grant funding.

Figure 5.1 presents revenue sources for all hospitals in 2019 and **Table 5.3** demonstrates how a hospital's payer mix would be calculated. Both dollar totals and percentages by source are reported.

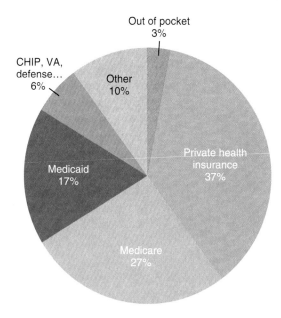

Figure 5.1 Hospital Revenues by Source, 2019

Data from Managed Care Fact Sheets. (n.d.). National expenditures by source. https://mcol.com

Grouping Revenue for Planning and Control

Grouping revenue by different classifications is an effective method for managers to use the information to plan and control operations. In the preceding paragraphs, we saw revenue reported by source; other classifications are now discussed.

Revenue Centers

A revenue center is one type of responsibility center in which managers and employees are responsible for generating revenues to meet a certain target. Actually, the responsibility in the healthcare setting is more for generating volume than for generating a specific revenue dollar amount, and the volume will, in turn, generate the dollars. Revenue centers tend to occur most often in special programs where volume is critical to the survival of the program.

Care Settings

Grouping revenue by care setting recognizes the different sites where services are delivered. The most basic grouping by care settings is inpatient versus ambulatory services. **Figure 5.2** shows the distribution of U.S. health expenditures.

Table 5.4 illustrates a six-way classification of care setting revenues within a health system. In this case, the performance of hospital inpatient, hospital outpatient, off-site clinic, skilled nursing facility, home health agency, and hospice can be tracked. Individual providers may wish to advertise this type of classification in a brochure or report to highlight the different types of healthcare services offered by the organization.

Table 5.4 reports Codman's revenues across care settings for 2021 and 2022 and the percentage growth in 2022.

Table 5.3 Statement of Revenue by Source

Payer	Year-to-Date Revenue	% Total Revenue
Private (self-pay)	$100,000	2.9%
Managed care	560,000	16.7%
Medicare	1,420,000	42.4%
Medicaid	820,000	24.5%
Commercial	400,000	12.0%
Other revenue	50,000	1.5%
Total	$3,350,000	100.0%

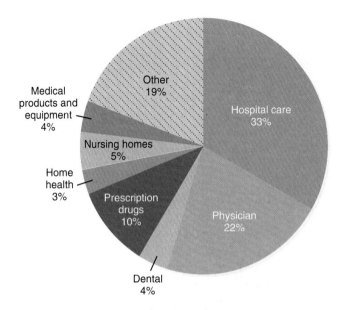

Figure 5.2 Revenues by Care Setting, 2019[12]

Data from Centers for Medicare and Medicaid Services. (n.d.). Table 7-Hospital care expenditures; levels, percent change, and percent distribution, by source of funds: Selected calendar years 1970-2019. https://www.cms.gov
/Research-Statistics-Data-and-Systems/Statistics-Trends-and-Reports/NationalHealthExpendData/NationalHealthAccountsHistorical

Table 5.4 Codman Medical Center 2021 and 2022 Revenues

Care Setting	2021		2022		
	$ (millions)	%	$ (millions)	%	Increase
Hospital Inpatient	$63.213	42.1%	$64.317	40.4%	1.7%
Hospital Outpatient	56.907	37.9%	62.088	39.0%	9.1%
Off-site Clinic	5.856	3.9%	6.368	4.0%	8.7%
Skilled Nursing Facility	12.162	8.1%	12.736	8.0%	4.7%
Home Health Agency	8.859	5.9%	10.189	6.4%	15.0%
Hospice	3.153	2.1%	3.502	2.2%	11.0%
Total Revenue	$150.150	100.0%	$159.200	100.0%	6.0%

Service Lines

In traditional cost accounting a product line is a grouping of similar products.[13] In the healthcare field, many organizations opt instead for "service line" terminology. A service line is a grouping of similar services. Strategic planning often revolves around setting goals for service lines including the type and volume of medical services to be provided, payer mix, and financial performance.

Hospitals

A number of hospitals have adopted the major diagnostic categories (MDCs) as service lines. One advantage of MDCs is that they are a universal designation in the United States. MDCs also have the advantage of possessing a standard definition. In another approach to service line classification, Codman Medical Center recently updated its strategic plan and settled on five inpatient service lines: (1) medical, (2) surgical, (3) women and children, (4) mental health, and (5) rehabilitation (neuro-ortho rehab) (**Table 5.5**).[14]

Long-Term Care

A continuing care retirement community (CCRC) can use its various levels of care as a starting point for revenue classification. CCRCs usually have four service lines, listed in the descending order of resident acuity: (1) skilled nursing facility, (2) nursing facility, (3) assisted living, and (4) independent living. The skilled nursing facility provides services for the highest level of resident acuity, and the independent living provides services for the lowest level of resident acuity. One adjustment to this approach includes isolating subacute services from

the remainder of skilled nursing facility services. Another adjustment involves splitting independent living into two categories, one for Housing and Urban Development (HUD)–subsidized independent housing and the other for private-pay independent housing. **Table 5.6** illustrates CCRC service lines by acuity level.

Home Care

Numerous categories of service delivery can be considered "home care." A practical approach was taken by one home care entity—part of a health system—that defined its "key functions." Key functions can in turn be converted to service lines (**Table 5.7**).

Physician Groups

Service delivery for physician groups will vary, of course, with the nature of the group itself. A generic set of service lines is presented in **Figure 5.3**.

Table 5.8 shows the breakdown of revenue for Salk Family Practice by services delivered. The

Table 5.5 Hospital Service Lines

Hospital Inpatient	2021 $ (millions)	% of Total	2022 $ (millions)	% of Total	% Increase
Medical	$17.953	28.4%	$18.459	28.7%	2.8%
Surgical	22.314	35.3%	22.768	35.4%	2.0%
Women and children	7.459	11.8%	7.268	11.3%	-2.6%
Mental health	4.298	6.8%	4.438	6.9%	3.2%
Other	11.189	17.7%	11.384	17.7%	1.7%
Total revenue	$63.213	100.0%	$64.317	100.0%	1.7%

Table 5.6 Skilled Nursing Facility Service Lines

Skilled Nursing	2021 $ (millions)	% of Total	2022 $ (millions)	% of Total	% Increase
Nursing facility	$4.269	35.1%	$4.598	36.1%	7.7%
Assisted living	5.205	42.8%	5.426	42.6%	4.2%
Independent living	2.688	22.1%	2.713	21.3%	0.9%
Total revenue	$12.162	100.0%	$12.736	100.0%	4.7%

Table 5.7 Home Health Service Lines

Home Health	2021 $ (millions)	% of Total	2022 $ (millions)	% of Total	% Increase
Diabetes	$1.409	15.9%	$1.640	16.1%	16.5%
Infusion therapy	2.321	26.2%	2.629	25.8%	13.3%
Maternity	1.019	11.5%	1.080	10.6%	6.0%
Mental health	0.682	7.7%	0.805	7.9%	18.0%
Wound care	1.754	19.8%	2.180	21.4%	24.3%
Other	1.674	18.9%	1.854	18.2%	10.8%
Total revenue	$8.859	100.0%	$10.189	100.0%	15.0%

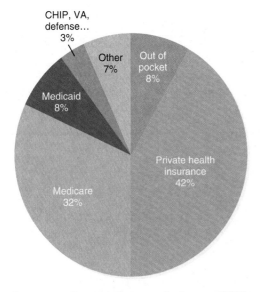

Figure 5.3 Physician Revenues by Source, 2019[15]

Data from Centers for Medicare and Medicaid Services. (n.d.). Table 9-Physician services expenditures; levels, percent change and percent distribution, by source of funds: Calendar years 1998-2019. https://www.cms.gov/Research-Statistics-Data-and-Systems/Statistics-Trends-and-Reports/NationalHealthExpendData/NationalHealthAccountsHistorical

major source of revenue is office visits and procedures accounting for 82.6% of revenue in 2021 and 84.4% in 2022.

Table 5.8 also shows the growth in C-ray and patient visit revenue from 2021 and the decline in lab tests. The physician and/or office manager may wish to investigate to determine how much of the change is due to changes in volume, reimbursement, or both and what implications the change may have on the future (e.g., will more X-ray equipment or space be needed?).

Other Service Designations

Other classifications may meet the needs of particular organizations. Columbia/HCA was reported to classify its services in a disease management approach. The classification consists of eight disease management areas: (1) cancer, (2) cardiology, (3) diabetes, (4) behavioral health, (5) workers'

Table 5.8 Salk Family Practice Service Lines

Services	2021 Revenue	% of Total	2022 Revenue	% of Total	% Increase
Office visits	$324,480	67.5%	$332,640	67.8%	2.5%
Procedures	$72,604	15.1%	$72,939	14.9%	0.5%
Lab tests	$16,224	3.4%	$15,900	3.2%	-2.0%
X-rays	$67,392	14.0%	$69,264	14.1%	2.8%
Total revenue	$480,700	100.0%	$490,743	100/0%	2.1%

compensation, (6) women's services, (7) senior care, and (8) emergency services.[16]

Other Types of Revenue Groupings

Other healthcare organizations may have revenue groupings that are not service lines. An entity that provides services is able to choose service lines as a method of grouping its revenue. But if the entity sells or makes a product (rather than providing services), its revenue will have to be classified differently. Two examples within the healthcare industry follow: a retail pharmacy and a pharmaceutical manufacturer.

Retail Pharmacy

A retail pharmacy's revenue primarily comes from sales. A typical retail pharmacy may group revenues into three major categories of sales:

prescription drugs, nonprescription (over-the-counter, or OTC) drugs, and other merchandise. "Other merchandise" would then have subcategories such as cosmetics, greeting cards, gifts, and so on.

Pharmaceutical Manufacturer

A pharmaceutical manufacturer's revenue groupings would likewise be specific to its type of healthcare business. This organization is producing a product rather than providing a service. Its major categories of revenues will probably be by type of drug manufactured. The next subcategory might then be either national versus international revenues or perhaps a classification of revenues by geographic region within the United States (i.e., East, South, Midwest, and West). In summary, the entity's revenue classification system, whatever it may be, must be consistent with the current structure and purpose of the organization.

WRAP-UP

Summary

Healthcare providers generate the overwhelming majority of their revenues from services to patients and hence should understand how these revenues are generated. A prime need is to understand who is receiving care as third-party payers reimburse providers at vastly different rates for the same services. Understanding Medicare reimbursement is vital as Medicare patients comprise the largest number of patients for most hospitals and physicians. Medicare inpatient revenue is based

on a fixed payment per admission, and physician revenue is based on relative value units (RVUs) determined by CPT code; in both cases, payments are significantly lower than commercial payers.

The difference between third-party allowable charges and the amount charged (price) is written off as a contractual allowance or discount and thus reduces revenue. Failure to write these amounts off and subsequent attempts to collect these amounts from patients (balance billing) are illegal.

Key Terms

Capitation Reimbursement
Cost Reimbursement
Discounted Fee for Service
Fee for Service

Managed Care
Medicaid
Medicare
Payer Mix

Per Case Reimbursement
Per Diem Reimbursement

Discussion Questions

1. Explain the difference between operating and nonoperating revenue.
2. Define contractual allowances and discounts and explain their impact on revenue.
3. Describe the difference in sources of revenue for hospitals and physicians (hospitals: 37% commercial insurance and 27% Medicare; physician: 42% commercial insurance and 32% Medicare).
4. Explain why revenue is grouped to facilitate planning and control.

Problems

1. Calculate the average revenue for CPT 99215 the provider will receive based on the payment rates in Table 5.1 and the payer mix in Table 5.2. If the average cost to provide the patient visit is $64.00, will the provider need nonoperating revenues to cover its costs?
2. Calculate the average revenue for CPT 99215 the provider will receive given the payment rates in Table 5.1 and the following payer mix. If the average cost to provide the patient visit is $64.00, will the provider need nonoperating revenues to cover its costs?

Payer	Payer Mix
Charge	8%
Medicare	45%
Medicaid	10%
Blue Cross	15%
Managed Care—Giant	10%
Managed Care—Sigma	5%
Managed Care—Unity	4%
Charity/No-pay	3%
	100%

3. Snowden Hospital is reviewing its inpatient services lines using the following table to calculate the year-to-year change in revenue (millions). Which services lines have the highest and lowest growth rates? Which services are growing faster than the average for inpatient services?

Inpatient Services	2022 Revenue	2023 Revenue
Internal medicine	$25.3	$26.1
Oncology	18.6	19.9
Cardiology	32.1	34.2
Neurology	12.7	13.1
Obstetrics	6.8	6.7
Pediatrics	9.5	9.8
General surgery	22.1	23.6
Mental health	13.4	12.6
Total revenue	$140.5	$146.0

4. Snowden Hospital is reviewing its outpatient services lines using the following table to calculate the year-to-year change in revenue (millions). Which services have the highest and lowest

growth rates? Which services are growing faster than the average for outpatient services?

Outpatient services	2022 Revenue	2023 Revenue
Emergency department	$18.9	$20.5
Same-day surgery	12.8	$13.5

Outpatient services	2022 Revenue	2023 Revenue
Clinic	6.7	$7.1
Physician practices	25.3	$28.7
Dialysis	14.6	$15.2
Lab and imaging services	4.5	$4.8
Total revenue	$82.8	$89.8

Notes

1. Texas Medical Association, American Medical Association, Texas Medical Foundation, and Texas Osteopathic Medical Association, *A Guide to Forming Physician-Directed Managed Care Networks* (Austin, TX: Texas Medical Association, 1994), 3.
2. Optum360°, *2017 Almanac of Hospital Financial and Operating Indicators* (Salt Lake City, UT: Author, 2016).
3. Mayo Clinic, 2018 990 Filing.
4. Optum360°, *2017 Almanac of Hospital Financial and Operating Indicators* (Salt Lake City, UT: Author, 2016).
5. Centers for Disease Control and Prevention, "Health Insurance Coverage," https://www.cdc.gov, accessed September 29, 2021.
6. N. Jagoda, "Social Security Reserves Estimated to Be Depleted Earlier Than Previously Expected," https://thehill.com, accessed September 29, 2021.
7. Health Care Financing Administration, *Health Care Financing Review: Medicare and Medicaid Statistical Supplement* (Baltimore, MD: U.S. Department of Health and Human Services, 1997), 8.
8. Ibid., 9.
9. D. I. Samuels, *Capitation: New Opportunities in Healthcare Delivery* (Chicago: Irwin Professional Publishing, 1996), 20–21.
10. MCOL, "Managed Care Fact Sheets," "National Expenditures by Source," https://mcol.com, accessed September 29, 2021.
11. Centers for Medicare and Medicaid Services, "Table 7 Hospital Care Expenditures; Levels, Percent Change, and Percent Distribution, by Source of Funds: Selected Calendar Years 1970–2019," https://www.cms.gov /Research-Statistics-Data-and-Systems/Statistics -Trends-and-Reports/NationalHealthExpendData /NationalHealthAccountsHistorical, accessed June 1, 2021.
12. D. E. Goldstein, *Alliances: Strategies for Building Integrated Delivery Systems* (Gaithersburg, MD: Aspen Publishers, Inc., 1995), 283; and Texas Medical Association, American Medical Association, Texas Medical Foundation, and Texas Osteopathic Medical Association, *A Guide to Forming Physician-Directed Managed Care Networks* (Austin, TX: Texas Medical Association, 1994), 4–6.
13. Centers for Medicare and Medicaid Services, "Table 2 National Health Expenditures; Aggregate, Annual Percent Change, Percent Distribution and Per Capita Amounts, by Type of Expenditure: Selected Calendar Years 1960–2019," https://www.cms.gov /Research-Statistics-Data-and-Systems/Statistics -Trends-and-Reports/NationalHealthExpendData /NationalHealthAccountsHistorical, accessed June 1, 2021.
14. When ICD-10 is fully implemented, it is possible that the term *major diagnostic categories* (MDCs) may have to be replaced with some other universal designation. Whether these hospitals will change the names of their service line designations to match the new titles is unknown at this point. We do know it will take time to decide upon such a change and then additional time to implement the change.
15. Centers for Medicare and Medicaid Services, "Table 9 Physician Services Expenditures; Levels, Percent Change and Percent Distribution, by Source of Funds: Calendar Years 1998–2019," https://www.cms.gov /Research-Statistics-Data-and-Systems/Statistics -Trends-and-Reports/NationalHealthExpendData /NationalHealthAccountsHistorical, accessed June 1, 2021.
16. A. Sharpe and G. Jaffe, "Columbia/HCA Plans for More Big Changes in Health-Care World," *Wall Street Journal*, 28 May, 1997, A8.

CHAPTER 6

Expenses

PROGRESS NOTES

After completing this chapter, you should be able to

1. Describe the major expenses for hospitals and physicians.
2. Explain how disbursements for services represent an expense stream (an outflow).
3. Explain how expenses are grouped for planning and control.

Overview: Expenses

Maximizing revenue is one way to improve the financial health of an organization; the other is minimizing **expenses**, and unlike revenue, expenses are within the control of every employee. Expenses are the **costs** incurred to produce goods and services and earn revenue. Every employee can take actions that reduce the amount of time and resources used to produce a good or service and/or improve the value of the good or service to customers.

Expenses are the costs of doing business. Just as revenues represent the inflow into the organization, expenses represent the outflow—a stream of expenditures flowing out of the organization. Examples of expenses include salary expense for labor performed, payroll tax paid on the salary, the cost of supplies, utility expense for electricity, gas, and interest expense for the use of money.

In fact, expenses are **expired costs**—costs that have been used up, or consumed, while carrying on business. Revenues and expenses affect

the net worth of an organization. The inflow of revenues increases net worth, whereas the outflow of expenses decreases net worth. For-profit organizations may use the term *equity* and nonprofit organizations may use the term *fund balance* rather than *net worth*. A nonprofit organization, by its nature, does not exist to make a profit and should not have equity. However, the principle of inflow and outflow remains the same. In the case of nonprofits, the inflow of revenues increases the fund balance, and the outflow of expenses decreases the fund balance (i.e., increasing the value of any organization requires that revenues exceed expenses).

Many managers use the terms *expense* and *cost* interchangeably. Expense in its broadest sense includes every expired (used-up) cost that is deducted from revenue. A narrower interpretation groups expenses into categories such as operating expenses, administrative expenses, and so on. Cost is the amount of cash expended, property transferred, services received, or liability incurred in consideration for goods or services received or to be received. As we have already said, costs can be either expired or unexpired. Expired costs are used up in the current period and are thus matched against current revenues. **Unexpired costs** are not yet used up and will be matched against future revenues.[1]

For example, an electric bill for $500 is recorded in the books of a clinic as an expense. The administrator sees the $500 as the cost of electricity for that month in the clinic and is correct in seeing the $500 as a cost because it has been used up (expired) within the month. On the other hand, a $50,000 invoice for equipment that will be used over the next five years is a cost but the expense is recognized over the life of the asset.

Confusion also exists in healthcare reporting over the terms *cost* and *charges*. Charges are the amounts billed to patients and a provider's revenues or inflows that increase the value of the organization. Costs are a provider's expenses or outflows that decrease the value of an organization. To a patient or their third-party payer, cost is the provider's charge highlighting the fact that a patient's cost (i.e., payment for services) is a provider's revenue.

Composition of Expenses

Generating revenues requires resources, and expenses categorize the amount of money spent on labor, supplies, equipment, buildings, and other inputs used to deliver services. Labor is the major expense of most healthcare providers; labor expense includes wages, health insurance, Social Security taxes, retirement, and unemployment taxes. Supplies include medical, office, and cleaning and maintenance. Equipment and building expenses include depreciation, interest expense, maintenance, insurance, and rents.

Hospital Expenses

Figure 6.1 provides a pie chart showing the breakdown of total expenses in 2022 for Codman Medical Center. Salaries and fringe benefits are 78% of total expense; note that fringe benefits are

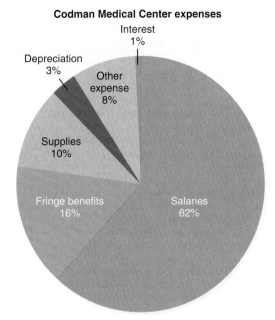

Figure 6.1 Hospital Expenses

25% of total salaries. Supplies are 10% and equipment and building expenses are 4%, 3% depreciation plus 1% interest expense. "Other" includes all other expenses that managers have deemed are too small to track separately (i.e., they do not warrant a distinct reporting category).

Physician Expenses

Figure 6.2 shows the breakdown of expenses for Salk Family Medicine for 2022. The major expense is again salaries, which constitute 48% of total expense. Other large expenses include occupancy (mortgage or rent) at 13% and supplies at 10%.

Figures 6.1 and 6.2 highlight that cost control must begin with labor as the smaller amounts spent on supplies, equipment, and facilities offer less potential to reduce the cost of health care. For example, reducing hospital labor expense by 1% could save the organization 0.78% versus reducing supply expense by 5%, which would net only 0.5% savings. The 1% reduction not only saves more money, it is much more likely to be achieved than the more ambitious 5% reduction.

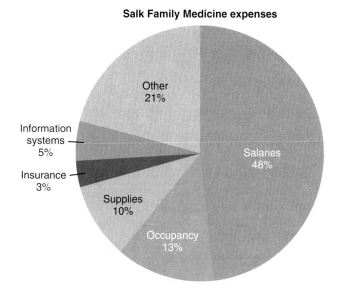

Figure 6.2 Physician Expenses

Disbursements for Services

There are two types of disbursements for services:

1. *Payment when expense is incurred.* If an expense is paid at the point when it is incurred, it does not enter the accounts payable account (i.e., a liability). In large organizations, it is rare to see payments when expenses are incurred. The only place where this usually occurs is the petty cash fund.

2. *Payment after expense is incurred.* In most healthcare organizations, expenses are paid at a later time and not at the point when the expense is incurred (e.g., supplies are received or repairs made and the vendor bills the organization). When this is the case, the expense is recorded in the accounts payable account. It is cleared from accounts payable when payment is made. One measurement of performance is "days in accounts payable," whereby the amount in accounts payable is divided by the average daily cash expense to determine how many days the organization takes to pays its bills. Most vendors expect payment in 30 days or less, so when days

in accounts payable exceeds 30, managers should examine why payment processing is taking so long.

Grouping Expenses for Planning and Control

Cost Centers

A cost center is one form of a responsibility center. In a responsibility center, the manager is responsible, as the name implies, for a particular set of activities. In a cost center, a particular unit of the organization is given responsibility for controlling costs of the operations over which it holds authority. The medical records division and the billing and collection office are two examples. A cost center might be a division, an office, or an entire department, depending on how the organization is structured. Cost center managers control the amount and type of resources used to provide work (i.e., how work is performed) and should identify the most efficient methods and ensure that they are used in a manner consistent with quality care.

In healthcare organizations, it is common to find departments as cost centers. This is often a logical way to designate a cost center because the lines of authority are generally organized by department. Cost centers can then be grouped into larger groups that have something in common, such as nursing and ancillary care, support services, and administration in hospitals. Within this method of grouping, the manager of a cost center may receive his or her own reports and figures, but not those of the entire group. The director or officer in charge of the larger

grouping receives a report that contains multiple cost centers (e.g., the chief nursing officer receives a report detailing the performance of all nursing units). The chief executive officer receives a report for the entire organization because he or she is ultimately responsible for overseeing the operations of all cost centers.

Table 6.1 illustrates this concept. It contains 20 different cost centers, all of which are revenue producing. The 20 cost centers are divided into

Table 6.1 Nursing Services and Other Professional Services Cost Centers

Nursing Services	2021	% of Total	2002	% of Total	Year-to-Year Change
Medical & surgical units	$390,000	76.5%	$405,000	76.0%	3.8%
Operating room	30,000	5.9%	33,000	6.2%	10.0%
Intensive care units	40,000	7.8%	44,000	8.3%	10.0%
OB–nursery	15,000	2.9%	15,000	2.8%	0.0%
Other	35,000	6.9%	36,000	6.8%	2.9%
Total expenses	$510,000	100.0%	$533,000	100.0%	4.5%
Ancillary Services					
Laboratory	$220,000	18.1%	$233,000	18.1%	5.9%
Radiology	139,000	11.4%	148,000	11.5%	6.5%
CT, MRI, and PET scans	18,000	1.5%	19,000	1.5%	5.6%
Pharmacy	128,000	10.5%	140,000	10.9%	9.4%
Emergency department	89,000	7.3%	94,000	7.3%	5.6%
Medical and surgical supply	168,000	13.8%	178,000	13.8	6.0%
Operating rooms	142,000	11.7%	150,000	11.7%	5.6%
Respiratory therapy	48,000	4.0%	50,000	3.9%	4.2%
Physical therapy	64,000	5.3%	65,000	5.1%	1.6%
EKG	16,000	1.3%	17,000	1.3%	6.3%
EEG	1,000	0.1%	1,000	0.1%	0.0%
Ambulance service	7,000	0.6%	7,000	0.5%	0.0%
Substance abuse	43,000	3.5%	45,000	3.5%	4.7%
Home health and hospice	120,000	9.9%	126,000	9.8%	5.0%
Other	12,000	1.0%	13,000	1.0%	8.3%
Total expenses	$1,215,000	100.0%	$1,286,000	100.0%	5.8%

two groups: nursing services and ancillary services. There are five cost centers in the nursing services group, ranging from operating room to obstetrics–nursery. There are 15 cost centers in the ancillary services group. In the hospital that uses the grouping shown in Table 6.1, however, not all of the 20 cost centers are departments. Some are divisions within departments. For example, EKG and EEG operate out of the same department but are two separate cost centers.

Table 6.2 shows 11 different cost centers that are not directly revenue producing. The dietary department yields some cafeteria revenue, but that revenue is not central to the major business of the organization, which is providing healthcare services. The 11 cost centers are divided into two groups: general services and support services. The six cost centers in the general services group happen to all be departments in this hospital. Other hospitals might not have security as a separate department. The other cost centers—dietary,

maintenance, laundry, housekeeping, and medical records—would be separate departments. The five cost centers in the support services group include general administration, health insurance, Social Security taxes, employee welfare, and retirement; the last four may be in one department. It is the prerogative of management to set up cost centers specific to the organization's own needs and preferences, so these four may be in a benefits department. It is the responsibility of management to make the cost centers match the proper lines of authority.

Table 6.2 illustrates two categories of healthcare expense: general services and support. A third related category is operations expense. An operations expense provides service directly related to patient care such as radiology and pharmacy. A general services expense provides services necessary to maintain the patient, but the service is not directly related to patient care; examples are laundry and dietary. **Support services expenses**, on

Table 6.2 General Services and Support Services Cost Centers

General Services Cost Center	2021	% of Total	2022	% of Total	Year-to-Year Change
Dietary	$97,000	33.0%	$100,000	32.8%	3.1%
Maintenance	92,000	31.3%	96,000	31.5%	4.3%
Laundry	27,000	9.2%	28,000	9.2%	3.7%
Housekeeping	43,000	14.6%	45,000	14.8%	4.7%
Security	5,000	1.7%	5,000	1.6%	0.0%
Medical records	<u>30,000</u>	<u>10.2%</u>	<u>31,000</u>	<u>10.2%</u>	<u>3.3%</u>
Total expenses	$294,000	100.0%	$305,000	100.0%	3.7%
Support Services Cost Center					
General administration	$455,000	55.4%	$480,000	55.5%	5.5%
Health insurance	24,000	2.9%	25,000	2.9%	4.2%
Social Security taxes	112,000	13.6%	118,000	13.6%	5.4%
Employee welfare	188,000	22.9%	197,000	22.8%	4.8%
Retirement	<u>43,000</u>	<u>5.2%</u>	<u>45,000</u>	<u>5.2%</u>	<u>4.7%</u>
Total expenses	$822,000	100.0%	$865,000	100.0%	5.2%

the other hand, provide support to both **general services expenses** and **operations expenses**. A support service expense is necessary for support, but it is neither directly related to patient care nor a service necessary to maintain the patient. Examples of support services are insurance and payroll taxes.

Diagnoses and Procedures

It is common to group expenses by **diagnoses** and **procedures** for purposes of planning and control. This grouping is beneficial because it matches costs against common classifications of revenues. Much of the revenue in many healthcare organizations is designated by either diagnoses or procedures. Medicare groups costs into cost centers by **major diagnostic categories (MDCs)**. The 26 MDCs serve as the basic classification system for 761 distinct **diagnosis-related groups (DRGs)**. Each DRG represents a category of patients whose resource consumption is approximately equivalent. DRGs are part of Medicare's prospective payment reimbursement methodology. **Table 6.3** provides a listing of the 26 MDCs.[2]

Given the large number of patients covered by Medicare, a hospital may choose to group its departments and cost centers by MDCs. One

Table 6.3 Major Diagnostic Categories

MDC	Description
0	Pre-MDC
1	Diseases and Disorders of the Nervous System
2	Diseases and Disorders of the Eye
3	Diseases and Disorders of the Ear, Nose, Mouth and Throat
4	Diseases and Disorders of the Respiratory System
5	Diseases and Disorders of the Circulatory System
6	Diseases and Disorders of the Digestive System
7	Diseases and Disorders of the Hepatobiliary System and Pancreas

MDC	Description
8	Diseases and Disorders of the Musculoskeletal System and Connective Tissue
9	Diseases and Disorders of the Skin, Subcutaneous Tissue and Breast
10	Diseases and Disorders of the Endocrine, Nutritional and Metabolic System
11	Diseases and Disorders of the Kidney and Urinary Tract
12	Diseases and Disorders of the Male Reproductive System
13	Diseases and Disorders of the Female Reproductive System
14	Pregnancy, Childbirth and Puerperium
15	Newborn and Other Neonates (Perinatal Period)
16	Diseases and Disorders of the Blood and Blood Forming Organs
17	Myeloproliferative Diseases and Disorders (Poorly Differentiated Neoplasms)
18	Infectious and Parasitic Diseases and Disorders (Systemic or unspecified sites)
19	Mental Diseases and Disorders
20	Alcohol/Drug Use or Induced Mental Disorders
21	Injuries, Poison and Toxic Effect of Drugs
22	Burns
23	Factors Influencing Health Status and Other Contacts with Health Services
24	Multiple Significant Trauma
25	Multiple Significant Trauma

Data from Centers for Medicare and Medicaid Services. (n.d.). Table 5—List of Medicare Severity Diagnostic-Related Groups (MS-DRGS), relative weighting factors and geometric and arithmetic mean length of stay—FY 2020 correction notice. https://www.cms.gov/Medicare/Medicare-Fee-for-Service-Payment/AcuteInpatientPPS/FY2020-IPPS-Final-Rule-Home-Page-Items/FY2020-IPPS-Final-Rule-Tables

hospital uses 27 cost center codes: the first 23 MDCs plus 4 other codes, "Special Drugs," "HIV," "Unassigned," and "Outpatient." The special drugs and HIV cost centers represent high-cost services that management wants to track separately. Unassigned is a default category and should have little assigned to it. Outpatient is a separate cost center at the preference of management.

Table 6.4 illustrates the grouping of costs for MDC 2, Diseases and Disorders of the Eye, cost center code 18. The DRG numbers range from 113 to 125; five DRGs record surgical care, 113 through 117, and five record medical care, 121 through 125.[3] Note that surgical care has a longer average length of stay and higher cost and thus has a higher weight than medical care. These costs can now be matched to their corresponding revenues.

Outpatient services are generally designated by Current Procedural Terminology (CPT) codes that provide a listing of descriptive terms and identifying codes for medical services and procedures performed. CPT codes are commonly used to group cost centers for outpatient services. Procedures are also used for purposes of grouping inpatient costs,

generally within a certain cost center. **Table 6.5** provides an example of reporting radiology department costs by procedure code. In this example, the procedure code is in the left column, the description of the procedure is in the middle column, and the total departmental cost for the procedure appears in the right column. These costs can now be readily matched to equivalent revenue.

Care Settings and Service Lines

Expenses can be grouped by care setting, which recognizes the different sites at which services are delivered. "Inpatient" versus "outpatient" is a basic type of care setting grouping. Expenses can also be classified by service lines, a method that groups similar services.[4]

When revenues are grouped by care setting or by service line, as discussed in the previous chapter, then expenses should also be grouped in

Table 6.4 DRGs in MDC 2

MS-DRG	MDC	TYPE	MS-DRG Title	Weight	Arithmetic Mean LOS
113	02	SURG	ORBITAL PROCEDURES W CC/MCC	2.1321	5.8
114	02	SURG	ORBITAL PROCEDURES W/O CC/MCC	1.1908	2.7
115	02	SURG	EXTRAOCULAR PROCEDURES EXCEPT ORBIT	1.4860	4.7
116	02	SURG	INTRAOCULAR PROCEDURES W CC/MCC	1.8910	6.0
117	02	SURG	INTRAOCULAR PROCEDURES W/O CC/MCC	1.0967	2.7
121	02	MED	ACUTE MAJOR EYE INFECTIONS W CC/MCC	1.2678	5.7
122	02	MED	ACUTE MAJOR EYE INFECTIONS W/O CC/MCC	0.7726	4.3
123	02	MED	NEUROLOGICAL EYE DISORDERS	0.7808	2.7
124	02	MED	OTHER DISORDERS OF THE EYE W MCC	1.3894	5.2
125	02	MED	OTHER DISORDERS OF THE EYE W/O MCC	0.7894	3.2

Table 6.5 Radiology Department Costs Classified by Procedure Code

Procedure Code	Procedure Description	Department Cost
557210	Ribs, Unilateral	$60,000
557230	Spine Cervical Routine	125,000
557280	Pelvis	33,000
557320	Shoulder	55,000
557360	Wrist	69,000
557400	Hip, Unilateral	42,000
557410	Hip, Bilateral	14,000
557430	Knee Only	62,000
	Total expense	$460,000

Table 6.6 Program Cost Center: Southside Homeless Intake Center

Program:	Southside Homeless Intake Center
Department:	Feeding Ministry
For the Month of:	January 2022
Food	$14,050
Dietary Supplies	200
Paper Supplies	300
Minor Equipment	50
Consultant Dietitian	50
Utilities	300
Telephone	50
Total expense	$15,000

the same way. In that way, matching of revenues and expenses can readily occur (i.e., are services recovering their costs?). A more detailed discussion of care settings and service lines with examples was presented in the preceding chapter.

Programs

A program can be defined as a project that has its own objectives and its own performance indicators. A program is often funded separately for a finite period of time and is expected to stand on its own. For example, funds from a grant might fund a specific project such as a three-year community outreach program to reduce obesity. Often programs—especially those funded separately from the revenue stream of the main organization—have to arrange their expenses in a special format that is specified by the entity that provides the grant funds.

Program expenses should be grouped in such a way that they are distinguishable from other operating expenses. An example of a program cost center is given in **Table 6.6**. This cost center example has received special funds and must be reported separately, as shown.

The major expense for providers is labor as health care is a service industry where patients often interact with one or more personnel to obtain care. While wages are the largest expense, the costs of fringe benefits, health insurance, payroll taxes, and retirement often amount to 20% or more of wages. The next highest expense for hospitals is often supplies, while physicians' next highest expense is often occupancy.

It is important to understand the difference between expenses and costs. Expenses are costs that correspond to the revenues generated during a period, whereas costs for equipment and building may be assigned to future revenues. It is also important to recognize that expenses represent an outflow of an organization's resources and reduce the value of the organization.

Given the magnitude of expenses incurred by a provider, it is vital that the expenses be grouped for planning and control. These groupings include cost centers that aggregate costs by manager and service lines, diagnoses, procedures, and programs to match revenue and expenses.

WRAP-UP

Summary

The major expense for providers is labor as health care is a service industry where patients often interact with one or more personnel to obtain care

Key Terms

Cost

Diagnoses

Diagnosis-Related Groups
  (DRGs)

Expenses

Expired Costs

General Services Expenses

Major Diagnostic Categories
  (MDCs)

Operations Expenses

Procedures

Support Services Expenses

Unexpired Costs

Discussion Questions

1. Describe the major expenses of hospitals and physician practice.
2. Explain the effect of expense (outflows) on an organization's net worth.
3. Explain how expenses are grouped in different ways for planning, controlling, and evaluating performance.

Problems

1. Snowden Hospital is reviewing its inpatient services lines using the following table to calculate the year-to-year change in expenses (millions). Which services lines have the highest and lowest growth rates? Which service line expenses are growing faster than the average for inpatient services?

2. Snowden Hospital is reviewing its inpatient services lines using the following table to calculate the year-to-year change in expenses (millions) by department. Which departments have the highest and lowest growth rates? Which departments' expenses are growing faster than overall expenses?

Inpatient Services	2022 Expenses	2023 Expenses
Internal medicine	$24.3	$24.8
Oncology	18.1	18.3
Cardiology	30.7	31.5
Neurology	12.5	12.8
Obstetrics	6.9	7.0
Pediatrics	9.1	9.4
General surgery	21.5	22.6
Mental health	13.2	13.8
Total expenses	$136.3	$140.2

Department	2021 Expenses	2022 Expenses
Laboratory	$10.9	$11.1
Radiology	13.3	13.5
Pharmacy	14.1	14.8
Emergency department	7.0	7.1
Operating rooms	9.7	10.1
Respiratory therapy	6.2	6.2
Nursing	35.3	36.3

Department	2021 Expenses	2022 Expenses
Physical therapy	3.5	3.6
Central supply	17.7	18.6
Administration	4.4	4.5
Finance	5.3	5.4

Department	2021 Expenses	2022 Expenses
Human resources	2.1	2.1
Housekeeping	<u>6.8</u>	<u>6.9</u>
Total expenses	$136.3	$140.2

Notes

1. S. A. Finkler, *Essentials of Cost Accounting for Health Care Organizations*, 2nd ed. (Gaithersburg, MD: Aspen Publishers, Inc., 1999).
2. Centers for Medicare and Medicaid Services, "Table 5.—List of Medicare Severity Diagnostic-Related Groups (MS-DRGS), Relative Weighting Factors and Geometric and Arithmetic Mean Length of Stay—FY 2020 Correction Notice," https://www.cms.gov/Medicare /Medicare-Fee-for-Service-Payment/AcuteInpatientPPS /FY2020-IPPS-Final-Rule-Home-Page-Items/FY2020 -IPPS-Final-Rule-Tables, accessed March 2, 2021.
3. Ibid.
4. G. F. Longshore, "Service-Line Management/Bottom-Line Management for Health Care," *Journal of Health Care Finance*, 24, no. 4 (1998): 72–79.

Understanding Costs and Managing Expenses

CHAPTER 7

Direct and Indirect Costs

PROGRESS NOTES

After completing this chapter, you should be able to

1. Explain the difference between direct and indirect costs.
2. Describe how indirect costs are allocated to revenue generating departments.
3. Explain how direct and indirect costs should affect managerial decisions and actions.
4. Describe the responsibilities of cost, profit, and investment center managers.
5. Explain the difference between product and period costs.

Overview: Direct and Indirect Costs

Departments serving patients in large healthcare organizations require support from multiple departments that do not generate revenue to complete their work. The support services include housekeeping, maintenance, billing and payroll services, human resources, accounting and finance, administration, and so on. The cost of non-revenue-generating departments must be recouped in revenue-producing departments to ensure that an organization's total revenues exceed its total expenses (i.e., the charges for services must cover the department's cost plus the costs of support services).

Direct costs can be specifically associated with a particular patient, work group, or department. The critical distinction for a manager is that the cost is under their control (i.e., they can increase or decrease the level of the expenditure). Whatever the manager is responsible for—that is, patient, work group, or department—is known as a *cost object*. The somewhat vague definition of a cost object is any unit for which a separate cost measurement is desired. It might help the manager to think of a *cost object* as a *cost objective* instead.[1] The important thing is that direct costs can be traced to a cost object. Indirect costs, on the other hand, cannot be specifically associated with a particular cost object. The cost to run the accounting and finance services is an example of indirect cost. Accounting and finance services are essential to the overall organization itself, but their cost is not specifically or directly associated with providing healthcare services. Indirect costs usually cannot be traced to the work performed by the patient-serving departments but are allocated or apportioned to revenue-producing departments.[2] **Figure 7.1** illustrates the direct–indirect cost distinction.

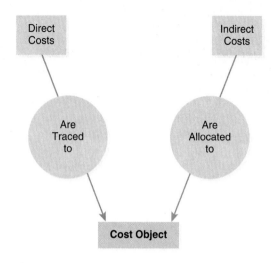

Figure 7.1 Assigning Costs to the Cost Object

It is helpful to recognize that direct costs are incurred for the sole benefit of a particular patient or department. As a rule of thumb, if the answer to the following question is "No," the cost is a direct cost: "If the operating unit, such as the emergency department, did not exist, would this cost be incurred?" When a department can be eliminated or a patient or group of patients do not receive care and the cost remains, it is an indirect cost. For example, eliminating the emergency department would zero out its expenses, but the cost of running accounting and finance services would remain the same.

Indirect costs are incurred for the overall organization and not for any one patient or department. Because they are shared, indirect costs are sometimes called **joint** or **common costs**. As a rule of thumb, if the answer to the following question is "Yes," the cost is an indirect cost: "Must this cost be allocated in order to be assigned to a revenue-producing department such as nursing or ancillary units?"

Allocating Indirect Costs

It is important for managers to recognize direct and indirect costs and how they are treated on reports. Two sets of examples illustrate the reporting of direct and indirect costs. The first example concerns a clinic and ambulance service cost center, and the second concerns a rehabilitation cost center.

Table 7.1 sets out the direct costs for a clinic and ambulance cost center. These costs are what the organization's managers believe can be traced to the specific operation of the clinic or ambulance service (i.e., direct costs). **Table 7.2** sets out the indirect costs that the organization's managers believe are not directly attributable to the specific operation of the ambulance service (i.e., $72,000 for general administration and $48,000 for facility costs). The decisions about what will and what will not be considered direct or indirect costs will almost always have been made for the manager.[3] What is important is that the manager understand two things: first, what costs are considered indirect, and second, how the indirect costs are allocated to revenue generating departments. Remember the rule of thumb discussed earlier in this chapter: If the answer to the following question is "No," the cost is a direct cost: "If the operating unit (i.e., the clinic and ambulance service) did not exist, would these costs be incurred?"

The allocation of indirect cost is based on total direct expenses; the ambulance service generates 16.7% of direct expenses, $100,000 ÷ $600,000, and thus is allocated 16.7% of general administrative and facility costs. The general administrative allocation is $12,000, $72,000 × 16.7%, and facility cost is $8,000, $48,000 × 16.7%. The clinic therefore is allocated the remaining 83.3%

Table 7.1 Ambulance and Clinic Direct Costs

	Ambulance	Clinic
Salaries and wages	$60,000	$325,000
Fringe benefits	12,000	71,500
Supplies	5,000	27,500
Repairs and maintenance	1,200	4,200
Utilities	5,000	22,900
Depreciation	15,000	43,900
Other	1,800	5,000
Total direct costs	$100,000	$500,000

Table 7.2 Ambulance and Clinic Indirect and Total Costs

	Ambulance	Clinic	Total
Total direct expenses	$100,000	$500,000	$600,000
Allocation rate (% direct cost)	16.7%	83.3%	100.0%
Total direct expenses	$100,000	$500,000	$600,000
Allocated administrative cost	12,000	60,000	72,000
Allocated facility cost	8,000	40,000	48,000
Total cost	$120,000	$600,000	$720,000

of these costs, 100% – 16.7%, $60,000 for administration and $40,000 for facility costs.

The total allocated indirect cost must equal the total cost in the support departments, and the revenues generated by the patient service departments must cover their direct and indirect costs for the organization to survive. **Table 7.3** represents a report with the direct and allocated indirect costs for the rehabilitation cost center. The report is divided into three types of therapy, physical, occupational, and speech therapy, with the total allocated indirect cost for three support departments, administration, accounting and finance, and information technology, whose costs are allocated on different bases. In this report, the manager can observe the differences between direct and indirect costs and the differences among the three types of therapies.

Markup indicates how much prices must be increased over direct expenses to cover the allocated costs. The allocation of indirect costs is provided in **Table 7.4**. Note that the "Allocated

Indirect Costs" in column 5 of Table 7.4 are the same as the "Allocated Indirect Costs" in column 3 of Table 7.3. Thus, Table 7.4 is a subsidiary report showing the allocation of indirect costs in the main report. The use of one or more supporting reports to reveal details behind the main report is quite common in managerial reports. The allocation of indirect costs subsidiary report details how indirect costs were distributed to the three revenue generating therapy departments.

Table 7.4 shows the expenses, administrative services, accounting and finance, and information technology included in the $185,000 indirect cost total. It also shows how each of these expenses was allocated to the physical, occupational, and speech therapy departments. Administrative service expense was allocated based on the number of patient visits, accounting and finance expense was allocated on the percent of direct costs, and information technology expense was allocated on the number of computers in service. The calculations for physical therapy are

Table 7.3 Rehabilitation Cost Center Direct and Indirect Costs

Revenue Department	Direct Expense	Allocated Indirect Costs	Total Cost	Markup
Physical therapy (PT)	$390,000	$97,500	$487,500	25.0%
Occupational therapy (OT)	210,000	45,000	255,000	21.4%
Speech therapy (ST)	150,000	42,500	192,500	28.3%
Total	$750,000	$185,000	$935,000	24.7%

Table 7.4 Indirect Costs Allocated to Rehabilitation Cost Center

Nonrevenue Department	Administration	Accounting and Finance	Information Technology	Total
Expense to Be Allocated	$50,000	$60,000	$75,000	$185,000
		Direct	Computers	
Allocation Basis	**Visits**	**Expense**	**in Service**	
Physical therapy (PT)	8,500	$390,000	10	
Occupational therapy (OT)	4,000	210,000	4	
Speech therapy (ST)	2,500	150,000	6	
Total	15,000	$750,000	20	
		% Direct	% Computers	
Allocation Rate	**% Visits**	**Expense**	**in Service**	
Physical therapy (PT)	56.7%	52.0%	60.0%	
Occupational therapy (OT)	26.7%	28.0%	20.0%	
Speech therapy (ST)	16.7%	20.0%	20.0%	
Total	100.0%	100.0%	100.0%	
		Accounting	Information	Allocated
Allocated Costs	**Administration**	**and Finance**	**Technology**	**Indirect Costs**
Physical therapy (PT)	$26,000	$34,000	$37,500	$97,500
Occupational therapy (OT)	14,000	16,000	15,000	45,000
Speech therapy (ST)	10,000	10,000	22,500	42,500
Total	$50,000	60,000	$75,000	$185,000

Administration: (8,500 PT visits ÷ 15,000 total visits) × $50,000 = $26,000
Accounting and finance: ($390,000 PT direct ÷ $750,000 total direct) × $60,000 = $34,000
Information technology: (10 PT computers ÷ 20 total computers) × $75,000 = $37,500
Total indirect costs allocated to physical therapy $97,500

Responsibility Centers

The allocation of indirect cost is often a contentious issue in organizations. The manager of physical therapy may believe it unfair that her department must carry $97,500 of the $185,000 total indirect costs and that the required 25% markup may make her services more expensive than competing providers. The indirect cost allocation reduces the profitability of her area by $97,500, and she may argue that a different allocation method should be used (e.g., allocating accounting and finance expenses on patient visits rather than direct costs would reduce the PT allocation and increase the allocation to OT and ST). These costs must be recouped to ensure that the organization earns a profit. We previously discussed revenue centers, where managers are responsible for generating revenue (or volume), and cost centers, where managers are responsible for managing and controlling costs. A *profit center* makes a manager responsible for both the volume and revenue (inflow) side and the expense (outflow) side of a department, division, unit, or program. In other words, the manager is responsible for setting prices and determining product mix (revenue) and input mix (cost).

We will examine the type of information a manager receives about his or her own responsibility center by reviewing the Westside Clinic operations. Westside Clinic offers two basic types of services: an ambulatory surgery center (ASC) and a rehabilitation center. Bill Emerson, the chief executive officer (CEO), is responsible for the overall profitability of Westside and supervises Joe Clark, director of the ambulatory surgery center; Bonnie Hackett, director of the rehabilitation center; and Denisha Jones, a part-time radiologist, who provides radiology services on an as-needed basis. **Figure 7.2** illustrates the managerial relationships.

To restate the relationships shown in Figure 7.2, Clark manages the ambulatory surgery

services profit center, and Hackett manages the profit center for rehabilitation services. These services represent the business of the Westside Clinic. Jones manages the radiology services cost center supporting the surgery and rehabilitation profit centers. Emerson, the CEO, manages the investment center that includes all of the functions just described plus the general and administrative support center.

Emerson receives the accounting report, shown in **Table 7.5**, that contains the net income for each **responsibility center** in the Westside operation. Indirect expenses are allocated based on direct expenses, so the ambulatory surgery center is allocated $41,892 of indirect expenses, ($155,000 ÷ $370,000) × $100,000).

Clark's report for the ambulatory surgery center shows $225,000 in revenue less the $155,000 of controllable expenses he is responsible for. The difference is labeled "Surplus." The surplus amounts to $70,000, $225,000 – $155,000; after $41,892 is deducted for indirect costs; the net income for the ambulatory surgery center is $28,108.

Hackett's rehabilitation center is the second line of Table 7.5. Her report shows $300,000 in revenues less $215,000 of controllable expenses she is responsible for. The difference is again labeled "Surplus." The surplus amounts to $85,000, $300,000 – $215,000, after allocated costs are deducted, $58,108, her net income is $26,892. Clark and Hackett should work to increase the profits of their area of responsibility

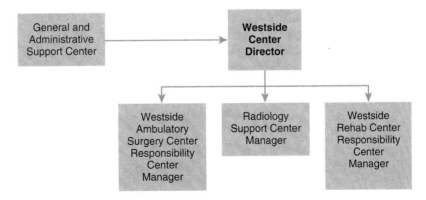

Figure 7.2 Lines of Managerial Responsibility at Westside Clinic

Courtesy of Resource Group, Ltd., Dallas, Texas.

Table 7.5 Income Statement by Responsibility Center

Responsibility Center	Revenue	Direct Expenses	Surplus	Allocated Expenses	Net Income	Profit Margin
Ambulatory surgical center	$225,000	$155,000	$70,000	$41,892	$28,108	12.5%
Rehabilitation center	$300,000	$215,000	$85,000	$58,108	$26,892	9.0%
General and administrative		$80,000	-$80,000			
Radiology		$20,000	-$20,000			
Net income	$525,000	$470,000	$55,000	$100,000	$55,000	10.5%

by increasing volume or revenue or reducing costs and be evaluated on the profit earned.

Jones's report for radiology services is at the bottom right of **Figure 7.3**. Her report shows the controllable expenses she is responsible for, which amount to $20,000. Her report shows only expenses because it is a cost enter, not a profit center. Therefore, Jones is responsible for expenses but not for volume or revenue; she should strive to reduce the cost per X-ray.

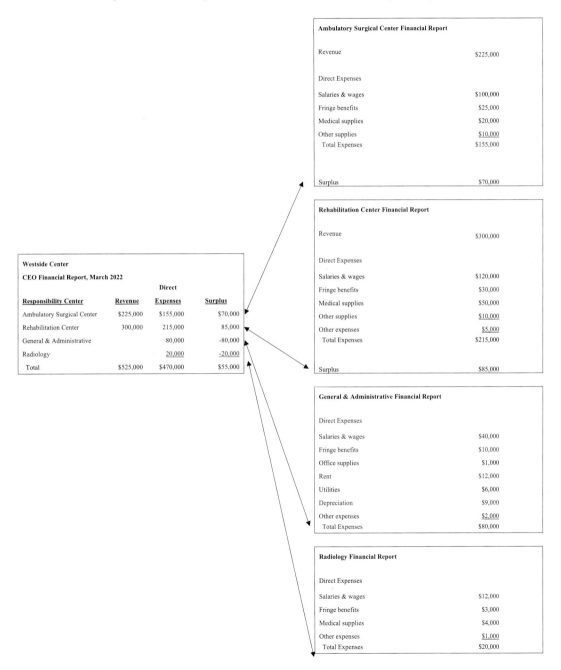

Figure 7.3 Westside Center Financial Reports by Responsibility Center

Emerson, the CEO, receives a report for the general and administrative (G&A) expenses, as shown second from the bottom on the right of Figure 7.3. This report shows the G&A controllable expenses that Emerson is responsible for at Westside, which amount to $80,000. The G&A report shows only expenses because it is an expense center, not a profit center. In his role of managing G&A expenses, Emerson is responsible for expenses but not for volume or revenue. In the case of G&A, Emerson should strive to ensure that G&A expenses are comparable to if not lower than those of similar organizations.

Emerson in his role of CEO is also responsible for the entire Westside operation. That is, the overall Westside operation is his investment center. Therefore, Emerson's financial report, reproduced on the left side of Figure 7.3, contains the results of both profit centers and the cost and expense centers. The surplus figures from Clark's and Hackett's reports are positive figures of $70,000 and $85,000, respectively (i.e., revenues exceed expenses). The expense-only figures from Emerson's G&A support center report and from Jones's radiology support center report are negative figures of $80,000 and $20,000, respectively. Therefore, to determine net income for the entire Westside operation, the $80,000 and the $20,000 expense figures are subtracted from the surplus figures to arrive at a net income of $55,000. Emerson should be evaluated on overall profit; he should ensure that future investments are made in the units that would yield the greatest financial benefit. Future investments could be sought to enhance the profitability of surgical or therapy services or lower the costs of G&A or radiology services.

Table 7.6 illustrates the effect of changing the allocation base to revenue.

Tables 7.5 and 7.6 show a negligible difference in the profit margins of the two revenue centers (e.g., the ambulatory surgical center margin falls from 12.5% to 12.1% when revenue is used as the allocation base). However, the importance of the allocation base should be judged by its effect on employee behavior. Allocating indirect cost based on revenue does not encourage Emerson or Hackett

to improve financial performance (i.e., reducing revenue to reduce allocated indirect expenses would reduce their profit margins). On the other hand, if indirect expenses were allocated on direct expenses, each would have an incentive to reduce unnecessary direct costs *and* lower their allocated costs. The change to direct expense rather than revenue reduces the ambulatory surgical center's allocation rate from 42.9% to 41.9% and increases its reported profit margin by 3.5%. As indirect cost allocation is a zero-sum game, the change increased the rehabilitation centers' allocation rate from 57.1% to 58.1% and reduced its profit margin by 3.5%; note that Westside's total profit remains at $55,000.

The bottom half of **Table 7.7** shows the potential impact of the change. The shift to direct expenses provides a real incentive to reduce direct costs. In this case, if the ambulatory surgery center director reduces his expenses by $4,650 (3.0%), his profit margin increases from 12.5% to 14.9%, a 19.2% increase. The improvement is due to the lower direct costs and a shift of an additional $740 of indirect costs to the rehabilitation cost center. Rehabilitation's profit margin is reduced by 2.8%, but Westside's overall profit increases from $55,000 to $59,650, an 8.5% increase. Allocation bases should be selected to encourage value-increasing actions from managers such as better utilization of staff, supplies, and equipment.

Although the lines of managerial responsibility will vary in other organizations, the relationships between and among investment, profit, and cost centers and overall supervision will remain as shown in this example.

Product and Period Costs

Product costs is a term that was originally associated with manufacturing rather than with services. The concept of product costs assumes that a product has been manufactured and placed into inventory while waiting to be sold. When that product is sold, the product is matched with revenue and recognized as a cost. Thus, *cost of sales* is the common usage for manufacturing firms.

Table 7.6 Income Statement by Responsibility Center (Revenue Allocation Base)

Department	Revenue	Allocation Rate (% rev)	Direct Expense	Allocated Indirect Expense	Total Cost	Net Income	Profit Margin
Ambulatory surgical center	$225,000	42.9%	$155,000	$42,857	$197,857	$27,143	12.1%
Rehabilitation center	$300,000	57.1%	$215,000	$57,143	$272,143	$27,857	9.3%
General and administrative	$0		$80,000	-$80,000	$0		
Radiology	$0		$20,000	-$20,000	$0		
Total	$525,000	100.0%	$470,000	$20,000	$470,000	$55,000	10.5%

Table 7.7 Impact of 3.0% Direct Expense Reduction in Ambulatory Surgery

Department	Revenue	Direct Expense	Allocation Rate (% exp)	Allocated Indirect Expense	Total Cost	Profit	Profit Margin
Ambulatory surgery	$225,000	$155,000	41.9%	$41,892	$196,892	$28,108	12.5%
Rehabilitation	$300,000	$215,000	58.1%	$58,108	$273,108	$26,892	9.0%
Total	$525,000	$370,000	100.0%	$100,000	$470,000	$55,000	10.5%

Department	Revenue	Direct Expense2	Allocation Rate (% exp2)	Allocated Indirect Expense	Total Cost	Profit	Profit Margin
Ambulatory surgery	$225,000	$150,350	41.2%	$41,152	$191,502	$33,498	14.9%
Rehabilitation	$300,000	$215,000	58.8%	$58,848	$273,848	$26,152	8.7%
Total	$525,000	$365,350	100.0%	$100,000	$465,350	$59,650	11.4%

Period costs, in the original manufacturing interpretation, are not connected with the manufacturing process. They are matched with revenue on the basis of when the cost is incurred (thus *period costs*). The term comes from the span of time in which matching occurs, known as *time period*.

Service organizations have no manufacturing process as such. The business of healthcare service organizations is service delivery, not the manufacturing of products. Although the overall concept of product versus period cost is not as vital to service delivery, the distinction remains important for healthcare managers to know.

In healthcare organizations, product cost can be viewed as traceable to the cost object of the

department, division, or unit. A period cost is not traceable in this manner. Another way to view this distinction is to think of product costs as those costs necessary to actually deliver the service, whereas period costs are costs necessary to support the existence of the organization itself.

Finally, medical supply and pharmacy departments do have inventories on hand. In their case, a product is purchased (rather than manufactured) and placed into inventory while waiting to be dispensed. When that product is dispensed, the product is matched with revenue and recognized as a cost of providing the service to the patient. Therefore, the product cost concept is important to managers of departments that hold a significant amount of inventory.

WRAP-UP

Summary

This chapter examined direct and indirect costs. Direct costs are those that are under the control of a manager, and indirect costs are incurred in other areas and are allocated to revenue-producing departments. The distinction between direct and indirect costs is important as indirect costs reduce the reported profitability of revenue-producing departments and are often beyond the control of their managers (i.e., their decisions and actions have no influence on the expenses allocated to their departments).

Managers of cost and expense centers should be evaluated on their ability to keep their expenses low as they cannot control patient volume or revenue. Managers of profit

centers should be evaluated on their ability to serve patients (volume), the prices and services offered (revenue), and maintenance of low expenses (i.e., they should be assessed on profit earned in their area). Managers of investment centers are responsible for an entire operation, so in addition to controlling volume, revenue, and expenses, they should also be assessed on where investments are made. Investment center managers should be assessed on whether their organization makes comparable profits to similar organizations. Chapter 8 explores fixed and variable costs (i.e., whether a cost changes with output) to recognize how much control a manager has over their direct costs.

Key Terms

Cost Object
Direct Cost
Indirect Cost

Joint Cost (common cost)
Period Cost
Product Cost

Responsibility Centers

Discussion Questions

1. Explain the difference between direct and indirect costs.
2. Explain how direct and indirect costs affect managerial decisions and actions.
3. Describe the responsibilities of cost, profit, and investment center managers.
4. Explain the difference between product and period costs.

Problems

1. Henry Hospital is reviewing the profitability of its nursing and ancillary services. The following table provides the revenue, direct expenses, and general and administrative costs. Allocate the general and administrative costs to the nursing and ancillary services based on revenue to calculate the net income and profit margin generated by each.

2. Henry Hospital is reviewing the profitability of its nursing and ancillary services. The table in problem 7–1 provides the revenue, direct expenses, and general and administrative costs, allocate the general and administrative costs to the nursing and ancillary services based on direct expenses to calculate the net income and profit margin generated by each.

	Nursing	Ancillary	Total
Revenue	$29,100,000	$55,900,000	$85,000,000
Total direct expenses	21,100,000	38,600,000	59,700,000
General and administrative cost			21,500,000
Net income			$3,800,000
Profit margin			4.5%

3. Barnard Surgical Associates, a for-profit outpatient surgery center, is instituting a profit-sharing program for physicians and other medical personnel. The profit-sharing program will distribute half of the fully allocated net income in each revenue line. Given the following table, allocate general and administrative costs to the three revenue lines based on revenue; calculate net incomes and profit margins and the amount of profit-sharing that will be distributed to medical staff.

4. Barnard Surgical Associates, a for-profit outpatient surgery center, is instituting a profit-sharing program for physicians and other medical personnel. The

profit-sharing program will distribute half of the fully allocated net income in each revenue line. Given the table in problem 7–3, allocate general and administrative costs to the three revenue lines based on direct expenses; calculate net incomes and profit margins and the amount of profit-sharing that will be distributed to medical staff. What are the increase and decrease in profit-sharing payments for employees in the three revenue lines based on the use of direct expenses rather than revenue (problem 7–3)? Which allocation base would you recommend to the owners of Barnard, and why?

Department	Revenue	Expense	Net Income
General surgery	$9.8	$6.6	$3.2
Orthopedic surgery	5.5	3.2	2.3
Reconstructive and cosmetic surgery	7.2	5.2	2.0
General and administrative	0.0	5.5	-5.5
Total	$22.5	$20.5	$2.0

Notes

1. C. Horngren et al., *Cost Accounting: A Managerial Emphasis*, 9th ed. (Englewood Cliffs, NJ: Prentice Hall, 1998), 70.
2. J. J. Baker, *Activity-Based Costing and Activity-Based Management for Health Care* (Gaithersburg, MD: Aspen Publishers, Inc., 1998).
3. D. A. West, T. D. West, and P. J. Malone, "Managing Capital and Administrative (Indirect) Costs to Achieve Strategic Objectives: The Dialysis Clinic Versus the Outpatient Clinic," *Journal of Health Care Finance*, 25, no. 2 (1998): 20–24.

CHAPTER 8

Cost Behavior and Break-Even Analysis

PROGRESS NOTES

After completing this chapter, you should be able to:

1. Describe the behavior of fixed, variable, semivariable, and semifixed costs.
2. Identify the efficient and profit-maximizing output.
3. Calculate fixed and variable costs using the high–low and scatter graph methods.
4. Calculate a contribution margin and break-even volume.
5. Assess profitability by service.

Overview: Fixed, Variable, and Semivariable Costs

Costs must be understood to ensure that revenues exceed expenses (i.e., one cannot know if the prices charged for services will cover costs when costs are unknown). A prime issue in management is understanding how costs should change with changes in output (e.g., when the output of a medical service increases by 10%, should the cost of the resources needed to produce it increase by 5%, 10%, or 15% or not at all?). For example, when patients require more medication, the cost of purchasing and dispensing medications should increase proportionally; on the other hand, an increase in the number of participants in a nutrition class may not increase

costs at all. One of Murphy's Laws state that expenditures always increase to meet income, but the role of management should be to ensure that expenditures only increase to the extent *needed* to provide quality care.

This chapter examines the differences between fixed, variable, **semivariable**, and **semifixed costs** because this knowledge is essential for resource scheduling, price setting, contract negotiations, service decisions, and investing in equipment, buildings, and land. A manager needs to understand how costs change with output to make good decisions about staffing levels, supply use, and equipment usage. Managers should also know the difference between fixed and **variable costs** to compute **contribution margins** and break-even points to determine whether planned services will generate sufficient revenue to cover their expenses.

Fixed costs are costs that do not vary in total when activity levels (or volume) of operations change—that is, more or fewer resources are not needed when output increases or decreases. **Table 8.1** shows the annual expenses for the Salk Family Medicine practice. Monthly rent for the practice is $2,000 per month, $24,000 per year, and that amount does not change, whether the number of patients (the activity level or volume) is low or high. Rent does not vary whether the practice is at capacity or empty (i.e., the two weeks per year it is closed for vacation); thus, rent is a good example of a fixed cost. The third column identifies the expenses that are expected to be fixed. Fixed costs include the physician salary, insurance, and information technology.

The nature of fixed cost is illustrated in **Figure 8.1**. The horizontal axis of the graph shows the number of patients treated per week at the Salk Family Medicine practice, and the vertical axis shows the weekly total fixed cost. In the graph, the total weekly fixed cost for the practice is $4,056, and that number does not change whether the number of patients (the activity level or volume) is low or high.

Variable costs, on the other hand, are costs that increase and decrease in direct proportion to changes in activity levels (or volume) of

operations. These costs are identified in the fourth column of Table 8.1. The best example of a variable cost is supplies; medical and office supplies should increase and decrease with the number of patients treated. In this case, the practice uses an average of $10.00 in supplies per patient, $8.00 for personal protective equipment, syringes, tongue depressors, and so on and $2.00 for forms, copies, and pens. Other expenses considered to be variable include staff salaries and information technology; the billing software charges $2.00 per claim. The behavior of total variable cost is illustrated in **Figure 8.2**. The horizontal axis of the graph shows the number of patients treated in a week at Salk Family Medicine, and the vertical axis shows total weekly variable cost. The graph shows that weekly variable cost for the practice changes proportionately with the number of patients (the activity level or volume).

The behavior of total cost, the sum of total variable and total fixed cost is illustrated in **Figure 8.3**. This graph is similar to Figure 8.2 except for the fact that total cost is $4,056 when no patients are seen and increases for every patient treated.

A third type of expense is semivariable. A semivariable cost varies with the activity levels (or volume) of operations, but not in direct proportion. The most frequent pattern of semivariable

Table 8.1 Identifying Fixed and Variable Costs

Expense	Total Cost	Fixed Cost	Variable Cost
Physician salary	$150,800	$150,800	
Staff salaries	117,700		$117,700
Supplies	53,500		53,500
Occupancy	24,000	24,000	
Insurance	7,800	7,800	
Other	15,000	15,000	
Information technology	15,900	5,200	10,700
Total expense	$384,700	$202,800	$181,900
		or $4,056	or $34
		per week	per patient

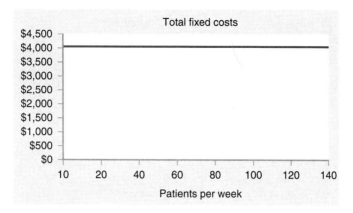

Figure 8.1 Fixed Costs—Salk Family Medicine

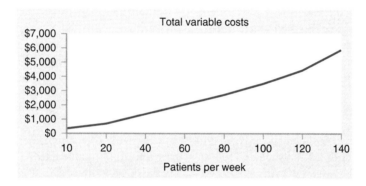

Figure 8.2 Variable Cost—Salk Family Medicine

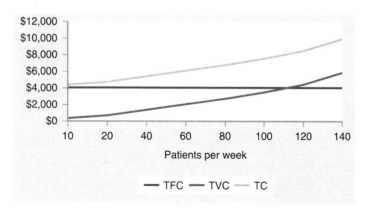

Figure 8.3 Total Cost—Salk Family Practice

costs is the step pattern, where the semivariable cost increases when output is produced and remains constant as output increases until output hits a level requiring additional resources, when cost rises again. The step pattern of semivariable costs is illustrated in **Figure 8.4**. The horizontal axis of the graph shows the number of patients in the ICU at Codman Medical Center. Staffing rules

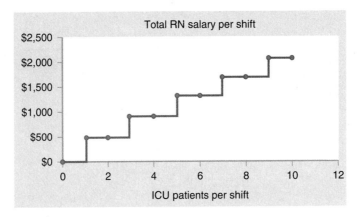

Figure 8.4 Semivariable (or Step) Cost—Codman Medical Center ICU

require one registered nurse (RN) for every two patients, so the cost line resembles stair steps—thus, the "step pattern" name for this configuration. In non-ICU nursing units, an RN may be able to handle six patients before additional RNs are needed.

A fourth type of cost is semifixed. Information technology cost was identified as a fixed and variable cost in Table 8.1; the medical record and billing software requires a weekly fee of $100 for access and a $2.00 charge for every reimbursement claim processed. Semifixed costs include utility and communication services, where users must pay a connection fee and a usage charge per

kilowatt hour, per cubic foot of gas used, or per gigabyte over a set limit.

A semifixed cost has a fixed component and a variable component based on usage. Staff wages are semifixed when employees are paid for 40 hours per week (the fixed component) and time and a half for every hour over 40 (the variable component).

It is important to know that there are two ways to think about fixed cost. The usual view is the flat line illustrated in Figure 8.1. That flat line represents the total weekly cost for the practice. The second view is based on **Table 8.2** and presented in **Figure 8.5**, the average fixed cost

Table 8.2 Salk Family Practice Weekly Costs

Patients per Week	TFC	TVC	TC	AFC	AVC	ATC	MC	TR	Profit
10	$4,056	$340	$4,396	$405.60	$34.00	$439.60	$34.00	$710	–$3,686
20	4,056	680	4,736	202.80	34.00	236.80	34.00	1,420	–3,316
40	4,056	1,360	5,416	101.40	34.00	135.40	34.00	2,840	–2,576
60	4,056	2,040	6,096	67.60	34.00	101.60	34.00	4,260	–1,836
80	4,056	2,720	6,776	50.70	34.00	84.70	34.00	5,680	–1,096
100	4,056	3,500	7,556	40.56	35.00	75.56	39.00	7,100	–456
120	4,056	4,440	8,496	33.80	37.00	70.80*	47.00	8,520	24**
140	4,056	5,880	9,936	28.97	42.00	70.97	72.00	9,940	4

* minimum ATC, ** maximum profit.

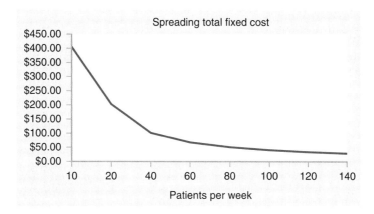

Figure 8.5 Average Fixed Cost

per patient. The average fixed cost is total fixed cost ÷ total patients. The line is no longer flat but declines as total fixed cost is spread over a larger number of patients.

We can also think about variable cost in two ways. The usual view of variable cost is the diagonal line rising from the bottom of the graph to the top, as illustrated in Figure 8.2. That steep diagonal line shows that total weekly cost varies in direct proportion to the number of patients treated. The second view is shown in **Figure 8.6**, average variable cost = total variable cost ÷ total patients. The line is no longer diagonal but is now flat because variable cost stays the same for each patient up to 80 patients per week (an average of

30 minutes per patient); after 80 patients, costs begin to increase.

When only 80 patients are seen, there is sufficient slack to handle all cases (i.e., when one or more patients require more than 30 minutes for care, adjustments can be made that will allow the practice to close at 5:00 p.m.). When 100 patients are scheduled, patients must be treated in 24 minutes or less. Invariably, more than 40 hours will be needed to complete treatment, and the practice will have to remain open after 5:00 p.m. Staff are then paid time and a half for every hour over 40 per week, and the average cost per patient increases. When more than 120 patients are treated, the increase in average variable cost

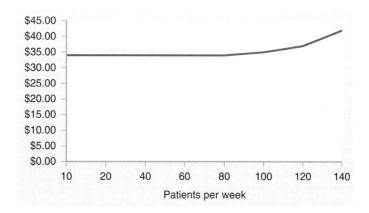

Figure 8.6 Average Variable Cost

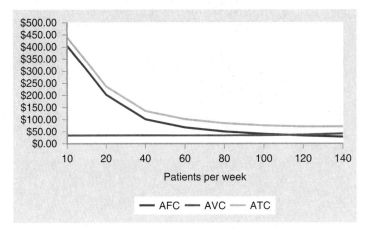

Figure 8.7 Average Total Costs

accelerates as it may be impossible to complete all tasks needed for a patient visit in 20 minutes.

Figure 8.7 clearly shows that the cost per patient is substantially higher when fewer than 100 patients per week are seen. Table 8.2 also reports **marginal cost**, the change in total cost resulting from increasing output. Marginal cost is the change in cost divided by the change in output; for example, the marginal cost of increasing the number of patients treated from 60 to 80 per week is ($6,776 − $6,096) ÷ (80 − 60), $680 ÷ 20 = $34.00. Marginal cost rapidly increases when more than 80 patients are treated in a week.

Identifying the Efficient Output and Profit-Maximizing Output

The efficient output level occurs where average total cost (ATC) is minimized—in Table 8.2 at 120 patients, $70.80. ATC is $75.56 at 100 patients as fixed costs are not spread over the optimal number of patients and $70.97 at 140 patients as variable costs increase.

The profit-maximizing output occurs when price is greater than or equal to marginal cost. Assume the average price is $71.00 per visit; at 120 patients, price exceeds the marginal cost of $47.00, and the practice earns $24.00 per week. If the

practice increases its patient load to 140 per week, price will not cover marginal cost, $72.00, and profit falls to $4 per week. Profit falls despite the fact the $71.00 price exceeds the ATC of $70.97.

The efficient output level and profit-maximizing level do not have to be the same; for example, assume the average price increases to $75.00. Salk would earn a profit of $504 per week at 120 patients and $564 with 140 patients despite ATC increasing to $70.97. A provider earns higher profits as long as the price they receive for services equals or exceeds their marginal cost regardless of whether it is operating efficiently.

Table 8.3 shows how costs change for three types of office visits. A brief office visit, CPT 99211, with no tests and only 10 minutes of physician and nurse time required, so the cost is only $42.95. A comprehensive visit, CPT 99215, requiring 60 minutes of physician and nurse time costs six times more for labor, $4.00 more in supplies, and $10.00 for testing. Providers should understand their costs to ensure that they are neither overpricing brief visits nor under-pricing comprehensive visits. Charging the "average" cost of $80.93 would produce a $46.99 loss per comprehensive visit and a $37.98 profit for brief visits. As long as the number of brief visits offsets the loss on comprehensive visits, the practice will be financially stable, but an increase in comprehensive visits could threaten the long-term survival of the practice.

Table 8.3 Office Visit with Variable Cost of Tests

Service Code (expected visit time)	CPT 99211 (10 min)	CPT 99213 (30 min)	CPT 99215 (60 min)
Lab tests	0	1	2
Physician	$9.66	$28.97	$57.94
RN	4.54	13.61	27.21
Receptionist	7.78	7.78	7.78
Supplies	8.00	10.00	12.00
Test processing	0.00	5.00	10.00
Billing	2.00	2.00	2.00
Overhead (rent, insurance...)	10.98	10.98	10.98
Total visit cost	$42.95	$78.34	$127.92

Determining Fixed and Variable Costs

It is important for planning that managers know how to determine fixed and variable costs because there are few costs that are purely fixed or variable. Pure fixed costs may include administrative salaries, rent, depreciation, and interest expense, and pure variable costs include supplies and food. Other expenses such as staff salaries, utilities, and maintenance generally require a minimum cost and increase when output increases. We briefly discuss two simple methods of determining fixed and variable costs before introducing the high–low method and the scatter graph methods.

The Predominant Characteristics and Step Methods

Both the predominant characteristics and the step method of analyzing mixed costs are quite simple. In the predominant characteristic method, the manager judges whether the cost is more fixed or more variable and treats all costs as fixed or variable. In the case of information technology expense, Table 8.1, the $16,328 could be consider entirely fixed (as overhead) or entirely variable, $2.93 per bill. The predominant method would favor treating the expense as variable since $10,700 of the total $16,328 is based on the $2.00 per bill charge.

In the step method, the manager examines the "steps" in the step pattern of mixed costs and decides when the costs appear to change; in the case of the registered nurse and receptionist, it would be at the point where more than 40 hours are needed to treat the patients (i.e., 107 patients per week). After 107 patients, the RN salary per patient (CPT 99213) would increase from $13.61 to $20.41, and the receptionist hourly salary would also increase by 50% due to the overtime premium. Both methods are subjective.

The High–Low Method

As the name implies, the high–low method of analyzing costs requires that the cost be examined at its highest and lowest output levels. To compute the amount of variable cost involved, the difference in cost between the maximum and minimum outputs is calculated and divided by the change in the output (or volume): variable cost = (cost at maximum output – cost at minimum output) ÷ (maximum output – minimum output). Two examples are examined.

The first example is for an employee cafeteria. **Table 8.4** contains the basic data required for the high–low computation.

With the formula described in the preceding paragraph, the following steps are performed:

1. Find the maximum output of 45,000 meals at a cost of $165,000 in September (see Table 8.4) and the minimum output of 20,000 meals at a cost of $95,000 in March.
2. Compute the variable rate per meal. Subtract the low cost from the high cost, $165,000 – $95,000 = $70,000, subtract the lowest output from the highest output, 45,000 – 20,000 = 25,000 meals, divide the difference in cost by the difference in number of meals, $70,000 ÷ 25,000 = $2.80.

Table 8.4 Employee Cafeteria Number of Meals and Cost by Month

Month	Number of Meals	Employee Cafeteria Cost
July 2021	40,000	$164,000
August	43,000	167,000
September—**high meals**	45,000	165,000
October	41,000	162,000
November	37,000	164,000
December	33,000	146,000
January	28,000	123,000
February	22,000	91,800
March—**low meals**	20,000	95,000
April	25,000	106,800
May	30,000	130,200
June 2022	35,000	153,000

	Cafeteria Cost	Number of Meals
Maximum output (September)	$165,000	45,000
Minimum output (March)	95,000	20,000
Difference	$70,000 ÷	25,000 = $2.80

3. Compute the fixed overhead rate as follows:

  a. At the highest cost:

Maximum cost	$165,000
Less: variable portion [45,000 meals × $2.80]	126,000
Fixed portion of cost	$39,000

  b. At the lowest cost:

Minimum cost	$95,000
Less: variable portion [20,000 meals × $2.80]	56,000
Fixed portion of cost	$39,000

Table 8.5 Number of Drug Samples and Cost for November 2022

Sales Representative	Number of Samples	Cost
Smith, J.—**high samples**	1,000	$5,000
Jones, A.	900	4,300
Baker, B.	850	4,600
Black, G.	975	4,500
Potter, T.	875	4,750
Conner, D.—**low samples**	750	4,200

  c. Proof: $39,000 is the fixed portion at maximum and minimum output.

The second example concerns drug samples and their cost. In this example, a marketing manager is concerned about the number of drug samples distributed by members of her staff. She uses the high–low method to determine the portion of fixed cost. **Table 8.5** contains the basic data required for the high–low computation.

Using the formula previously described, the following steps are performed:

1. Identify the highest sample volume, 1,000 (see Table 8.5), the corresponding cost, $5,000, and the lowest sample volume, 750, and its corresponding cost, $4,200.
2. Compute the variable rate per sample: subtract the low cost from the high cost, $5,000 − $4,200 = $800, subtract the lowest volume from the highest volume, 1,000 − 750 = 250 samples, divide the difference in cost by the difference in number of samples, $800 ÷ 250 = $3.20, cost per sample.

	Cost	Number of Samples
Highest volume	$5,000	1,000
Lowest volume	4,200	750
Difference	$800 ÷	250 = $3.20

3. Compute the fixed overhead rate as follows:

a. At the highest cost:

Maximum cost	$5,000
Less: variable portion	
[1,000 samples × $3.20]	3,200
Fixed portion of cost	$1,800

b. At the lowest cost:

Minimum cost	$4,200
Less: variable portion	
[750 samples × $3.20]	2,400
Fixed portion of cost	$1,800

c. Proof: $1,800 is the fixed portion at maximum and minimum output.

The high–low method is an approximation that is based on the relationship between the highest and the lowest output levels, and the computation assumes a straight-line relationship. The advantage of the high-low method is its simple computation.

The Scatter Graph Method

The scatter graph method is more accurate than the high–low method previously described. It uses a graph to plot all points of data rather than simply the highest and lowest figures used by the high–low method. Generally, cost will be on the vertical axis of the graph, and volume will be on the horizontal axis. All points are plotted, each point being placed where cost and volume intersect for the observation. A regression line is then fitted to the plotted points. The regression line basically represents the average—or a line of averages. The average total fixed cost is found at the point where the regression line intersects with the cost (horizontal or Y) axis.

Two examples are examined; they are the high–low examples previously calculated. **Figure 8.8** presents the cafeteria data. The costs for cafeteria meals have been plotted on the graph; the regression line has been fitted to the plotted data points, and the equation for the best-fitting line was reported using Excel's Insert Trendline function. The regression line strikes the cost (horizontal or Y) axis at $28,726 and represents the fixed cost portion of the mixed cost (i.e., the minimum cost to operate the cafeteria). The balance (or total cost less the fixed cost portion) represents the variable portion.

The regression line again strikes the cost axis at $28,726, the minimum expected cost. The balance (total cost less the fixed cost portion) represents the variable portion; in this case, the cost per meal is expected to be $3.32 for every meal.

The second example also matches the previous high–low example. **Figure 8.9** presents the drug sample data. The costs for drug samples have been plotted on the graph, and the regression line has been fitted to the plotted data points.

The fixed cost for drug samples was calculated as $2,666 and increased by $2.12 for every sample distributed. You should notice that the high–low and scatter graph methods did not

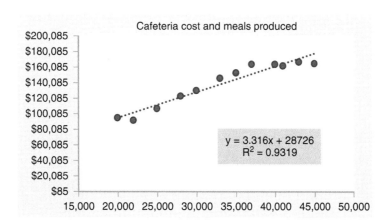

Figure 8.8 Employee Cafeteria Scatter Graph

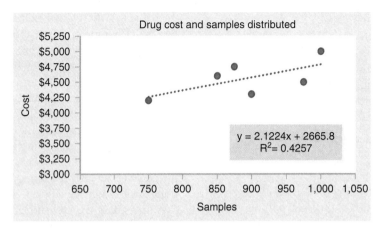

Figure 8.9 Drug Sample Scatter Graph for November 2022

produce identical estimates. In the cafeteria example, the high–low method calculated a fixed cost of $39,000 and cost per meal of $2.80, and the scatter graph calculated $28,726 and $3.32. Given the difference, a manager could decide to use an average cost of $3.06 per meal, ($2.80 + $3.32) ÷ 2, or assess and use the estimate that they believe more accurately reflects the economic reality of meal production. The point is you now know how to calculate fixed and variable costs. Practice exercises are included at the end of the chapter. The following section will demonstrate how you can use this information in financial decision-making.

Contribution Margin and Cost-Volume-Profit and Profit-Volume Ratios

A manager should know how to translate their understanding of costs and output into expected financial performance (i.e., expected profit). Fixed and variable cost information assists the manager in understanding and controlling operations. The first step in such analysis is the computation of the contribution margin. Assume a newly graduated pediatrician wants to open a practice and expects her variable costs will be $300,000, $60 per visit assuming 5,000 patient visits, and fixed

costs will be $175,000 in the first year and wants to determine the volume of patients needed to cover her expenses if she receives $100 per visit.

Contribution Margin

The contribution margin based on 5,000 visits is calculated as:

	5,000 Visits	% Net Revenue
Net revenues	$500,000	100%
Less: variable cost	300,000	60%
Contribution margin	$200,000	40%
Less: fixed cost	175,000	35%
Operating income	$25,000	5%

The contribution margin of $200,000 or 40%, is net revenues less variable cost. The contribution margin represents how much revenue from the sale of goods and services can be used to pay fixed costs and increase profit after fixed costs are covered.

Cost-Volume-Profit (CVP) Ratio or Break-Even

The **break-even point** is the number of units of a good or service that must be sold to produce a contribution margin (i.e., net revenues less variable costs) equal to fixed costs. When operations exceed the break-even point, an excess of revenues over expenses (profit) is realized, but if output does not reach the break-even point, expenses will exceed revenues, and a loss will be realized.

Managers should recognize that there are two ways of expressing the break-even point: either by an amount per unit or as a percentage of net revenues. If the contribution margin is expressed as a percentage of net revenues, it is often called the **profit-volume (PV) ratio**. A PV ratio example follows this **cost-volume-profit** (CVP) computation.

The CVP example is given in **Figure 8.10**. The data points for the chart come from the contribution margin as computed above.

Four lines were first drawn to create the chart: total cost, total fixed cost, total variable cost, and total revenue. At 5,000 patient visits, total fixed cost is $175,000, total variable cost is $300,000, and total revenue is $500,000; a $25,000 profit is earned. The break-even point appears at the point where the total cost line intersects the total revenue line. The break-even formula is TFC ÷ (Price − AVC). The break-even point for the practice is 4,375 visits, $175,000 ÷ ($100 − 60). At 4,375 visits, the provider will have no profit or loss; total fixed cost is $175,000, total variable cost is $262,250, and total revenue is $437,250. The wedge shape to the left of the break-even point is the potential loss when visits fall below 4,375, whereas the narrower wedge to the right is potential profit when output exceeds 4,375. CVP charts illustrate the relationships between cost, revenue, and volume to assess the feasibility of operations. Can sufficient output be sold to sustain the organization?

Profit-Volume (PV) Ratio

Remember that the second method of expressing the break-even point is as a percentage of net revenues and that if the contribution margin is expressed as a percentage of net revenues, it is called the profit-volume (PV) ratio. **Figure 8.11** illustrates the effect of reducing variable cost; if AVC can be reduced from $60 to $50, the break-even point falls to 3,500 visits. The physician or office manager can thus determine what actions are necessary to ensure that revenue will equal expenses when fewer than 4,375 patient visits are likely.

Revenue per visit	$100.00	100%
Less variable cost per visit	60.00	60%
Contribution margin per visit	$40.00	40%
Fixed costs per period	$175,000	

$40.00 contribution margin per visit divided by $100 price per visit = 40% PV ratio

On the chart, the profit pattern is illustrated by a line drawn from the beginning level of fixed costs to be recovered ($175,000 in our case). When the diagonal line begins at $175,000, its intersection with the break-even or zero line is at $437,250 in revenue (see left-hand dotted line on chart). We can prove the $175,000 versus $437,250 relationship as follows. Each dollar of revenue reduces

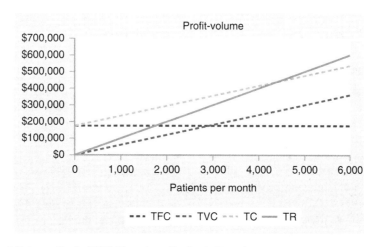

Figure 8.10 Cost-Volume-Profit (CVP) Chart for a Pediatric Practice

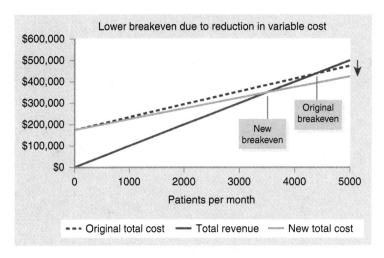

Figure 8.11 Profit-Volume Chart for a Pediatric Practice

the potential loss by $0.40 (or 40%). Fixed costs are fully recovered at a revenue level of $437,250, proved by dividing $175,000 by 0.40 equals $437,250. This can be written as follows:

0.40R = $175,000
　R = $437,250 [$175,000 ÷ 0.40 = $437,250]

The PV chart is very effective in planning because only two lines are necessary to show the effect of changes in volume. Both PV and CVP are useful when working with the effects of changes in break-even points and revenue volume assumptions.

Assessing Services by Volume and Profitability

Understanding profitability is essential for decision-making, should prices be increased, costs reduced, and/or services expanded or contracted? We will conclude this chapter by examining profitability across major diagnostic categories (MDC) that organize inpatient care by body system. **Table 8.6** shows profitability and the percent of total inpatient cases by MDC.

Figure 8.12 shows the same information as Table 8.3 but places it into a scatter diagram. The diagram highlights that pregnancy care (MDC 14)

Table 8.6 Operating Margin and Patient Volume by MDC

MDC	Operating Margin	% Admissions
MDC 4: Respiratory	2.5%	8%
MDC 5: Circulatory	3.5%	23%
MDC 6: Digestive	2.8%	7%
MDC 14: Pregnancy	6.7%	9%
MDC 17: Neoplasms	4.3%	7%
MDC 19: Mental	1.9%	10%
MDC 12/13: Genitourinary	1.2%	6%

has the highest profitability, 6.7%, while cardiology (MDC 5) serves the highest number of patients, 23%; both are substantially higher than other MDCs. Four of the remaining five MDCs produce profits of 1.2% to 2.9% and account for between 6% and 10% of patients.

An analysis similar to Figure 8.12 is helpful to decide what actions should be taken to improve current profitability (i.e., increasing prices, reducing expenses, increasing or reducing patient volume) and guide future investment.

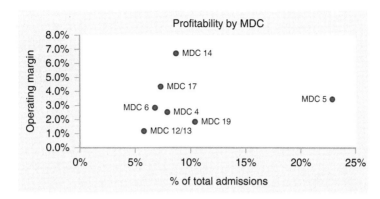

Figure 8.12 MDC Profitability and Volume Matrix

WRAP-UP

Summary

It is vital that managers understand cost behavior so they can determine how cost should change with output and whether their department is operating efficiently. Efficiency occurs when the department reaches the minimum cost per output, however, it may be desirable for the department to operate at a cost above minimum when revenue exceeds marginal cost. That is, a department can maximize profit at an output level above the minimum cost output.

The first step to utilizing cost information is to calculate fixed and variable costs. Four methods were demonstrated: predominant characteristics, step, high–low, and scatter graph. Each may arrive at different numbers for fixed and variable

cost, so managers must use their knowledge to determine which supplies the best information for their operation.

Managers should calculate their contribution margin and break-even volume. That is, given fixed and variable costs, can the department generate sufficient revenue to break even or earn a profit? **Break-even analysis** is vital when a provider has little control over pricing and must rely on cost control to sustain operations. Finally, providers should assess the profitability of their major services or service lines to understand where money is earned or lost and plan service volumes and prices.

Key Terms

Break-Even Analysis
Break-Even Point
Cost-Profit-Volume Ratio
Contribution Margin

Fixed Cost
Marginal Cost
Profit-Volume Ratio
Semifixed Cost

Semivariable or Step Cost
Variable Cost

Discussion Questions

1. Describe the behavior of fixed, variable, semivariable, and semifixed costs.

2. Explain where the efficient output and profit-maximizing output occur.

3. Explain how the high–low and scatter graph methods determine fixed and variable costs.
4. Explain the purpose of calculating contribution margins and break-even volumes.

5. What is the purpose of assessing patient volume and profitability by service?

Problems

1. The CEO of Henry Hospital wants to know the per patient cost on 2 South, a medical nursing unit. Using the following table, calculate total cost, average fixed cost, average variable cost, and average total cost. What is the most efficient output level for the unit?

Patients per Month	TFC	TVC
0	$350,000	$0
150	350,000	75,000
300	350,000	150,000
450	350,000	225,000
600	350,000	300,000
750	350,000	375,000
900	350,000	450,000

2. The CEO of Henry Hospital also wants to know the per patient cost on 2 North, a surgical nursing unit. Using the following table, calculate total cost, average fixed cost, average variable cost, and average total cost. What is the most efficient output level for the unit?

Patients per Month	TFC	TVC
0	$350,000	$0
150	350,000	75,000
300	350,000	150,000
450	350,000	225,000
600	350,000	300,000
750	350,000	425,000
900	350,000	600,000

3. The CEO of Barnard Surgical Associates has received an offer from a large managed care payer to direct its enrollees to the facility for outpatient surgery. Using the following table, calculate the fixed and variable costs for an outpatient surgery patient using the high–low method. If the managed care payer is offering to pay $700 per surgery, what is your recommendation to the CEO?

Month	Total Patients	Total Cost
January	600	$650,000
February	510	615,000
March	625	663,000
April	607	662,000
May	655	688,000
June	621	671,000
July	637	664,000
August	649	669,000
September	602	651,000
October	633	667,000
November	650	675,000
December	545	623,000

4. The CEO of Barnard Surgical Associates has received an offer from its state Medicaid program offering the practice $500 per outpatient surgery. Using the table in Problem 8–3, calculate the fixed and variable costs for an outpatient surgery patient using a scatter graph with a trend line. What is your recommendation to the CEO?

5. Calculate the breakeven quantity (BE_Q) for the Blundell Blood Center if it incurs $350,000 in monthly fixed costs and $50 in average variable cost per blood draw and receives $110 per pint. Create an income statement at the calculated BE_Q and if 560 and 610 pints are drawn.

6. Using the following table, assess the profitability by MDC. Calculate the profit margin and the percent of revenue for each MDC. Create a scatter graph with profit margin on the *x*-axis and percent of revenue on the *y*-axis. Explain what the scatter graph indicates about the relationship between profit margin and revenue.

Major Diagnostic Category	Total Revenue	Operating Income
MDC 4: Respiratory	$5,000,000	$300,000
MDC 5: Circulatory	8,000,000	700,000
MDC 6: Digestive	5,700,000	250,000
MDC 14: Pregnancy	2,700,000	−100,000
MDC 17: Neoplasms	6,500,000	600,000
MDC 19: Mental	2,400,000	150,000
MDC 12/13: Genitourinary	3,300,000	100,000

Managing Staffing and Salaries: Methods, Operations, and Regulations

PROGRESS NOTES

After completing this chapter, you should be able to:

1. Describe the difference between productive time and nonproductive time.
2. Calculate full-time equivalents to annualize staff positions and FTE staffing requirements.
3. Calculate full-time equivalents to fill a scheduled position.
4. Calculate wage expense based on staffing.
5. Calculate employee turnover rates.
6. Describe regulatory requirements that affect staffing.

Overview: Staffing and Salaries

The greatest opportunity for managers to reduce costs lies in salaries. Salaries are the largest expense for healthcare providers, so efficient scheduling, effective oversight of staff, and retention of staff are essential to delivering quality care and avoiding unnecessary cost. Labor expenses, including salaries, fringe benefits, and professional fees, account for 67.9% of total hospital expenses.[1] In physician practices, labor expenses comprise approximately 48% of total practice expenses. One of the foundations of Lean Six Sigma is **load leveling**—that is, ensuring that employees are neither over- or underworked. Appropriate **staffing** ensures timely and efficient high-quality care that increases patient and employee satisfaction.

Assume Codman Medical Center employs two shifts of eight full-time personnel to prepare and deliver meals to patients and employees during weekdays, Monday through Friday. **Figure 9.1** shows the staffing level and the demand for meals (i.e., the number of employees needed to prepare and deliver meals). Weekend

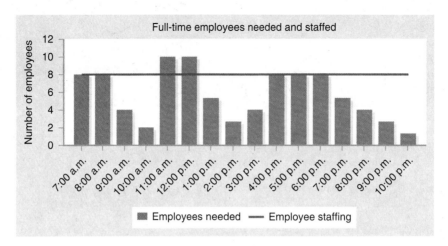

Figure 9.1 Previous Food Service Staffing

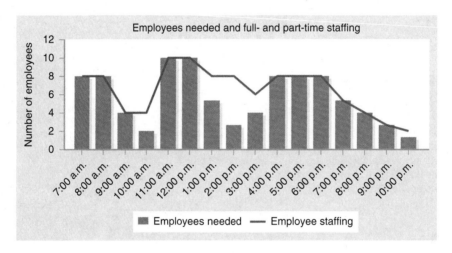

Figure 9.2 Revised Food Service Staffing

staffing uses a single 12-hour shift model due to the lower number of patients and employees on Saturday and Sunday.

The problem is immediately apparent. For the majority of hours between 7:00 a.m. and 11:00 p.m., Codman has too little work to keep eight people fully employed. Employees are fully employed from 7:00 a.m. to 9:00 a.m. and from 4:00 p.m. to 7:00 p.m., five of 16 paid hours. The demand for meals exceeds capacity, (i.e., employees are overworked) between 11:00 a.m. and 1:00 p.m., and multiple patient complaints are received about delays in receiving lunch and cold food. Many food service businesses use part-time

employees to better match capacity and demand. **Figure 9.2** shows the recently revised staffing plan based on 10 full-time employees and four or fewer part-time employees during peak periods.

The new staffing model ensures that enough personnel are working to meet the demand at all three peak periods and reduces idle time. Idle time could not be entirely eliminated due to a guaranteed eight-hour day for full-time employees and minimum four-hour shifts for part-time employees. The revised staffing plan also eliminated hours where required work exceeded the number of employees working. The move from an all full-time to a combination full-time and part-time model reduced paid hours and salary expense by 18.9%.

In most businesses, a position is filled when the employee works an eight-hour day, from 9:00 a.m. to 5:00 p.m., five days a week, generally Monday through Friday. In health care, many positions must be filled, or covered, 24 hours a day, seven day a week. Patients need care on Saturday and Sunday as well as around the clock, 24 hours a day, Monday through Friday.

Thus, healthcare employees work in shifts. The shifts are often eight-hour shifts, requiring three shifts to provide 24-hour coverage. Some facilities now use 12-hour shifts, so only two 12-hour shifts are needed per day. The manager is responsible for seeing that an employee is present and working for each position and every shift. Of course, ensuring that 10 full-time and four part-time employees are on duty requires a staff of more than 14 due to planned and unplanned absences. Therefore, it is necessary to understand and use the staffing measurement known as the **full-time equivalent (FTE)**. Two different approaches are used to compute FTEs: the annualizing method and the scheduled-position method. Full-time equivalent is a measure of the number of people paid for 2,080 hours per year (i.e., 52 weeks × 40 hours per week) to express the equivalent of an employee (*annualized*) or a position (*staffed*) for the full time required. We examine both methods in this chapter.

FTEs for Annualizing Positions

Annualizing is necessary because each employee is eligible for benefits such as holidays, vacation days, and sick days and will not be on duty for 2,080 hours per year, the total number of hours paid by the organization. Annualizing allows the full cost of the position to be computed through a burden approach. In the burden approach, the net hours desired are inflated, or burdened, to arrive at the gross number of paid hours that will be needed to obtain the desired number of net hours on duty from the employee.

Productive Versus Nonproductive Time

Productive time equates to an employee's net hours on duty performing the functions in his or her job description. **Nonproductive time** is paid time when the employee is not on duty—that is, not producing goods or services—including paid vacation days, holidays, personal leave days, and/or sick days.[2]

Table 9.1 illustrates productive time (work or on-duty days) versus nonproductive time (days paid for but not worked). The Curie Imaging Center provides imaging services 364 days per year (closed Christmas Day) with scheduled business hours from 8:00 a.m. through 5:00 p.m. In Table 9.1, Dominique Rand, a radiology technician, is paid for 260 days per year (52 weeks × 5 days per week) but works only 230 days per year. The remaining 30 days are holidays (10 days), sick days (10 days), and vacation days (2 weeks or 10 days), nonproductive time.

The 364 paid days would be sufficient to provide all scans if demand only required one radiology tech per day, but Curie's business manager projects 20,000 scans will be needed and each scan takes an average of 30 minutes, so 1,250 productive days are needed. **Table 9.2** shows the number of FTEs Curie needs to employ.

Curie needs 5.43 FTEs to fulfill radiology technician functions. The manager has three scheduling options. She can employ 6 FTEs, 5 FTEs and approve overtime, or 5.43 FTEs (i.e., employ 0.43 part-time FTE). The bottom of Table 9.2 examines the cost of each option assuming a wage of $40,000. The most efficient option is the use of one or more part-time employees to meet the 0.43 FTE needed for a total salary expense of $217,391. The second-best option is approving overtime. Paying time and a half for 0.43 FTEs adds an additional $8,696, but no additional nonproductive time is incurred. Assuming each of the five FTEs is scheduled to work overtime known days each week (e.g., Monday and Tuesday), they may like the additional income. A sixth full-time rad tech should be hired when demand increases to require more than 5.67 FTEs. When more than 5.67 FTEs are needed, it is less expensive to hire

Table 9.1 Staffing Requirements

1. Total days in business year	364	
2. Days worked by D. Rand	260	5 days per week × 52 weeks = 260 days
3. During the year Rand gets paid for:		
Holidays	10	
Sick days	10	* all days may or may not be taken
Vacation days	10	
Total nonproductive days	30	
4. Net paid days worked	230	
5. Additional days needed to provide scans:		
Weekends	104	2 days per week × 52 weeks = 104 days
Rand's holidays	10	
Rand's sick days	10	
Rand's vacation days	10	
Total part-time days	134	
6. Total days scans are provided	364	230 FT + 134 PT

Table 9.2 Calculation of Needed Productive Days

Productive Days Needed:		
Total scans	20,000	
Scans per day	16	
Required days	1,250	
Required FTEs	5.43	1250 ÷ 230 productive days per FTE

Expected Salary Expense:		
Staffing Option	**Expense**	**% Increase**
6 FTEs	$ 240,000	10.4%
5 FTEs + overtime	$ 226,087	4.0%
5.43 FTEs	$ 217,391	0.0%

a sixth FTE than to pay overtime (i.e., 0.67 FTE × 1.5 wage = 1.0 FTE). The least efficient option is to employ six techs as 0.57 FTE would be idle and salary expense would increase by $22,609 or 10.4% over employing part-time workers.

The choice of staffing and scheduling should depend on the operation. A food service department with known peaks in demand—breakfast, lunch, and dinner—could use fixed part-time employees during demand surges. An emergency department that must service patients on an unpredictable and as-needed basis could use overtime and/or on-call staffing. The Curie Imaging Center may choose to rely on overtime until demand justifies hiring an additional FTE when a qualified part-time technician cannot be employed.

FTE for Annualizing Positions Defined

For purposes of annualizing positions, the definition of FTE is as follows: the equivalent of one full-time employee paid for one year, including both productive and nonproductive (vacation, sick, holiday, etc.) time. Two employees working half-time for one year would be the same as one FTE (e.g., 2 employees × 20 hours per week × 52 weeks = 2,080 hours).

Staffing Calculations to Annualize Positions

Exhibit 9.1 contains a two-step process to perform the staffing calculation by the annualizing method. The first step computes the net paid days worked. In this step, the number of paid days per year is first arrived at; then paid days not worked are deducted to arrive at net paid days worked. The second step of the staffing calculation converts the net paid days worked to a factor. In the example in Exhibit 9.1, the factor ranges from 1.6323 to 1.6545. This calculation is for a 24-hour around-the-clock staffing schedule. Thus, the 364 in the step 2 formula equates to a 24-hour staffing expectation.

Exhibit 9.2 illustrates a master staffing plan for a surgical nursing unit at Codman Medical Center. The demand for nursing services is higher during the day when patients must be prepared for tests, procedures, and therapies and given meals and declines during evening and overnight hours when patients are often sleeping. Exhibit 9.2 shows that the need for RNs falls during the evening and night shifts, and they are replaced with LPNs. CNA staffing, like that of RNs, also declines in the evening and night hours.

Exhibit 9.1 Basic Calculation for Annualizing Master Staffing Plan

Step 1: How Many Net Paid Days Are Worked?

(a) A *business year* has 364 days.

(b) In this example, the employee works five days per week. The other two days off are not paid for. Thus, two days off per week times 52 weeks equals 104 *nonpaid days*.

(c) Therefore, the number of *paid days per year* equals 364 less 104, or 260 days.

(d) But not all paid days per year are worked. In this example, each employee (RN, LPN, and certified nurse assistant [CNA]) receives 35 *personal leave days*. The personal leave days are intended to include holidays, sick leave, and vacation days.

(e) In addition, these employees are entitled to *continuing professional education (CPE) days*. These are also paid days not worked; RNs are paid for five days per year; LPNs, three days; and CNAs, two days.

(f) Therefore the *net paid days worked* are as follows:

$$RN = 260 \text{ days} - 35 \text{ personal leave} - 5 \text{ education} = 220$$

$$LPN = 260 \text{ days} - 35 \text{ personal leave} - 3 \text{ education} = 222$$

$$CNA = 260 \text{ days} - 35 \text{ personal leave} - 2 \text{ education} = 223$$

Step 2: How Are Net Paid Days Worked Converted to a Factor?

The factor is calculated by dividing total days in the business year (364) by the net paid days worked, as follows:

$$RN = 364/220 = 1.6545$$

$$RN = 364/222 = 1.6396$$

$$RN = 364/223 = 1.6323$$

Courtesy of J. J. Baker and R. W. Baker, Dallas, Texas.

Exhibit 9.2 Master Staffing Plan for Nursing Unit

Eight-hour shifts	RNs	LPNs	CNAs
Day shift	3	1	6
Evening shift	2	2	5
Night shift	1	2	2
24-hour total	6	5	13

Number of Employees Required to Fill a Position: Another Way to Calculate FTEs

The calculation of the number of FTEs by the scheduled position method—in other words, to fill a position—is used in planning, organizing, controlling, and evaluating resource use. **Exhibit 9.3** sets out the schedule and the FTE computation. A summarized explanation of the calculation in Exhibit 9.3 is as follows. One full-time employee (as shown) works 40 hours per week. One eight-hour shift per day multiplied by seven days per week equals 56 required hours. Therefore, to cover seven days per week, or 56 hours, requires 1.4 times a 40-hour employee, 56 hours ÷ 40 hours = 1.4 FTEs.

Staffing Calculations to Fill Scheduled Positions

The term *staffing*, as used here, means the assignment of staff to fill scheduled positions. The staffing measure used to compute coverage is also called the FTE. It measures the proportion of one single full-time employee required to fill the required hours (i.e., full-time equivalent) for a position. For example, the cast room has to be staffed 24 hours a day, seven days a week because it supports the emergency room and therefore has to provide service at any time. In this example, the employees are paid for an eight-hour shift. The three shifts required to fill the position for 24 hours are called the day shift (7:00 a.m. to 3:00 p.m.), the evening shift (3:00 p.m. to 11:00 p.m.), and the night shift (11:00 p.m. to 7:00 a.m.).

It takes seven days to fill the day shift cast room position from Monday through Sunday, as required. Seven days is 140% of five days, 7 ÷ 5 = 1.4. The FTE for the day shift cast room position is 1.4 when a seven-day schedule is required.

Exhibit 9.3 Staffing Requirements Example

Emergency department scheduling for eight-hour shifts: 24-hour scheduling

	Shift 1	Shift 2	Shift 3		
	Day	Evening	Night	=	Total
Position:					
Emergency room intake to cover position seven days per week	1	1	1	=	3, 8-hour shifts
Equals FTEs of:	1.4	1.4	1.4	=	4.2 FTEs

One full-time employee works 40 hours per week. One eight-hour shift per day times seven days per week equals 56 hours on duty. Therefore, to cover seven days per week or 56 hours requires 1.4 times a 40-hour employee, 56 hours ÷ 40 hours = 1.4 or 1.4 FTEs.

This method of computing FTEs uses a basic 40-hour work week. Some institutions may use a 37.5-hour work week (to account for two 15-minute breaks per day) or another standard. The method computes a figure that will be necessary to fill the position for the desired length of time, measuring this figure against the standard work week. For example, if the standard work week is 40 hours and a receptionist position is to be filled for just 20 hours per week, then the FTE for that position would be 0.5 FTE, 20 hours to fill the position divided by the 40-hour standard work week. **Table 9.3** illustrates the difference between a standard work year at 40 hours per week and 37.5 hours per week.

A Demand-Based Approach to Staffing

The calculation of needed FTEs is based on some measure of output, whether you manage radiology, patient accounting, the cafeteria, or another area in which your employees are paid to produce services (i.e., images, bills, meals, etc.). Returning to the Curie Imaging Center, Curie employs six full-time radiology technicians to produce 20,000 images per year. Note that Table 9.1 documents the number of days needed to keep a rad tech on-site during business hours. The manager estimates that each image takes an average of 30 minutes to

complete; thus, 10,000 productive hours will be needed to complete all images.

Tying Cost to Staffing

In the case of the annualizing method, the factors of 1.6323 to 1.6545 have the organization's vacation, holiday, sick pay, and other nonproductive days accounted for in the formula. (Review Exhibit 9.2 to check this fact.) Therefore, this factor is multiplied by the base hourly rate (the net rate) paid to compute cost.

In the case of the scheduled position method, however, the FTE figure of 1.4 will be multiplied by the burdened hourly rate. The burden on the hourly rate reflects the vacation, holiday, sick pay, and other nonproductive days accounted for in the formula. (Review Exhibit 9.3 to see the difference.) The scheduled position method is often used in the forecasting of new programs and services.

Actual cost is attached to staffing in the accounting books and records through a subsidiary journal and a basic transaction record. **Table 9.4** illustrates a subsidiary journal in which employee hours worked for a one-week period are recorded. Both regular and overtime hours are noted. The hourly rate, base pay, and overtime premiums are noted, and gross earnings are computed. Deductions for federal income tax,

Table 9.3 Calculations to Staff the Operating Room

Job Position	Number of FTEs	Number of Annual Hours Paid at 2,080 Hours*	Number of Annual Hours Paid at 1,950 Hours**
Supervisors	2.2	4,576	4,290
Technicians	3.0	6,240	5,850
RNs	7.7	16,016	15,015
LPNs	1.2	2,496	2,340
Aides & orderlies	1.0	2,080	1,950
Clerical staff	1.2	2,496	2,340
Totals	16.3	33,904	31,785

* 40 hours per week × 52 weeks = 2,080
** 37.5 hours per week × 52 weeks = 1,950

Table 9.4 Example of a Payroll Register

| Employee Number | Name | Hours Worked | | | | | | Gross Earnings | Deductions | | | Net Pay |
		Regular	Over-time	Total	Rate	Base Pay	Overtime Premium		Federal Income Tax	Social Security	Medicare	
1071	J. F. Green	40	2	42	$14.00	$588.00	$14.00	$602.00	$90.30	$37.32	$8.73	$465.65
1084	C. B. Brown	40		40	14.00	560.00		560.00	84.00	34.72	8.62	432.66
1090	K. D. Grey	40		40	10.00	400.00		400.00	60.00	24.80	6.16	309.04
1092	R. N. Black	40	5	45	10.00	450.00	25.00	475.00	71.25	29.45	6.89	367.41

Deduction calculations for J. F. Green based on gross earnings of $602.00*

Deduction	$90.30	$37.32	$8.73
Rate	15.00%	6.20%	1.45%

* The federal income tax rate is based on withholding and income level, 6.2% Social Security tax is levied on first $142,800 earned as of 2021, and 1.45% Medicare tax applies to all income.

Social Security payroll tax, and Medicare payroll tax were calculated and deducted from gross earnings to compute the net pay for each employee in the final column. In the real world (i.e., your paycheck), additional deductions for state income tax, employee retirement contributions, and employee health insurance premiums are taken.

Table 9.5 illustrates a time card for one employee for one week. This type of record, whether it is generated by a time clock or an electronic entry, is the original record upon which the payroll process is based. Thus, it is considered a basic transaction record. In this example, time in and time out are recorded daily. The resulting regular and overtime hours are recorded separately for each day worked. Although the appearance of the time card may vary or be recorded within a computer instead of on hard copy, the essential transaction is the same: The recording of daily time is where the payroll process begins.

Table 9.6 presents an emergency department staffing report. Actual productive time is shown in columns 1 and 2, with regular time in column 1 and overtime in column 2. Nonproductive time is shown in column 3, and columns 1, 2, and 3

are totaled to arrive at column 4, labeled "Total Paid (Actual) Hours." The final actual figure is the FTE figure in column 5; since this is a two-week pay period, column 4 is divided by 80 hours to calculate FTE.

We can tell from this line item that the second method of computing FTEs—the FTE computation to fill scheduled positions—has been used in this case. Columns 6 through 9 report budgeted time and FTEs, and columns 10 through 12 report the variance between actual hours and FTEs and budgeted hours and FTEs.

The emergency department was 1.7% over budget on paid hours and FTEs for the pay period ending September 20, 2022. The higher-than-expected hours total should be examined in two ways. The first is determining if this is a one-time variance or a continuing variance. What was the variance for the pay period ending September 4, and what is the variance for the current year? One-time variations do not warrant the same scrutiny as continuing variances.

The second examination should identify the job code(s) accounting for the higher hours. In the current pay period, unit coordinators, job

---

Table 9.5 **Example of a Time Record**

Curie Imaging Center

| Employee: | J. F. Green | | | Employee No. | 1071 | | |
| Department: | 3 | | | Week ending: | June 10, 2022 | | |

| Day | Regular | | | | Overtime | | Hours | |
	In	Out	In	Out	In	Out	Regular	Overtime
Monday	8:00	12:01	1:02	5:04			8	
Tuesday	7:56	12:00	12:59	5:03	6:00	8:00	8	2
Wednesday	7:57	12:02	12:58	5:00			8	
Thursday	8:00	12:00	1:00	5:01			8	
Friday	7:59	12:01	1:01	5:02			8	
Saturday								
Sunday								
Total regular hours							40	

Table 9.6 Comparative Hours Staffing Report

Position	Job Code	Actual Regular Hours (1)	Overtime Hours (2)	Actual Non-productive Hours (3)	Total Actual Paid Hours (4)	Actual Paid FTEs (5)	Budgeted Productive Hours (6)	Budgeted Non-productive Hours (7)	Budgeted Total Hours (8)	Budgeted FTEs (9)	Variance Hours (10)	Variance FTEs (11)	% Variance Hours (12)
Manager nursing service	11075	80.0	0.0	0.0	80.0	1.0	69.8	10.2	80.0	1.0	0.0	0.0	0.0%
Supervising charge nurse	11403	383.2	0.1	79.0	462.3	5.8	456.0	64.0	520.0	6.5	57.7	0.7	11.1%
Medical assistant	12007	6.2	0.0	0.0	6.2	0.1	0.0	0.0	0.0	0.0	-6.2	-0.1	100.0%
Staff RN	13401	2010.5	32.8	285.8	2329.1	29.1	2012.8	240.8	2253.6	28.2	-75.5	-0.9	-3.4%
Relief charge nurse	13403	81.9	4.3	0.0	86.2	1.1	0.0	0.0	0.0	0.0	-86.2	-1.1	100.0%
Orderly/transporter	15483	203.8	38.0	20.0	261.8	3.3	279.8	35.3	315.1	3.9	53.3	0.6	16.9%
ER tech	22483	244.6	27.5	67.9	340.0	4.3	336.2	34.5	370.7	4.6	30.7	0.3	8.3%
Secretary	22730	58.1	0.0	0.0	58.1	0.7	50.5	5.9	56.4	0.7	-1.7	0.0	-3.0%
Unit coordinator	22780	555.1	35.6	74.9	665.6	8.3	505.4	53.8	559.2	7.0	-106.4	-1.3	-19.0%
Preadmission testing clerk	22818	0.0	6.5	0.0	6.5	0.1	0.0	0.0	0.0	0.0	-6.5	-0.1	100.0%
Patient registrar	22873	617.5	78.6	105.7	801.8	10.0	718.2	57.8	776.0	9.7	-25.8	-0.3	-3.3%
Lead patient registrar	22874	0.0	0.0	0.0	0.0	0.0	73.8	6.2	80.0	1.0	80.0	1.0	100.0%
Patient registrar (weekend)	22876	36.7	0.0	0.0	36.7	0.5	0.0	0.0	0.0	0.0	-36.7	-0.5	100.0%
Overtime	29998	0.0	0.0	0.0	0.0	0.0	38.5	0.0	38.5	0.5	38.5	0.5	100.0%
Department totals		4277.6	223.4	633.3	5134.3	64.3	4541.0	508.5	5049.5	63.1	-84.8	-1.2	0.0%

code 22780, were paid 106.4 more hours than budgeted, 19.0% over budget. Unit coordinators were budgeted for 7.0 FTEs and 8.3 FTEs were paid. The manager of nursing services should examine why the additional time was needed. RNs also were paid for 75.5 hours more than budgeted, but their percent variance was only 3.4%. The ED manager should consider the number of ED patients served and their severity when assessing the appropriateness of the variance (i.e., were more hours needed due to more and/or sicker patients?). The budget and variance portions of this report structure will be more thoroughly discussed in Chapters 14 and 15.

A final examination should consider if the right people are doing the right jobs. Managers can reduce staffing costs by ensuring the lowest-paid person qualified to do a task performs the work and more highly skilled and compensated employees perform more complex work. For example, the ED may employ RNs, LPNs, and CNAs. To minimize costs, it is vital that RNs do not routinely handle tasks that can be accomplished by CNAs. Similarly, from a quality and safety standpoint, CNAs should not be performing work that should be completed by RNs.

Measuring Employee Turnover

In summary, hours worked and pay rates are essential ingredients of staffing plans, budgets, and forecasts. Appropriate staffing is the responsibility of the manager. Another factor increasing healthcare cost is employee turnover; when employees leave an organization, expenses are incurred to recruit and train new employees. Employee turnover is the number of new hires in a year divided by total FTEs. Employee turnover is a constant in organizations; turnover arises from geographical relocation, career opportunity, family issues, retirement, dissatisfaction of the employee with the employer, dissatisfaction of the employer with the employee, commute time, scheduling, and workload, among other reasons. Determining when turnover is excessive is difficult, but analysis should be done to determine turnover rates, the cost of turnover,

the reason for turnover, and the actions that should be taken. Benchmarking is a first step toward assessing the acceptability of turnover rates, and benchmarks should be identified by job classification. For example, Nursing Solutions Inc. reports that the annual turnover rate for certified nursing assistants [CNAs] was 19.2% higher than registered nurses [RNs], 27.5% versus 18.7%, in 2020.[3]

Overall staff turnover in **Table 9.7** is 20.2%, 13 ÷ 64.3. Staff RNs account for the highest number of hires, five, and have a turnover rate of 17.2%, 5 ÷ 29, lower than the department and the 18.7% national benchmark. Patient registrars had the highest turnover percent, 40%, 4 ÷ 10. Simple turnover rates provide a partial picture of turnover; understanding whether turnover is excessive requires assessing average employee length of service and other variables. Departments with high average length of service should have higher turnover rates as employees retire. Four of the most common reasons for leaving a job are career advancement, personal reasons (own health or need to care for a child or parent), poor relationship with supervisor, and better pay. Three of the four top reasons for employee separations are within the control of managers; the exception is personal reasons.

Senior managers should first examine what they can do to create career advancement tracks within the organization when advancement is a common reason for employee resignations. Second, they should explore whether poor relationships with supervisors are similar across departments (i.e., if the rate of problems with supervisors is similar across departments, it may be dismissed as simple interpersonal differences between people). On the other hand, if one or more departments have a substantially higher rate of employees citing poor supervisor relations as the reason for their departure, it may warrant examining the supervisors' behavior. As for pay, managers should again identify whether this is an across-the-board problem or particular to a few occupations. When limited to a few occupations, managers should determine whether raises are needed to recruit and/or retain certain professionals.

Table 9.7 Employee Turnover

Position	Job Code	FTEs	Hires	Turnover Rate
Manager nursing service	11075	1.0	0	0.0%
Supervisor charge nurse	11403	5.8	1	17.2%
Medical assistant	12007	0.1	0	0.0%
Staff RN	13401	29.1	5	17.2%
Relief charge nurse	13403	1.1	0	0.0%
Orderly/transporter	15483	3.3	1	30.3%
ED technician	22483	4.3	1	23.3%
Secretary	22730	0.7	0	0.0%
Unit coordinator	22780	8.3	1	12.0%
Preadmission testing clerk	22818	0.1	0	0.0%
Patient registrar	22873	10.0	4	40.0%
Lead patient registrar	22874	0.0	0	0.0%
Patient registrar (weekend)	22876	0.5	0	0.0%
Overtime	29998	0.0	0	0.0%
Department totals		64.3	13	20.2%

Regulatory Requirements Regarding Staffing

As if staffing a healthcare organization wasn't complex enough because of the need to cover positions 24 hours a day, there are regulatory requirements that impact staffing configurations.

The IMPACT Act Staffing Report Requirements

This complexity is no more apparent than in the 2016 skilled nursing facility staffing requirements embodied in P.L. 113-185, the Improving Medicare Post-Acute Care Transformation Act of 2014 (the IMPACT Act). In essence, the Centers for Medicare and Medicaid Services (CMS) required expanded reporting on nursing home staffing.

Regulatory Specifics About Staffing Reports

The first set of regulatory specifics is contained in the Final Rule for the FY 2016 Prospective Payment System under the heading "Staffing Data Collection."[4] The regulation had its genesis in the Affordable Care Act, P.L. 111-148. Section 1128I(g) that specifies nursing homes are required to "electronically submit...direct care staffing information, including information for agency and contract staff, based on payroll and other verifiable and auditable data in a uniform format according to specifications established by the Secretary in consultation with (stakeholders)."[5]

The direct care staffing information submitted to CMS then appears on the Nursing Home Compare website.[6] Note the phrase "verifiable and auditable data." Previously, facilities could self-report such staffing information, but this information did not have to be "verifiable and auditable."

Additional Reporting Requirements

Additional requirements are also spelled out in the statute. Specifications in the CMS regulation state that the following must be included in the report:

- The category of work a certified employee performs, such as whether the employee is a registered nurse, licensed practical nurse, licensed vocational nurse, certified nursing assistant, therapist, or other medical personnel
- Resident census data
- Information on resident case mix
- Information on employee turnover and tenure
- The hours of care provided by each category of certified employees per resident per day[7]

This information must be reported on a regular basis. Also, information for agency and contract staff must be kept separate from the information submitted for employee staffing.

We draw your attention to the two phrases requiring the following: the category of work a certified employee performs and the hours of care provided by each category of certified employees per resident per day. What can your organization do to ensure compliance with these requirements that is both "verifiable and auditable"?

For example, which documentation within your system should be retained? To what level of detail should it be retained, and for how long? What guidance can be found, either from government sources or from your professional organizations? And if such guidance is made available, how do your own records compare? What adjustments or additions should be made?

We can also expect that these specific requirements will evolve over time. While the first set of regulatory specifics is set out within the FY 2016 PPS final rule, we can expect that refinements to these requirements will be forthcoming over each succeeding year, as experience provides evidence for the needed adjustments.

Funding Provided for Report Improvements

The IMPACT Act provides a one-time allocation of $11 million to implement these improvements to the Nursing Home Compare website.[8] Additional details about the Nursing Home Compare website and its 5-Star Rating appear in the chapter titled "Standardizing Measures and Payment in Post-Acute Care: New Requirements."

From a public domain perspective, Medicare.gov/Nursing Home Compare serves as a useful reference enabling consumers to assess staffing results among Medicare- and Medicaid-participating nursing homes. Staffing data are submitted by the facility and are adjusted for the needs of nursing home residents.

State Certificate-of-Need (CON) Laws and Regulations

Additional regulatory sources have had an impact on staffing. Central to health planning in the United States are **Certificate-of-Need (CON)** regulations. To place CON in its proper context, a brief overview of health planning is in order.

Health Planning Background

Shortly after Medicare was enacted into law in 1965, the Comprehensive Health Planning and Services Act (CHP) was passed in 1966. It was noteworthy insofar as it encouraged states to use health planning to remedy geographic disparities in access to care (i.e., prevent additional investment in equipment and facilities in adequately served areas). This was an application of planning that went beyond just allocating funds for hospital construction in underserved areas as in the historically important Hospital Survey and Construction Act of 1946, popularly known as the Hill–Burton Act.[9]

Planning was carried out by state-level CHP-A agencies and local CHP-B agencies. The former were charged with developing a statewide, comprehensive plan for the delivery of health services in each state; the latter were responsible for assessing the health services needs of populations in their designated areas, determining the availability of resources, and developing a plan that specified what was required to meet those needs.[10]

While it is beyond the scope of this text to analyze in depth why the CHP program didn't deliver as promised, suffice it to say that it had no resource development component. Resources that were necessary to meet a community's needs had to be sought outside the CHP program's parameters. In effect, then, CHP's impact on staffing was immeasurable.

Congress sought to rectify CHP's shortcomings by enacting the National Health Planning and Resources Development Act in 1974. The act created state-level organizations that were charged with developing and implementing the state health plan. Operationally, though, it was the health systems agencies (HSAs), local organizations, that served a regulatory function. They were charged with developing annual plans to improve health services in their regions.[11]

The Certificate-of-Need (CON) Program

The regulatory leverage that states used to act on proposals for changes in health services was (and is) the Certificate-of-Need (CON) program. The program was originally aimed at hospitals and nursing homes that were permitted to spend funds on services, equipment, and facilities only if a need had been identified in the HSA plan for their region. The basic assumption underlying CON regulation is that excess capacity (in the form of duplication of equipment, facility overbuilding...) directly produces healthcare price inflation.[12] The 1974 law required all 50 states to have a structure in place involving the submitting of proposals and obtaining approval from a state health planning agency.

In 1986, the National Health Planning and Resources Development Act was repealed, along with its federal funding. Despite numerous changes since, 36 states retain some type of CON program, law, or agency according to the National Conference of State Legislatures.[13] These states tend to concentrate activities on outpatient facilities and long-term care. This is largely due to the trend toward freestanding, physician-owned facilities that constitute an increasing segment of the healthcare market.

How Do CON-Related Regulations Affect Staffing?

State CON-related regulations affect staffing across different types of facilities. For example, when a hospital CON is filed seeking approval for a new surgical wing, staffing needs must be included in the application along with facility and equipment requirements. When a nursing home wants to expand its bed capacity, new staff such as RNs, LPNs, and possibly even therapists will be required. When a home care agency seeks to increase its geographic reach and expand its program capacity, new nursing-related and social work staff is required.

A prime example of state regulatory requirements on minimum staffing levels in nursing homes may be found in Nursing Home Staffing Standards in State Statutes and Regulations.[14] It depicts minimum staffing standards for skilled nursing or nursing facilities. For example, for every state it lists three variables:

1. A Sufficient Staff Statement (i.e., licensed to meet the needs of individual residents)
2. Staff Requirement (i.e., RN, LPN/LVN per hour/per bed)
3. Direct Care Requirements (e.g., two people on duty at all times)

This site is a useful planning tool to ensure the right amount of and type of staff are on duty.

WRAP-UP

Summary

Full-time employees are paid for 2,080 hours per week, but the time available for productive work is significantly lower. As you saw, nonproductive time—holiday, sick, and vacation time—can consume 240 or more available hours. Managers must understand the difference to ensure that work is completed effectively and efficiently.

Managers must also understand the demand for work to efficiently schedule employees, including how much time it should take to complete work. Two methods to schedule employees were demonstrated: annualized full-time equivalents and full-time equivalents. Managers should also be capable of calculating the effect on salary expense of different staffing models.

In addition to efficient scheduling, managers should minimize the cost of hiring and training employees. One method is to reduce the number of voluntary resignations. **Employee**

turnover rates should be regularly reviewed to determine if excessive turnover is occurring and the actions necessary to reduce turnover.

The chapter concluded with a review of regulatory requirements that affect staffing. Managers should ensure that their staff have the required credentials to provide care, the minimum required staff levels are in place, and all mandatory reporting requirements are met.

There is no greater opportunity for managers to reduce expenses through effective management than labor given the amount of money spent on personnel. Managers should ensure that workers have the proper skills and compensation, can perform their duties effectively and efficiently, are properly staffed to meet demand and regulatory requirements, and are producing services with minimum time and error (working to their potential).

Key Terms

Certificate of Need (CON)
Employee Turnover Rate
Full-Time Equivalents (FTEs)

Load Leveling
Nonproductive Time
Productive Time

Staffing

Discussion Questions

1. Describe the difference between productive time and nonproductive time.
2. Describe the elements that determine an employee's gross earnings and net pay.
3. Explain why managers should monitor employee turnover rates.
4. Describe regulatory requirements that affect staffing.

Problems

1. The director of laboratory services at Henry Hospital is assessing his staffing requirements. The hospital processes 1,440,000 lab tests per year. A lab tech can process 500 per day and earns $50,000 per year. (a) Calculate the number of productive days and FTEs needed. (An FTE is 230 productive days per year.) (b) Calculate the cost to meet this need using full-time only, full-time

plus overtime for any fractional FTE, and full-time and part-time employees. What staffing method produces the lowest expense, and how much would be saved over the most expensive method?

2. The head nurse on 2 South at Henry Hospital is assessing his RN staffing requirements. The unit serves 5,750 patients per year. One RN can oversee four patients per shift. RNs earns $75,000 per year. (a) Calculate the number of productive days and FTEs needed. (An FTE is 230 productive days per year.) (b) Calculate the cost to meet this need using fulltime only, full-time plus overtime for any fractional FTE, and full-time and part-time employees. What staffing method produces the lowest expense, and how much would be saved over the most expensive method?

3. Henry Hospital is seeing high turnover in the hospital, and the chief nursing officer (CNO) has undertaken a review of turnover in her departments. The following table provides the number of FTEs and new hires in the past 365 days for 2 North, a surgical nursing unit. Calculate the turnover rate for the unit and each position. Which positions have the highest and lowest turnover rates?

Position	FTE	Hires
Head nurse and supervisors	3	1
RN	18	1
LPN	8	3
CNA	8	2
Clerical	6	1
	43	8

4. Henry Hospital is seeing high turnover in the hospital, and the chief nursing officer (CNO) has undertaken a review of turnover in her departments. The following table provides the number of FTEs and new hires in the past 365 days for the intensive care unit (ICU). Calculate the turnover rate for the unit and each position. Which positions have the highest and lowest turnover rates? Compare the turnover rates for 2 North (in problem 3) and ICU. If you were the CNO, which department would you focus turnover reductions efforts, and why?

Position	FTE	Hires
Head nurse and supervisors	3	1
RN	27	4
LPN	14	3
CNA	10	3
Clerical	8	1
	62	12

Notes

1. Statista, "U.S. Hospital Costs by Type of Expense in Percent 2016," https://statista.com, accessed September 29, 2021.
2. J. J. Baker, *Prospective Payment for Long-Term Care: An Annual Guide* (Gaithersburg, MD: Aspen Publishers, Inc., 1999).
3. 80 FR 46462 (Aug. 4, 2015).
4. Nursing Solutions Inc., "2021 NSI National Health Care Retention and RN Staffing Report," https://nsnursingsolutions.com, accessed September 29, 2021.
5. 80 FR 46462 (Aug. 4, 2015).
6. "What Is Nursing Home Compare?," Medicare.gov, http://www.medicare.gov/nursinghomecompare/About/What-Is-NHC.html.
7. 80 FR 46462.
8. SSA Sec. 1819(i).
9. R. I. Field, *Health Care Regulation in America: Complexity, Confrontation, and Compromise* (New York, NY: Oxford University Press, 2007).
10. P. L. Barton, *Understanding the U.S. Health Services System*, 4th ed. (Chicago, IL: Health Administration Press, 2010).
11. Field, *Health Care Regulation*.
12. Ibid.
13. National Conference of State Legislatures, "CON—Certificate of Need State Laws," http://www.ncsl.org/research/health/con-certificate-of-need-state-laws.aspx, accessed June 9, 2016.
14. C. Harrington, "Nursing Home Staffing Standards in State Statutes and Regulations," http://ltcombudsman.org/uploads/files/support/Harrington-state-staffing-table-2010_(1).pdf, accessed June 12, 2016.

CHAPTER 10

Managing Supplies, Equipment, and Facilities

PROGRESS NOTES

After completing this chapter, you should be able to:

1. Describe the interrelationship between inventory and cost of goods sold.
2. Explain the effect of LIFO and FIFO methods on the value of inventory and net income.
3. Calculate and interpret inventory turnover, inventory loss ratio, and economic order quantity.
4. Calculate the depreciation expense and net book value of a fixed asset.
5. Explain the four methods of calculating depreciation and their effect on asset book values and net income.
6. Explain the difference between an asset's useful and productive lives and why utilization of assets is more important than the reported depreciation expense.

Overview: Supplies, Equipment, and Facilities

Increasing the value of an organization requires maximizing the difference between revenues and expenses. Supplies, equipment, and buildings are the next highest healthcare expenses after labor. Supply and **inventory** expenses and equipment and building depreciation account for approximately 10% and 4% of total hospital costs, respectively. Managers can reduce supply costs by optimizing the amount of supplies held in inventory. Depreciation allocates the cost of equipment and facilities over the asset's useful life to match revenues with expenses and ensure that charges cover the total cost of providing care. Managers should ensure that an organization has the amount of supplies, equipment, and buildings that minimizes treatment costs as more or less assets than needed increase expenses and may undermine care.

Inventory in Healthcare Organizations

"Inventory" includes all the items (goods) held by an organization for sale or to be used to produce goods or services in the normal course of its business. Inventory is an asset owned by the company. It appears on the balance sheet as a current asset because the items held in inventory are expected to be used or sold within a 12-month period.

Types of Inventory in Healthcare Organizations

Healthcare organizations and departments invest in inventory to diagnosis and treat patients. All pharmacies—hospital-based, retail brick-and-mortar, or mail order—maintain a stock of medications to ensure that patients have the drugs they need when they are needed. Hospital gift shops maintain a stock of gifts, flowers, cards, snacks, and so on to meet the demands of patients, visitors, and employees. All managers should strive to avoid the costs associated with over- or understocking inventory.

The cost of holding too much inventory includes the acquisition cost (i.e., how much is paid to acquire goods). A hospital may invest $1,000,000 in medications; if it pays 5% interest to borrow funds, an additional $50,000 is added to the annual cost to run the pharmacy. A second cost is storage and handling. Room must be built to store drugs and personnel must be paid to put drugs into and remove them from storage. The greater the level of inventory, the higher the facility and handling costs. Finally, supplies go bad and/or may be lost or stolen (i.e., inventory shrinkage). The National Retail Federation estimates that the cost to retailers of inventory shrinkage is 1.33% of sales.[1] On the other hand, when too little inventory is held, an organization will be unable to meet customer demand and sales will be lost. In health care, stock outages could delay treatment, increase treatment cost, and/or have catastrophic consequences on patient health.

In manufacturing companies, inventory typically consists of three types of items: raw materials, work in progress, and the finished goods to be sold.

We might think that most inventory items for sale in a healthcare organization are not manufactured but are finished goods (e.g., pharmaceuticals, pacemakers, and so on). However, consider this example: The hospital cafeteria purchases flour, eggs, butter, and so on (raw materials), mixes the ingredients (work in progress), and produces a cake (finished goods) for sale or as the dessert in a patient meal. Another example is a pharmacy that compounds drugs.

Turning Inventory into the Cost of Goods Sold

Completed inventory items ("finished goods") are either sold or used to provide care. The sale or use of an item moves it out of inventory and recognizes its cost. When the item is recognized as cost, it becomes "cost of goods sold." Different terminology may be used; in some organizations, cost of goods sold is called "cost of sales." For a business such as a retail pharmacy, the cost of inventory sold to its customers is the single largest expense of the business.

Recording Inventory and Cost of Goods Sold

Recording inventory and cost of goods sold is a five-step process, **Table 10.1**.

1. Beginning inventory (inventory at the start of the period) is determined.
2. Purchases during the period are recorded.
3. Purchases are added to beginning inventory to calculate the "cost of goods available for sale."
4. Ending inventory (inventory at the end of the period) is determined.

Table 10.1 Estimating Ending Inventory and the Cost of Goods Sold

Beginning inventory	$1,000,000	Step 1
Purchases	500,000	Step 2
Cost of goods available for sale	$1,500,000	Step 3
Ending inventory	700,000	Step 4
Cost of goods sold	$800,000	Step 5

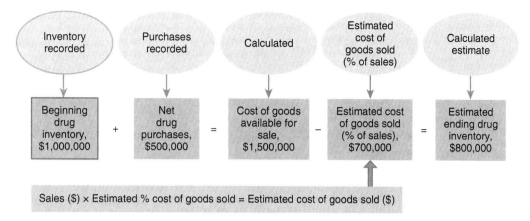

Figure 10.1 Estimating the Ending Pharmacy Inventory

5. Ending inventory is subtracted from the "cost of goods available for sale" to calculate the "cost of goods sold."

Figure 10.1 illustrates the steps to record inventory transactions. Purchases added to inventory typically include "freight in," or the shipping costs to deliver the items to you. Any discounts received on the purchases should be subtracted from the purchase cost. Thus, the purchases become "net purchases"—that is, net of discounts. Ending inventory may be determined by a physical count or an estimate; estimating the ending pharmacy inventory is shown in the next section.

Estimating the Ending Pharmacy Inventory

Certain healthcare organizations (or departments) require accounting for inventory. The most common example in health care is the pharmacy. Internal monthly statements of the pharmacy are not usually expected to reflect the results of an actual physical inventory unless your organization has an electronic inventory program—and that is another story. So what to do? **Figure 10.2** illustrates the solution.

The computations contained in Figure 10.2 are described as follows:

1. Add net drug purchases for the period to the beginning drug inventory, thus arriving at the cost of goods (drugs) available for sale.

2. Compute an estimated cost of goods (drugs) sold. To do this:

- First, find the amount of net sales (sales after allowances, discounts, rebates, etc.) for the period.
- Second, find the percent of net sales that represents cost of goods (drugs) sold in a prior period. This percentage figure is your estimated assumption, and it will probably come from the previous year's financial report. For example, $12,000,000 net sales and $8,400,000 cost of goods (drugs) sold equals 70% cost of goods sold [drugs] for last year. The 70% is the estimated assumption for this calculation.
- Third, apply this estimated assumption to the net sales for the period. For example, if the month's drug sales amounted to $1,000,000, multiply it by 70% to arrive at $700,000 for the estimated cost of goods (drugs) sold this month.

3. Finally, compute the estimated ending drug inventory. We subtract the cost of goods (drugs) sold (per step 2) from the cost of goods (drugs) available for sale (per step 1) to arrive at the "Estimated Ending Drug Inventory" for the monthly internal report.

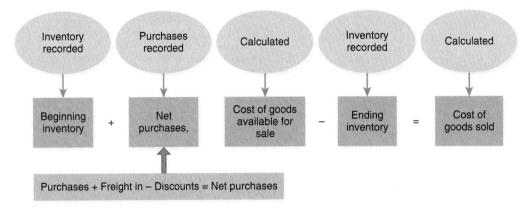

Figure 10.2 Recording Inventory in the Accounting Cycle

Gross Margin Computation

Gross margin equals revenue from sales less the cost of goods sold. Gross margin is often expressed as a percentage. Thus, a pharmacy's gross margin might appear as follows:

Sales	100%
Cost of goods (drugs) sold	70%
Gross margin	30%

An organization's gross margin percentage should be compared to industry standards to determine the appropriateness of pricing. An excessively high margin may be a competitive disadvantage if it drives patients to lower-priced providers and a low margin reduces net income.

Inventory Methods

The two most commonly used inventory valuation methods are first-in, first-out and last-in, first-out. The method chosen affects the reported net income on the income statement and the value of inventory on the balance sheet.

First-In, First-Out Inventory Method

The **first-in, first-out (FIFO)** inventory method recognizes the first costs placed into inventory as the first costs moved out into cost of goods sold when a sale occurs. Under FIFO, the ending inventory value is higher because the oldest and generally lower-priced purchases are deducted from inventory; ending inventory is thus based on the costs of the latest purchases, which we assume will be higher priced.

Last-In, First-Out Inventory Method

The **last-in, first-out (LIFO)** inventory method recognizes the latest, or last, costs placed into inventory as the first costs moved out into cost of goods sold when a sale occurs. Under LIFO, the ending inventory value will be lower because when the most recent and higher price purchases are deducted from inventory, ending inventory is based on the cost of the earliest purchases, which we assume will be lower priced. **Table 10.2** illustrates the difference between FIFO and LIFO on inventory value and net income.

Table 10.2 demonstrates the financial effects of LIFO and FIFO methods. Using LIFO, the cost of sales increases 33.3% as the most recent and higher-priced supplies were deducted from inventory. The higher cost of sales results in a 50% reduction in reported net income. For a non-profit organization, this change may have no real impact as the inventory valuation method has no impact on the physical quantity of supplies held but reduces the reported value of inventory and net income. Inventory valuation has a real impact on for-profit, taxed organizations as the $20 or 50% reduction in net income reduces taxes paid

Table 10.2 FIFO and LIFO Inventory

Cost of Sales	Assumptions	FIFO	LIFO	
Beginning Inventory	10 units × $6	$60	$60	
Plus: Purchases	10 units × $8	$80	$80	
Cost of Goods Available for Sale		$140	$140	**Assumption**
Less: Ending Inventory	10 units × $8	$80	$60	10 units × $6
Cost of Sales		$60	$80	+33.3%
Sales (Revenue)	10 units × $20	$200	$200	
Salaries		$100	$100	**Change**
Cost of Sales		$60	$80	+33.3%
Net Income (or Earnings Before Tax)		$40	$20	−50.0%
Income Tax (20%)		$8	$4	−50.0%
Earnings After Tax		$32	$16	−50.0%

by $4 for an organization paying a 20% tax rate. FIFO leads to lower reported supply expenses, higher inventory value, and higher net income as supplies were removed from inventory based on older, lower prices.

Weighted Average Inventory Method

The weighted average inventory method is based on the weighted average cost of inventory during the period. The weighted average inventory method is also called the "average cost method." The weighted average inventory cost is determined as follows: divide the cost of goods available for sale by the number of units available for sale. In Table 10.2, the weighted average supply expense would be $7 [(10 units × $6) + (10 units × $8)] ÷ 20 units. Reported inventory value and net income would be $10 lower than FIFO and $10 higher than LIFO.

No Method: Inventory Never Recognized

This inventory method is no method at all—that is, inventory is never recognized. For example, a physician's office may expense all drug purchases as supplies at the time of purchase and never count such drugs as inventory. This treatment might be justified when such supplies are a small percentage of total practice expenses. However, if the physician is purchasing expensive drugs and administering them in the office (e.g., infusing expensive drugs), then not recognizing these drugs being held as inventory on the financial statements is misleading.

Inventory Tracking

Perpetual Inventory System

With a perpetual inventory system, the healthcare organization keeps a continuous, or perpetual, record for every individual inventory item. Thus, the amount of inventory on hand can be determined at any time. A real-time system is a variation of the perpetual inventory system, where inventory is reduced at the time of sale or use and increased when supplies are received.

A perpetual inventory system requires a specific identification method for each inventory item. Bar codes to scan items into inventory when received and remove them as they are used on patients is often used for this purpose. You are most likely to find a perpetual inventory system in the pharmacy department of a hospital.

Periodic Inventory System

With a periodic inventory system, the healthcare organization does not keep a continuous record that identifies every individual inventory item on hand. Instead, at the end of the period, staff physically count the inventory items on hand. Then the cost per item is attached to the inventory counts to arrive at the cost of the inventory at the end of the period (the ending inventory).

Necessary Adjustments

Shortages

When the periodic inventory results are compared to the inventory balance on the financial statements, it is common to find that the actual physical inventory amount is less than the amount recorded on the books due to spoilage or theft. This difference, or shortage, is commonly termed *shrinkage*. The inventory amount on the books must then be reduced to the actual amount per the periodic inventory, and the resulting shrinkage cost must be recorded as an expense.

Obsolete Items

Most inventories will inevitably contain obsolete items. For example, the pharmacy inventory will contain drugs that have "sell by" or "use by" expiration dates. Obsolete inventory items should be discarded and their cost removed from the value of inventory on hand and recorded as an expense.

Inventory Distribution Systems

The ability to track inventory is directly impacted by the type of documentation required for removing items from inventory. Different types of inventory require different types of distribution systems. Thus, removing an item from a particular type of inventory needs documentation that varies according to the level of permission and scrutiny required.

Distribution Using Sign-Off Forms

For example, drawing light bulbs from the maintenance department inventory often does not require a high level of permission and/or scrutiny due to the low cost of the item. In one facility's inventory distribution method, such a requisition for light bulbs must always be attached to a maintenance department work order. Some responsible person has signed off on this work order, and it shows the reason for the inventory request. This method not only allows for inventory tracking but also indicates who was responsible for generating the order.

The distribution system for high-cost medical devices or drugs held in inventory typically requires a different type of requisition. The inventory requisition is usually triggered by a doctor's order, and more than one level of sign-off is typically required before the device is delivered to the operating room. Thus, tracking this inventory item may require multiple steps.

Distribution Using Robotic Technology

It should be noted that there are some characteristics that differentiate the pharmaceutical inventory from the rest of a hospital's inventory control mechanisms. The unit-dose drug distribution system is a particular example. In unit-dose dispensing, medication is dispensed in a package that is ready to administer to the patient. Unit-dose dispensing of medication was developed in the 1960s to support nurses in medication administration and to reduce the waste of expensive medications.[2]

Robotic Automation

The unit-dose system provides many safeguards and advantages in delivering medications, but it is highly labor intensive. Automation has been developed to support the patient care advantages of the system at a decreased cost, with some pharmacies using robotics for the bin-filling process.

Advantages of the robotic cart-filling method include improved accuracy in medication dispensing and accounting. Disadvantages include high startup costs resulting from needed facility renovations, ongoing support costs, space requirements, and limited robot capacity.[3]

Cost/Benefit of a Robot

Capital expense or lease costs for robotic technology are high, limiting their use to larger hospitals. However, Gebhart reports robots cost $12 per hour versus $18 for a pharmacy tech.[4]

The decision to purchase and implement an automated bin fill system should be based on an analysis of the financial benefits, return on investment, and potential for demonstrated improvements in service quality and patient care. Although the cost of a robot continues to decrease, information systems and other support costs will remain high enough to make the decision to purchase or lease a robot hard to justify in many cases.

Calculating Inventory Turnover: Why, EOQ

Inventory turnover is a ratio that shows how fast inventory is sold, or "turns over." The question is: Are managers stocking an appropriate level of supplies? A low turnover rate may indicate excessive inventory holdings (and potentially a high number of obsolete items), and a high turnover rate may indicate unnecessary work to continuously order supplies and/or stockout problems.

The computation requires two steps. **Table 10.3** illustrates the sequence.

Step 1. Compute "Average Inventory":

Beginning Inventory, $1,000,000, January 1, 2022 plus Ending Inventory, $700,000, December 31, 2022, divided by two equals Average Inventory, $850,000.

Step 2. Compute "Inventory Turnover":

Annual Cost of Goods Sold ($800,000 × 12 months), $9,600,000, divided by Average Inventory, $850,000, equals Inventory Turnover, 11.3. Inventory turns over 11.3 times per year or the entire inventory is replaced every 32.3 days, 365 days ÷ 11.3.

An organization's inventory turnover ratio should be compared to industry standards to determine if too much or too little inventory is maintained. For example, assume the average hospital pharmacy holds one month of inventory, $800,000, but your department maintains a two-month inventory, $1,600,000, an excess inventory of $800,000. The hospital will incur an unnecessary cost of $40,000 per year if the cost of funds is 5% due to the higher investment in inventory.

Economic Order Quantity

The economic order quantity (EOQ) model is designed to calculate the amount of supplies that should be purchased per order to minimize total inventory cost. EOQ determines the order quantity that balances ordering costs that decrease when more supplies are ordered and the higher

Table 10.3 **Calculating Inventory Turnover**

Beginning inventory	$1,000,000	
Ending inventory	700,000	
Average inventory	$850,000	Step 1: (Beginning + Ending Inventory) ÷ 2
Cost of goods sold	$9,600,000	
Inventory turnover	11.3	Step 2: CGS ÷ Average inventory
Days in inventory	32.3	

holding costs associated with holding larger inventories.

The EOQ formula is:

$$Q^* = \text{square root } (2DC_o/C_h)$$

Where:

D = annual demand
C_o = ordering cost per order
C_h = holding cost, cost per supply unit (C) × carrying rate (I, % of unit cost)

Assume a hospital implants 624 pacemakers a year (D) with an average cost of $800 (C) and a holding cost of 20% (I). The cost to process a purchase order is $50 (CO). The EOQ is 19.7 pacemakers per order, = SQRT((2 × 624 × $50)/($800 × 20%)). **Table 10.4** demonstrates how total cost changes based on the number of pacemakers ordered.

Note that ordering slightly more or less than the economic order quantity of 20 units (plus or minus five units per order) does not significantly increase inventory costs, but extremely small and large orders impose large and unnecessary costs on the organization. **Figure 10.3** graphically shows the lowest cost order quantity and the change in cost when more or fewer pacemakers are ordered.

Managers should also understand that 32 supply orders will be placed per year, 624 ÷ 19.7, and orders should be made every 11.6 days, 365 days ÷ 31.6, or when inventory hits 4 units based the average daily use of 1.7, 624 pacemakers ÷ 365 days, and a two-day delivery from the vendor. The point is managers should strive to reduce inventory costs by holding the optimal amount of supplies. Insufficient inventory leads to excessive ordering and potential stockouts; excess inventory increases the investment in inventory, storage and handling costs, holding costs, and losses due to spoilage and/or theft. Understanding how supply expense should be measured, inventory turnover, EOQ, and the **inventory loss ratio** is the first step to reducing supply costs.

Inventory Loss Ratio

As noted earlier, inventory is lost due to spoilage (or obsolescence), misplacement, unrecorded use, and theft, so the estimated amount in inventory may not agree with actual inventory. Managers should routinely conduct a physical count to determine what is in stock and determine the inventory loss ratio. The inventory loss ratio calculates the expense of supplies purchased but neither sold or recorded as used.

Assume that a physical count of inventory on December 31, 2022, calculates inventory at

Table 10.4 Economic Order Quantity

Q	Orders per Year	Total Co	Total Ch	Total Cost	% Above Q*	Excess Cost
5	124.8	$6,240	$400	$6,640	210.1%	$3,480
10	62.4	$3,120	$800	$3,920	124.1%	$760
15	41.6	$2,080	$1,200	$3,280	103.8%	$120
Q* 20	31.2	$1,560	$1,600	$3,160	100.0%	$0
25	25.0	$1,248	$2,000	$3,248	102.8%	$88
30	20.8	$1,040	$2,400	$3,440	108.9%	$280
35	17.8	$891	$2,800	$3,691	116.8%	$531
40	15.6	$780	$3,200	$3,980	125.9%	$820

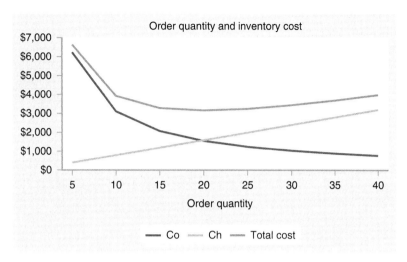

Figure 10.3 Minimizing Inventory Cost

$680,000 rather than the estimate of $700,000. The inventory loss ratio is 2.9%, ($700,000 − 680,000) ÷ $700,000, and accounting records should be reduced to reflect actual inventory.

Estimated Ending Inventory	$700,000	
Actual Inventory	$680,000	
Inventory Loss Ratio	2.9%	($700,000 − 680,000) ÷ $700,000

Sherman reports that the average inventory loss is 1.44% and recommends multiple methods to reduce inventory loss.[5] Loss prevention methods include assigning responsibility to a single person, restricting access to inventory, improving inventory processes (e.g., double-checking high-value inventory withdrawals), and automating inventory transactions to reduce human error.

Equipment and Facilities Depreciation

Healthcare delivery requires the use of high-cost equipment and buildings that must be purchased and maintained. **Depreciation** recognizes the wear and tear on long-term assets due to use or age and spreads the cost of fixed assets over their useful life. Depreciation expense reduces net income and hopefully organizations will set aside this money for the eventual replacement of equipment and buildings as they wear out. More important than the level of expense reported is the utilization of equipment and buildings. Managers should strive to ensure that these assets are used as fully as possible.

Fixed Assets and Depreciation Expense

Fixed assets, also known as long-term assets, are reported below current assets on the balance sheet because they will not be converted into cash in the coming 12 months. The purchase of a fixed asset is a capital expenditure. Capital expenditures involve the acquisition of assets that are long-lasting and high cost such as equipment and buildings.

We recognize the cost of owning equipment and buildings through depreciation expense. When the cost is spread, or allocated, over a period of years, each year's income statement reports a portion of the acquisition cost as depreciation expense.

Useful Life of the Asset

The useful life determines the period over which the fixed asset's cost will be spread. For example, a magnetic resonance imaging (MRI) can cost $2,000,000 and have a useful life of five years, so depreciation expense is recognized in each of the five years, $400,000 per year, $2,000,000 ÷ 5 years, until its value is zero.

Salvage Value

Before depreciation expense can be calculated, we need to know whether the fixed asset will have **salvage value** at the end of the depreciated period. Salvage value, also known as residual value or scrap value, represents any expected cash value of the asset at the end of its useful life (i.e., what it can be sold for). If the MRI is expected to have a salvage value of $250,000 at the end of its five-year useful life, then $1,750,000 will be spread over the five-year life as depreciation expense, $350,000 per year, and the $250,000 will remain undepreciated at the end of that time.

Book Value of a Fixed Asset and the Reserve for Depreciation

The Reserve for Depreciation

Depreciation expense over the years is accumulated into the reserve for depreciation. In other words, the reserve for depreciation holds the cumulative amount of depreciation expense that has been recognized over time starting with the date that the fixed asset was acquired. Another way to think about this is to view the reserve for depreciation as holding all the depreciation expense that has been recorded over the **useful life of the asset**.

Interrelationship of Depreciation Expense and the Reserve for Depreciation

Depreciation expense for the year is recorded in the income statement and reduces net income.

At the same time, the expense is added to the reserve for depreciation on the balance sheet. These amounts should balance each other—that is, when $350,000 is recognized as depreciation expense in the income statement, then $350,000 should be added to the reserve for depreciation on the balance sheet reducing the reported value of the asset by $350,000. This interrelationship is illustrated in **Figure 10.4**.

Net Book Value of a Fixed Asset

The net **book value** (also known as book value) of a fixed asset is a balance sheet figure that represents the remaining undepreciated portion of the fixed asset cost. The term derives from value recorded on the books—thus *book value*.

The net book value of a fixed asset is computed as follows:

- Determine the original cost of the fixed asset on the balance sheet (i.e., its purchase price).
- Subtract the reserve for depreciation, (i.e., the accumulated depreciation expense that has been recognized since the asset was purchased).

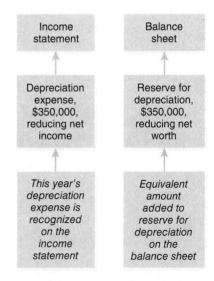

Figure 10.4 Interrelationship of Depreciation Expense and Reserve for Depreciation in the Accounting Cycle

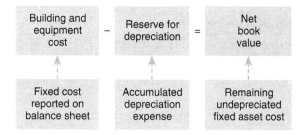

Figure 10.5 Net Book Value Computation

- The difference equals the net book value at that point in time (**Figure 10.5**).

Note that fully depreciated fixed assets may still remain on the books if they are still in use. A fully depreciated fixed asset, of course, means that the depreciable cost has been exhausted because all the depreciation expense over the asset's useful life has been recognized. Thus, the net book value would be either zero or the salvage value of the asset (e.g., a building with a 20-year life with no salvage value that is still in use after 20 years would have a zero value on the balance sheet).

Four Methods of Computing Book Depreciation

Just as *book value* means the value that is recorded on the organization's balance sheet, *book depreciation* means depreciation that is recorded on the income statement. *Tax depreciation*, on the other hand, is depreciation that is computed for tax purposes and is reflected on the applicable tax returns of the organization. Tax depreciation

methods are discussed in the final section of this chapter. Managers will most likely be using book depreciation in their planning, control, and decision-making activities. Four methods of computing book depreciation are described in the following sections.

Straight-Line Depreciation Method

The **straight-line depreciation** method assigns an equal or even amount of depreciation expense over each year (or period) of the asset's useful life. The expense is thus spread evenly—or in a straight line—over the life of the asset. **Table 10.5** illustrates the straight-line depreciation method applied to a fixed asset costing $2,000,000 with a five-year useful life and no salvage value. The depreciation expense would thus equal $400,000 for each of the five years, $2,000,000 ÷ 5 years.

Table 10.6 illustrates the straight-line depreciation method applied to a fixed asset costing $2,000,000 with a five-year useful life

Table 10.5 Straight-Line Depreciation: Five-Year Life with No Salvage Value

Year	Cost to Be Depreciated	Depreciation Expense	Accumulated Depreciation	Book Value
1	$2,000,000	$400,000	$400,000	$1,600,000
2	$2,000,000	$400,000	$800,000	$1,200,000
3	$2,000,000	$400,000	$1,200,000	$800,000
4	$2,000,000	$400,000	$1,600,000	$400,000
5	$2,000,000	$400,000	$2,000,000	$0

Table 10.6 Straight-Line Depreciation: Five-Year Life with Salvage Value

Year	Acquisition Cost	Cost to Be Depreciated	Depreciation Expense	Accumulated Depreciation	Book Value
1	$2,000,000	$1,750,000	$350,000	$350,000	$1,650,000
2	$2,000,000	$1,750,000	$350,000	$700,000	$1,300,000
3	$2,000,000	$1,750,000	$350,000	$1,050,000	$950,000
4	$2,000,000	$1,750,000	$350,000	$1,400,000	$600,000
5	$2,000,000	$1,750,000	$350,000	$1,750,000	$250,000

Table 10.7 Sum-of-the-Years' Digits Depreciation: Five-Year Life with No Salvage Value

Year	Years' Digits	Cost to Be Depreciated	Depreciation Expense	Accumulated Depreciation	Book Value
1	5	$2,000,000	$666,667	$666,667	$1,333,333
2	4	$2,000,000	$533,333	$1,200,000	$800,000
3	3	$2,000,000	$400,000	$1,600,000	$400,000
4	2	$2,000,000	$266,667	$1,866,667	$133,333
5	1	$2,000,000	$133,333	$2,000,000	$0
	15		$2,000,000		

and a $250,000 salvage value. The depreciation expense would thus equal $350,000 for each year because we must leave $250,000 at the end of the asset's five-year life, $2,000,000 − $250,000 = $1,750,000 ÷ 5 years.

If the asset was acquired in the second half of the year, in some cases only a half-year of depreciation will be recognized in year 1. If this is the case, the remaining half-year of depreciation will be recognized in year 6 in order to fully depreciate the asset.

Accelerated Book Depreciation Methods

As the name implies, accelerated book depreciation methods write off more depreciation in the first part of the asset's useful life. Thus, they "accelerate" recognizing depreciation expense. Three accelerated depreciation methods are briefly described here.

Sum-of-the-Years' Digits Method

The **sum-of-the-years' digits (SYD) accelerated depreciation** method computes depreciation by multiplying the depreciable cost of the asset by a fraction. The fraction is computed as follows:

- The numerator of the SYD fraction starts with the asset's useful life expressed in years and decreases by one each year thereafter. For an asset with a five-year useful life, the numerators are 5, 4, 3, 2, and 1 respectively.
- The denominator of the SYD fraction is the sum of the years' digits of the asset's life. For an asset with a five-year useful life, the sum is 15, 5 + 4 + 3 + 2 + 1.
- Depreciation for year 1 is then $2,000,000 × (5 ÷ 15), $666,667. Subsequent years depreciation is calculated by reducing the numerator by 1, year 2, (4 ÷ 15), year 3, (3 ÷ 15), and so on (**Table 10.7**).

Assuming the for-profit Curie Imaging Center earns a net income of $800,000 before depreciation, **Table 10.8** compares net income and taxes based on straight-line and sum-of-the-years' digits depreciation. Net income in year 1 under straight-line depreciation would be $400,000, $800,000 – $400,000. Under the accelerated sum-of-the-years' digits depreciation, net income falls to $133,333, $800,000 – $666,667, a reduction of $266,667. If the center pays a tax rate of 20%, it would reduce its year 1 tax by $53,333.

As both depreciation methods must expense the same $2,000,000 over five years, net income and taxes increase every year as the accelerated depreciation expense decreases. At the bottom of the table, you can see that both methods are equal, but Curie would benefit by reducing its tax payments by $80,000 in the first two years and paying $80,000 more in the last two years (i.e., having money in your pocket today is better than receiving money in four or five years).

Double-Declining Balance Method

The **double-declining balance (DDB) accelerated depreciation** method computes depreciation by multiplying the asset's net book value at the beginning of each year by a constant percentage, or factor, based on the asset's useful life. In the case of DDB, the constant factor is twice the straight-line rate (thus *double-declining*). In the case of an asset with a five-year useful life, straight-line depreciation percentage is 20%, (1 ÷ 5); the double-declining rate is 40%, 20% × 2, but unlike straight-line depreciation, the percentage is multiplied by remaining book value rather than acquisition cost minus salvage value.

Table 10.9 illustrates the computation for each year of a five-year useful life with no salvage value.

- Year 1 depreciation is $2,000,000 × 0.40 = $800,000. Accumulated depreciation for year 1 also equals $800,000 and is subtracted

Table 10.8 Comparison of Straight-Line and Sum-of-the-Years' Digits Depreciation Methods

Year	Net Income Straight-Line	Net Income Sum-of-the-Years' Digits	Change in Taxable Income	Tax Savings (Increase)
1	$400,000	$133,333	$266,667	–$53,333
2	$400,000	$266,667	$133,333	–$26,667
3	$400,000	$400,000	$0	$0
4	$400,000	$533,333	($133,333)	$26,667
5	$400,000	$666,667	($266,667)	$53,333
Total	$2,000,000	$2,000,000	$0	$0

Table 10.9 Double-Declining Balance Depreciation: Five-Year Life with No Salvage Value

Year	Cost to Be Depreciated	Depreciation Expense	Accumulated Depreciation	BookValue
1	$2,000,000	$800,000	$800,000	$1,200,000
2	$1,200,000	$480,000	$1,280,000	$720,000
3	$720,000	$288,000	$1,568,000	$432,000
4*	$432,000	$216,000	$1,784,000	$216,000
5	$216,000	$216,000	$2,000,000	$0

from the $2,000,000 cost to arrive at the net remaining undepreciated cost, or net book value, of $1,200,000 at the end of year 1.

- Year 2 depreciation is $1,200,000 × 0.40 = $480,000. The year 2 depreciation of $480,000 is added to the accumulated depreciation for a total of $1,280,000, $800,000 + $480,000. The $1,280,000 is subtracted from the $2,000,000 cost to arrive at the net remaining undepreciated cost, or net book value, of $720,000 at the end of year 2.
- Year 3 depreciation is $720,000 × 0.40 = $288,000. The year 3 depreciation of $288,000 is added to the accumulated depreciation for a total of $1,568,000, $1,280,000 + 288,000. The $1,568,000 is subtracted from the $2,000,000 cost to arrive at the net remaining undepreciated cost, or net book value, of $432,000 at the end of year 3.

The declining balance method has a peculiarity in that it switches back to the straight-line method at the point where the straight-line computation yields a higher annual depreciation than the declining balance computation. Thus, as we arrive at year 4 in this example, we must test the double-declining computation against the straight-line computation.

- To compute year 4 double declining, the factor of 0.40 is multiplied times the net book value of $432,000 to arrive at DDB depreciation expense of $172,800.
- To compute year 4 depreciation by the straight-line method, the remaining net book value of $432,000 is divided by the remaining two years of useful life, $216,000.
- Since the year 4 straight-line depreciation expense $216,000 is greater than the year 4 DDB expense, $172,800, $216,000 is used for years 4 and 5.

The point at which the straight-line method overtakes the declining balance method varies, of course, with the method and the number of years of useful life for the asset.

Units of Production Depreciation Method

The **units of production (UOP) or units of service depreciation** method assigns a fixed amount of depreciation to each unit of output or service produced by the equipment. *Units of production* is a manufacturer's term for manufacturing a product, so *units of service* may more properly describe the output of medical equipment providing healthcare services.

Instead of a useful life in years, equipment depreciated by the UOP method is assigned an expected amount of units of output, and then the number of units of output produced each year over the asset's useful life is depreciated. **Table 10.10** illustrates the UOP method. The depreciation per unit of service is computed as follows:

- The total depreciable units of service over five years are determined to be 5,000 units. The equipment cost to be depreciated of $2,000,000 is divided by 5,000 units to arrive at depreciation of $400.00 per unit.

Table 10.10   Units of Production Depreciation: Five Years of Service with No Salvage Value

Year	Output	Cost to Be Depreciated	Depreciation Expense	Accumulated Depreciation	Book Value
1	800	$2,000,000	$320,000	$320,000	$1,680,000
2	900	$2,000,000	$360,000	$680,000	$1,320,000
3	1000	$2,000,000	$400,000	$1,080,000	$920,000
4	1100	$2,000,000	$440,000	$1,520,000	$480,000
5	1200	$2,000,000	$480,000	$2,000,000	$0
	5000		$2,000,000		

- Units of service in year 1 are expected to be 800 scans. Thus, 800 scans × $400 per unit = equals $320,000 year 1 depreciation.
- Units of service in year 2 are expected to be 900 scans. Thus, 900 scans × $400 per unit = equals $360,000 year 2 depreciation. The computation continues in this manner until the total 5,000 units of service are exhausted and the equipment is fully depreciated.

In the depreciation examples it was assumed the MRI would be exhausted after five years or 5,000 scans, but the asset may continue to provide service. In fact, we hope that proper care and maintenance will extend assets' productive lives. On the other hand, technological advancements may render the continued use of an asset undesirable and may make it advantageous to purchase newer assets that require fewer supplies or utilities than to continue to use current equipment. Depreciation reduces net income and should be "set aside" for replacement; when depreciation is used for other purposes or distributed to owners in for-profits, then funds may be insufficient to acquire new equipment.

Utilization of Fixed Assets

Depreciation is often calculated based on the passage of time rather than output, but in terms of value, the critical issue is utilization (i.e., how many patients benefit from equipment and facilities). There is a clear economic benefit from using fixed assets to their potential, spreading the overhead to reduce the average cost to deliver services, as seen in Chapter 8.

Assume Codman Memorial Hospital has just replaced 200 inpatient beds with a new building costing $200,000,000 and an expected life of 20 years. Straight-line depreciation will report a cost of $10,000,000 a year for the next 20 years. More important than the depreciation expense is how

many of these beds will be occupied on a daily basis. Total patient days available are 73,000 (365 days × 200 beds) per year. Depreciation per patient day will be $152.21 when **occupancy** (beds filled ÷ beds available) averages 90%, $10,000,000 ÷ 65,700 days. If 100 beds are not needed, occupancy is only 50%, depreciation per patient day increases 80% to $273.97, $10,000,000 ÷ 36,500 days. Managers often track **census**, the number of occupied beds per day, to assess resource use. Are 180 of 200 beds routinely occupied (90%) or 140 beds (70%)? How beds are used is more controllable (and important) than the amount of depreciation recognized. Given that Medicare reimburses hospitals per inpatient case, managers should ensure that beds are filled and regularly turn over. Unnecessarily prolonging hospitalization to increase occupancy will reduce the fixed cost per patient day, increase variable costs, and have no effect on revenue and thus is not an effective means to improve financial performance.

Similarly, physicians should track utilization of their exam rooms (patient encounters per day, RVUs, and so on), and managers of ancillary departments should track use of their machines (e.g., how many MRIs are performed during a year, and what is the machine capacity?). Managers should maximize uptime, the number of hours equipment is available to provide service, by ensuring that timely and effective maintenance is performed. Unscheduled downtime not only reduces revenue; it also inconveniences patients.

Turnover ratios are another way to gauge asset productivity. **Total asset turnover** is annual revenue divided by total assets (i.e., the number of dollars of revenue generated by each dollar invested in assets). Managers should track turnover ratios over time to determine whether assets are becoming more or less productive so action can be taken to the amount of revenue generated by each dollar of assets when needed.

WRAP-UP

Summary

Managers should recognize that how supplies, equipment, and buildings are used is more important than the amounts invested in these assets and reported expenses. Minimizing expenses is one way of ensuring that total revenue exceeds total cost and assets can be replaced as they wear out. As we saw, there are multiple ways to reduce supply expenses, including ordering optimal quantities and minimizing inventory losses due to theft, obsolescence, or other factors.

We also saw that inventory valuation methods, while having no real effect on inventory, can significantly change reported supply expense. LIFO inventory methods increase supply expense and lower net income which will lower taxes for for-profit organization. FIFO methods, on the other hand, lower supply expense, increase net income, and increase taxes for for-profit organizations. Managers should recognize that LIFO (FIFO) may result in reported inventory values that are lower (higher) than the current value of the items in inventory.

Depreciation is designed to recognize the loss in value of fixed assets due to age or use. Like inventory valuation, depreciation methods affect reported expense, net income, and the book value of assets. Accelerated depreciation recognizes higher expense in the early years of an asset's life, thus lowering net income; in later years, depreciation expense falls, and reported net income increases. For-profits organizations may elect accelerated depreciation to postpone taxes. Managers should note that straight-line and accelerated methods ultimately result in the same total depreciation over the life of the asset. Managers should be familiar with inventory and depreciation methods to understand financial reports, but ultimately the value of the organization will be determined by how well supplies, equipment, and buildings are used, minimizing service times and defects and timely maintenance, rather than accounting methods.

Key Terms

Book Value
Census
Depreciation
Double-Declining Balance (DDB) Depreciation
First In, First Out (FIFO)
Inventory

Inventory Loss Ratio
Inventory Turnover
Last In, First Out (LIFO)
Occupancy
Salvage Value
Straight-Line Depreciation

Sum-of-the-Years' Digits (SYD) Depreciation
Total Asset Turnover
Units of Production (Units of Service) Depreciation
Useful Life of an Asset

Discussion Questions

1. Describe the interrelationship between inventory and cost of goods sold.
2. Explain the effect of LIFO and FIFO methods on value of inventory and net income.
3. Explain the purpose of inventory turnover and inventory loss ratios.
4. Explain the two major inventory costs and how the economic order quantity (Q^*) minimizes the total inventory cost.
5. Explain how an asset's net book value is calculated.
6. Explain the effect on asset book values and net income between straight-line and double-declining balance deprecation.
7. Explain why utilization of assets is more important than the reported depreciation.

Problems

1. Given sales of 100 units generating $90,000 in revenue and the following table with beginning inventory and purchases, calculate ending inventory and the cost of goods sold under (a) LIFO and (b) FIFO methods.

	Units	Per Unit Cost	Total Cost
Beginning inventory	500	$50	$25,000
Purchases	400	$50	$20,000
	100	$65	$6,500
	400	$80	$32,000
Total	1,400		$83,500

2. An outpatient clinic's beginning pharmacy inventory was $25,000, its cost of goods sold for the year was $600,000, and ending inventory was $83,500. Calculate inventory turnover and how often orders should be placed?

3. Given a supply item that costs $50 with annual demand of 1200 units, a holding cost of 10%, and an ordering cost of $100, calculate the Economic Order Quantity (EOQ). How many orders will be needed per year and how often should orders be placed?

4. The reported ending inventory for 2 South based on beginning inventory plus restocking less documented use is 1,000 units and $5,000. The actual ending inventory based on a physical count is 960 units and $4,800. Calculate the Inventory Loss Ratio. What actions can be taken to reduce inventory loss?

5. Create depreciation schedules for a $100,000 machine with a four-year life that will have no salvage value at the end of its useful life under (a) straight-line, (b) double-declining-balance, (c) sum-of-the-years' digits, and (d) units of production depreciation methods with year 1 output of 2,275, year 2 output of 2,425, year 3 output of 2,575, and year 4 output of 2,725. The schedule should report cost to be depreciated, depreciation expense, accumulated depreciation, and book value for each year. What depreciation method produces the highest and lowest year 1 depreciation expense?

6. Given a straight-line depreciation expense of $25,000 and the following table of output, calculate the depreciation expense per output. How much more expensive is low output, 2,275, compared to high output, 2,725?

Depreciation expense (straight-line) $25,000

Output	Depr per Output
2,275	_____
2,425	_____
2,525	_____
2,725	_____

Notes

1. National Retail Federation, "National Retail Security Survey 2018," http://www.nrf.com, accessed July 27, 2021.
2. Agency for Healthcare Research and Quality, "National Healthcare Disparities Report 2013, Chapter 10— Access to Health Care," http://www.ahrq.gov/research/findings/nhqrdr/nhdr13/chap10.html, accessed May 2014.
3. L. F. Wolper, *Health Care Administration: Managing Organized Delivery Systems* (5th ed.) (Sudbury, MA: Jones & Bartlett Publishers, 2011).
4. F. Gebhart, "The Future of Pharmacy Automation," *Drug Topics Journal*, 163, no. 7 (2019).
5. F. Sherman, "How to Calculate Inventory Shrinkage," https://bizfluent.com, accessed April 22, 2021.

PART IV

Reporting and Measuring Financial Performance

CHAPTER 11

Financial Statements, Reporting Organizational Financial Performance

PROGRESS NOTES

After completing this chapter, you should be able to:

1. Explain the purpose and structure of income statements.
2. Explain the purpose and structure of balance sheets.
3. Explain the purpose and structure of the statement of changes in net worth.
4. Explain the purpose and structure of the statement of cash flows.

Overview: Financial Statements

Financial information serves the same role in ensuring the health of an organization that vital signs play in assessing and improving patient health. When physicians and nurses collect vital signs, they are seeking information on basic physiologic functions (i.e., is a patient in good health?). A patient's temperature should range from 97.8 to 99.5 degrees; higher temperature may indicate fever and low temperature hypothermia. Treatment should be based on how far the patient's temperature varies from the desired range and the direction of difference. Similarly, pulse measures the sufficiency and consistency of cardiac output

and should range between 60 and 100 beats per minute. Respiration should be 12 to 16 breaths per minute; higher rates may indicate fever and illness. Blood pressure above 140 may increase the chance of heart attack or stroke. Finance should provide the information patient care and support services managers need to assess the use of resources. Like vital signs, managers need to know how to interpret financial information and what actions should be taken to improve financial performance.

Prior chapters defined assets, liabilities, revenues, and expenses; financial statements summarize each to report the status of an organization and the performance of its management. Did managers invest wisely, use liabilities effectively, sell valued goods and services, and minimize expenses? It is not our intention to convert you into an accountant. Therefore, our discussion of the major financial statements will center on the concept of each report and not on the **accounting** entries necessary to create the statement. The first concept we will discuss is that of cash versus accrual accounting. In **cash basis accounting**, a transaction does not enter the books until cash is either received or paid out. In accrual accounting, revenue is recorded when it is earned—not when payment is received—and expenses are recorded when they are incurred—not when they are paid.[1] Most healthcare organizations operate on the accrual basis.

There are four major financial statements, and you should think of them as a set. They include the **income statement** (a.k.a. the statement of revenue and expense), the **balance sheet**, the statement of fund balance or net worth, and the statement of cash flows. The financial statements we are about to examine were prepared using the accrual method. The goal of financial statements is to determine the financial health of an organization. Is the organization robust, earning more money than it spends? Does it have more assets than liabilities, and can it continue to operate into the future? Even when the answers to each of these questions is yes, managers should determine if adjustments could improve financial health. In the long run, every organization must bring in more money than it spends to continue operations.

The Income Statement

The income statement addresses the question of whether an organization is generating more revenue than its expenses. The formula for a very condensed income statement is:

Total Revenue − Total Expenses = Net Income

An income statement covers a period of time rather than one single date or point in time (e.g., revenue and expenses between January 1, 2022, and December 31, 2022). As you will see, the income statement begins by reporting revenue followed by the expenses incurred during the period

to generate the operating income. Net nonoperating gains (losses) are then added to or subtracted from operating income to determine net income.

Table 11.1 sets out the result of operations for Westside Clinic for two years. Performance in 2021 is shown in column 2, and performance in 2022, the current period, is shown in column 3. To direct managers' attention to large changes, column 4 calculates the change in revenue and expenses between the two years, and column 5 calculates the year-to-year percent change, column 4 divided by column 2, 2021, the base year. Operating revenues, which are revenues received from the organization's primary business, are reported first. Operating expenses, the costs incurred to generate the operating revenue, are next, with the difference being income from operations. Then "Nonoperating Gains (Losses)" are reported, including revenue from donations, investments, rents, and non-patient care service. The sum of income from operations and nonoperating gains is Net Income and gains in excess of expenses (losses) and will be reported as the increase (decrease) in fund balance on the balance sheet and statement of changes in fund balance.

The first thing most people look at on the income statement is the bottom line. Net income increased by $18,000 and 34.6% over the prior year. The increase was driven by a $15,000 or 30% increase in income from operations and an additional $3,000 in interest income, a nonoperating gain. While some people may conclude that the higher net income demonstrates that things are going well and no further examination is needed, managers should dig deeper to understand why financial performance improved.

Income from operations increased due to managers' ability to increase revenues more than expenses. Revenue increased by $100,000, 5.4%, when expenses increased by $85,000, 4.7%. Obviously, the organization's future will be secure if managers can continue increasing revenue by more than expenses. When reviewing this income statement, we should note that expenses are categorized by the area they are incurred. This breakdown allows us to assess expense growth by area (i.e., are growth rates appropriate or should cost increases be examined in areas with higher than

Table 11.1 Westside Clinic Income Statement

Revenue	For the December 31, 2021	Year Ending December 31, 2022	$ Change	% Change
Net Patient Service Revenue	$1,850,000	$1,950,000	$100,000	5.4%
Total Operating Revenue	$1,850,000	$1,950,000	$100,000	5.4%
Operating Expenses				
Medical/surgical services	$575,000	$600,000	$25,000	4.3%
Therapy services	806,000	850,000	44,000	5.5%
Other professional services	75,000	80,000	5,000	6.7%
Support services	220,000	230,000	10,000	4.5%
General services	60,000	65,000	5,000	8.3%
Depreciation	40,000	40,000	0	0.0%
Interest	24,000	20,000	−4,000	−16.7%
Total Operating Expenses	$1,800,000	$1,885,000	$85,000	4.7%
Operating Income	$50,000	$65,000	$15,000	30.0%
Nonoperating Gains (Losses)				
Interest Income	$2,000	$5,000	$3,000	150.0%
Net Nonoperating Gains	$2,000	$5,000	$3,000	150.0%
Net Income	$52,000	$70,000	$18,000	34.6%

average growth?). Expenses grew on average by 4.7%, but we see growth rates of 8.3% in General Services and 6.7% in Other Professional Services. Management should determine the cause(s) of the higher growth (i.e., higher workload, higher wages or prices, and whether action is necessary). Identifying the cause(s) of expense increase may warrant a different reporting format. **Table 11.2** reorganizes the information in Table 11.1 by type of expense rather than where the expense was incurred.

Format 2 breaks expenses into salaries, fringe benefits, and supplies and allows managers to pinpoint the expenses increasing more than the

4.7% average. In this case, the highest increase came in supply expense that increased $26,000 and 14.9%. Managers should again determine why supply expense increased three times faster than total expense. Is the cause higher workload; higher prices for medical, office, and/or other supplies; or inventory loss due to spoilage or theft? The purpose of the income statement is to assess financial performance in an accounting period and provide managers with the information they need to maintain or improve performance.

Figure 11.1 provides a faster means of assessing financial performance; it reports income from operations for the past four years. Income from

Table 11.2 Westside Clinic Income Statement, Format 2

Revenue	For the December 31, 2021	Year Ending December 31, 2022	$ Change	% Change
Net Patient Service Revenue	$1,850,000	$1,950,000	$100,000	5.4%
Total Operating Revenue	$1,850,000	$1,950,000	$100,000	5.4%
Operating Expenses				
Salaries and wages	$1,215,000	$1,262,000	$47,000	3.9%
Fringe benefits	347,000	363,000	16,000	4.6%
Supplies	174,000	200,000	26,000	14.9%
Depreciation	40,000	40,000	0	0.0%
Interest	24,000	20,000	-4,000	-16.7%
Total Operating Expenses	$1,800,000	$1,885,000	$85,000	4.7%
Operating Income	$50,000	$65,000	$15,000	30.0%
Nonoperating Gains (Losses)				
Interest Income	$2,000	$5,000	$3,000	150.0%
Net Nonoperating Gains	$2,000	$5,000	$3,000	150.0%
Net Income	$52,000	$70,000	$18,000	34.6%

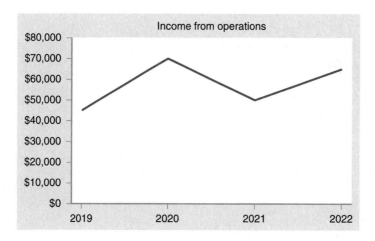

Figure 11.1 Westside Clinic Operating Income, 2019 through 2022

operations should be expected to fluctuate from year to year as it has between 2019 and 2022. The run chart demonstrates that management has consistently generated between $45,000 and $70,000 more revenue than expenses from patient care. A question that managers should ask is whether this return is sufficient to provide enough funds to replace equipment and assets in the future.

Exhibit 11.1 provides a list of questions to deepen your understanding of the financial performance reported on the income statement (the past) and what future performance may be.

The Balance Sheet

The balance sheet records the resources, cash, supplies, equipment, and buildings that employees have to deliver patient care versus the income statement, which focuses on revenues and expenses. Managers should determine whether net income and cash holdings are sufficient to replace organizational resources when they wear out. The balance sheet records what an organization owns, what it owes, and what it is worth (though the terminology uses *fund balance* rather than *net worth* or *equity* for nonprofit organizations). The total of

Exhibit 11.1 **Checklist for Review of the Income Statement**

1. What are the periods, the number of months and year(s), reported on the income statement?
2. Are there large discrepancies in balances between the prior year operations and the current year operations?
3. Did total operating revenue increase over the prior year?
4. Did total operating expenses increase, decrease, or stay about the same? Is any particular line item unusually large or small?
5. Did income from operations increase, decrease, or stay about the same?
6. Are there unusual nonoperating gains or losses?
7. Did net income increase, decrease, or stay about the same as the prior year?

what the organization owns, its assets, must equal the combined total of what the organization owes and what it is worth, its liabilities and net worth. This balancing of the elements in the balance sheet can be visualized as

$$Assets = Liabilities + Net\ Worth$$

or

$$Net\ Worth = Assets - Liabilities$$

The balance sheet is stated at a particular point in time, typically the end of a fiscal year (e.g., assets and liabilities on December 31, 2022). A common analogy is that a balance sheet is like a snapshot: It freezes the figures and reports them as of a certain date versus the income statement that reports performance over a month, quarter, or year.

Table 11.3 reports a single date rather than "For the years ending" at the top of the statement; a balance sheet is a snapshot of Westside Clinic's assets and liabilities on December 31 of each year. The current year is in column 3, and the prior year is in column 2. Total assets for 2022 amount to $1,147,000. Total liabilities and net worth also amount to $1,147,000 (i.e., the balance sheet balances). The total liabilities amount to $729,000 and net worth is $418,000, which of course equals total assets, $1,147,000.

Three types of assets are shown: current assets; property, plant, and equipment; and other assets. Current assets are supposed to be convertible into cash within one year and are always listed first on the balance sheet. Property, plant, and equipment and other assets (investments in this case) are long-term assets or non-current items.

Two types of liabilities are shown: current liabilities first and long-term debt second. Current liabilities are those expected to be paid within the next year, while long-term debt is not due within a year. Most long-term debt is due over a period of many years. The amount of long-term debt that will be due within the next year, $52,000, has been subtracted from the long-term debt amount and moved up into the current liabilities section, consistent with the concept of "current."

Table 11.3 Westside Clinic Balance Sheet

Assets	For the December 31, 2021	Year Ending December 31, 2022	$ Change	% Change
Current Assets				
Cash & cash equivalents	$145,000	$190,000	$45,000	31.0%
Accounts receivable (net)	300,000	310,000	10,000	3.3%
Inventories	20,000	25,000	5,000	25.0%
Prepaid Insurance	3,000	5,000	2,000	66.7%
Total Current Assets	$468,000	$530,000	$62,000	13.2%
Property, Plant, & Equipment				
Equipment (net)	$180,000	$190,000	$10,000	5.6%
Buildings (net)	300,000	285,000	−15,000	0.0%
Land	100,000	100,000	0	0.0%
Net Property, Plant, & Equipment	$580,000	$575,000	−5,000	−0.9%
Investments	32,000	42,000	10,000	31.3%
Total Assets	$1,080,000	$1,147,000	$67,000	6.2%
Liabilities				
Current Liabilities				
Current maturities of long-term debt	$48,000	$52,000	$4,000	8.3%
Accounts payable & accrued expenses	302,000	310,000	8,000	2.6%
Total Current Liabilities	$350,000	$362,000	$12,000	3.4%
Long-term debt	430,000	419,000	−11,000	−2.6%
Less Current maturities of long-term debt	−48,000	−52,000	−4,000	8.3%
Net long-term debt	$382,000	$367,000	−$15,000	−3.9%
Total Liabilities	$732,000	$729,000	−$3,000	−0.4%
Net Worth	$348,000	$418,000	$70,000	20.1%
Total Liabilities and Net Worth	$1,080,000	$1,147,000	$67,000	6.2%

Once again, because our intent is not to make an accountant of you, we will not be discussing generally accepted accounting principles (GAAP). Financial accounting and the resulting reports intended for third-party use must be prepared in accordance with GAAP. However, managerial accounting for internal purposes within an organization does not have to adhere to GAAP. One of the requirements of GAAP is that unrestricted fund balances be separated from restricted fund balances on the statements, so you may see two appropriate line items (restricted and unrestricted) in the fund balance section.

Exhibit 11.2 provides a series of questions for reviewing the balance sheet to deepen your understanding of the organization's current financial position and where it may be in the future.

Statement of Changes in Net Worth

Any monies earned or lost during a fiscal year increase or decrease the net worth of the organization and its owners. Remember that the formula for the income statement is

Total Revenue − Total Expenses = Net Income

The net income flows back into the fund balance or equity as seen in the statement of changes in net worth. **Table 11.4** shows a balance of $348,000 at the beginning of 2022 and adds income from operations, $65,000, and nonoperating gains (i.e., interest income), $5,000, to arrive at the $418,000 balance at the end of the year.

If you refer back to the balance sheet, you will see the $418,000 balance at the end of 2022. You should think of the income statement, balance sheet, and **statement of changes in net worth** as locked together, with the statement of changes in net worth being the mechanism that links the other two statements.

The $5,000 in nonoperating income earned by Westside Clinic is small, many health systems earn millions from donations and investments. Ellison reported that while many hospitals lost money in 2020 due to COVID, HCA reported a profit of $3.8 billion; Kaiser Permanente, $6.4 billion; and UPMC, $1.1 billion due to higher investment returns and other factors.[2] Westside's managers and employees grew the organization's net worth by 20.1% and ensured it will have more funds to work with in the future. There is one more major report—the statement of cash flows—and we will examine it next.

The Cash Flow Statement

We must revisit the concept of **accrual basis accounting** to understand why a statement of cash flows is necessary. If cash is not paid or received when revenues and expenses are entered on the books—the usual situation in accrual accounting—what happens? The revenue is not recorded as cash but rather as an accounts receivable. Likewise, when expenses are not paid in cash, they are recorded as an accounts payable on the balance sheet. The organization has neither received nor paid cash. Another characteristic of accrual accounting is the recognition of depreciation. For example, a capital asset, a piece of equipment, is purchased for $100,000 and has a usable life of five years. Therefore, $20,000 in depreciation expense is recognized every year for five years until the $100,000 investment is fully depreciated. Depreciation is recognized each year

---

Exhibit 11.2 Checklist for the Balance Sheet Review

1. What is the date on the balance sheet?
2. Are there large discrepancies in balances between the prior year and the current year?
3. Did total assets increase over the prior year?
4. Did current assets increase, decrease, or stay about the same?
5. Did land, plant, and equipment increase or decrease significantly over the prior year?
6. Did current liabilities increase, decrease, or stay about the same?
7. Did long-term debt increase or decrease significantly over the prior year?
8. Did net worth increase, decrease, or stay about the same?

Table 11.4 Westside Clinic Statement of Changes in Net Worth

	For the December 31, 2021	Year Ending December 31, 2022	$ Change	% Change
Net Worth First of Year	$296,000	$348,000	$52,000	17.6%
Income from Operations	50,000	65,000	$15,000	30.0%
Net Nonoperating Gain	2,000	5,000	$3,000	150.0%
Net Worth End of Year	$348,000	$418,000	$70,000	20.1%

as an expense, but it is not a cash expense (i.e., no money flows out of the organization). It is possible that a profitable organization may be unable to invest in supplies, equipment, and buildings or pay its bills due to a lack of cash. The statement of cash flows is designed to highlight the cash that flows into and out of an organization and the cash employees have to work with.

Table 11.5 reports the cash flows for 2021 and 2022. In effect, this statement takes the accrual basis statements and converts them to a cash flow for the period through a series of reconciling adjustments for noncash transactions. Understanding the cash/noncash concept makes sense of this statement. The starting point is the income from operations, the subtotal from the income statement. Depreciation is added back, and changes in asset and liability accounts, both positive and negative, are recognized. Increases (decreases) in current assets, accounts receivable, inventories, and prepaid expenses reduce (increase) cash (i.e., the organization invests more of its cash in these assets, reducing its cash holdings). Similarly, increases (decreases) in current liabilities, accounts payable and current maturities of long-term debt, accounts receivable, inventories, and prepaid expense increase (reduce) cash.

Next, capital and related financing activities are addressed. Westside purchased $35,000 in new equipment, a cash outflow, and received $33,000 in loan financing, a cash inflow; the net effect on cash was −$2,000. Organizations must replace and improve their equipment and facilities to stay in business. Westside also paid off $48,000 of its long-term obligations, a cash outflow. The sum of capital and financing transaction reduced cash by $50,000.

The last section accounts for investing activities. Westside obtained $5,000 in interest income, an inflow, and purchased $10,000 in investments, an outflow. The sum of investing activities is a net outflow of $5,000. The result is a net increase in cash and cash equivalents of $45,000—+$100,000 from operations, −$50,000 from capital and financing, and −$5,000 from investing. The $45,000 is added to the cash balance at the beginning of the year, $145,000, to arrive at the cash balance at the end of the year, $190,000. Refer back to the balance sheet and you will find that the cash balance at the end of 2022 is indeed $190,000. The fourth major report—the statement of cash flows—interlocks with the other three major reports.

The four major reports fit together; each makes its own contribution to reporting financial performance and understanding organizational performance and financial strength requires you to understand the information conveyed by each report.

Table 11.5 Westside Clinic Statement of Cash Flows

	For the December 31, 2021	Year Ending December 31, 2022	$ Change	% Change
Operating Activities				
Income from Operations	$50,000	$65,000	$15,000	30.0%
Adjustments to reconcile income from operations to net cash flows from operating activities				
Depreciation and amortization	$40,000	$40,000	$0	0.0%
Changes in asset and liability accounts				
Accounts receivable	–$20,000	–$10,000	$10,000	–50.0%
Inventories	–5,000	–5,000	0	0.0%
Prepaid expenses and other assets	–1,000	–2,000	–1,000	100.0%
Accounts payable and accrued expenses	4,000	8,000	4,000	100.0%
Current maturities of long-term debt	0	4,000	4,000	—
	$68,000	$100,000	$32,000	47.1%
Cash Flows from Capital and Related Financing Activities				
Acquisition of equipment	–$30,000	–$35,000	–$5,000	16.7%
Proceeds from loan for equipment	20,000	33,000	13,000	—
Repayment of long-term obligations	–35,000	–48,000	–13,000	37.1%
Net Cash Flows from Capital and Related Financing Activities	–$45,000	–$50,000	–$5,000	11.1%
Cash Flows from Investing Activities				
Interest income received	$2,000	$5,000	$3,000	150.0%
Investments purchased (net)	0	–10,000	–10,000	—
Net Cash Flows from Investing Activities	$2,000	–$5,000	–$7,000	–350.0%
Net Increase (Decrease) in Cash and Cash Equivalents	$25,000	$45,000	$20,000	80.0%
Cash and Cash Equivalents, Beginning of Year	$120,000	$145,000	$25,000	20.8%
End of Year	$145,000	$190,000	$45,000	31.0%

WRAP-UP

Summary

The purpose of financial statements is to document the financial health of an organization and highlight where improvement can be achieved. The income statement documents financial performance over a fiscal period, often one year. Were employees able to generate more revenue than expenses and the amount of nonoperating revenues? No organization can continue if it loses money year after year, so managers must ensure that revenues not only cover expenses but also provide sufficient resources to improve and expand operations.

The balance sheet reports on the relationship assets and liabilities. Management's first job is to ensure that assets exceed liabilities by a sufficient amount so the organization can reinvest in operations and obtain debt at a reasonable cost. Managers' second job is to increase an organization's net worth. Improving net worth requires managers to assess the type of assets held and how they are financed (i.e., are assets productive, and are they acquired at the lowest cost?). The statement of changes in net worth ties together the income statement and balance sheet; it summarizes the reason why net worth is increasing or decreasing—that is, is the change due to income from operations or nonoperating income?

Finally, the statement of cash flows examines the cash generated or consumed from operations, financing activities, the purchase or sale of assets, the assumption or repayment of debt, and investment activities. An organization may find itself without cash to pay bills when revenue exceeds expenses and assets exceed liabilities, so the **cash flow statement** reports on the sources, uses, and availability of cash. The goal of the statement of cash flows is to document changes in cash and encourage managers to maintain adequate cash holdings so purchases can occur when needed and bills are paid when they are due. Understanding the information on the four major financial statements is necessary to obtain an accurate assessment of an organization's prior performance and where it should go in the future.

Key Terms

Accrual Basis Accounting
Balance Sheet
Cash Basis Accounting
Cash Flow Statement
Income Statement
Statement of Changes in Net Worth

Discussion Questions

1. Explain the purpose and structure of income statements.
2. Explain the purpose and structure of balance sheets.
3. Explain the purpose and structure of the statement of changes in net worth.
4. Explain the purpose and structure of the statement of cash flows.

Problems

1. The following table provides the income statement for the Hale Medical Group. Calculate total expenses and net income. Calculate the dollar and percent change for each line item. What is the difference in growth rates between revenues and total expenses, and if this difference continues, what will happen to future net income? Which area's expenses have the highest and lowest growth rates?

Revenue	For the December 31, 2021	Year Ending December 31, 2022
Net Patient Service Revenue	$5,000,000	$5,200,000
Total Operating Revenue	_____	_____
Operating Expenses		
Internal Medicine	$2,500,000	$2,620,000
Oncology	950,000	1,000,000
Obstetrics/Gynecology	500,000	520,000
Administration	650,000	700,000
Depreciation	30,000	30,000
Interest	25,000	30,000
Total Operating Expenses	_____	_____
Income from Operations	_____	_____
Nonoperating Gains (Losses)		
Interest Income	$10,000	-$15,000
Net Nonoperating Gains	$10,000	-$15,000
Net Income	_____	_____

2. The following table provides the Hale Medical Group's income statement by expense item (rather than area of responsibility in problem 1). Calculate total expenses and net income. Calculate the dollar and percent change for each line item. What type of expenses have the highest and lowest growth rates?

Revenue	For the December 31, 2021	Year Ending December 31, 2022
Net Patient Service Revenue	$5,000,000	$5,200,000
Total Operating Revenue	_____	_____

(continues)

Revenue	For the December 31, 2021	Year Ending December 31, 2022
Operating Expenses		
Salaries and wages	$3,500,000	$3,670,000
Fringe benefits	600,000	660,000
Supplies	500,000	510,000
Depreciation	30,000	30,000
Interest	25,000	30,000
Total Operating Expenses	_____	_____
Income from Operations	_____	_____
Nonoperating Gains (Losses)		
Investment Income	$10,000	–$15,000
Net Nonoperating Gains	$10,000	–$15,000
Net Income	_____	_____

3. Given the following table with Hale Medical Group's income from operations, total operating revenue, and total operating expenses from 2019 through 2022, create a line chart and describe the trend in revenues, expenses, and income from operations. Note that a combo chart with income from operations on the secondary axis will provide a better picture of operations.

	2019	2020	2021	2022
Income from Operations	$250,000	$300,000	$345,000	$300,000
Total Operating Revenue	$4,800,000	$4,900,000	$5,000,000	$5,200,000
Total Operating Expenses	$4,550,000	$4,600,000	$4,655,000	$4,900,000

4. The following table provides the balance sheet for the Hale Medical Group. Calculate the growth rate for each line item. What is the difference in growth rates between total assets, total liabilities, and net worth? Which types of assets and liabilities have the highest growth rates?

Assets	For the December 31, 2021	Year Ending December 31, 2022
Current Assets		
Cash and cash equivalents	$300,000	$400,000
Accounts receivable (net)	450,000	490,000
Inventories	35,000	40,000
Prepaid Insurance	10,000	12,000
Total Current Assets	_____	_____
Property, Plant, and Equipment		
Equipment (net)	$200,000	$220,000
Buildings (net)	375,000	350,000
Land	200,000	200,000
Net Property, Plant, and Equipment	$775,000	$770,000
Investments	32,000	42,000
Total Assets	_____	_____
Liabilities		
Current Liabilities		
Current maturities of long-term debt	$40,000	$40,000
Accounts payable	25,000	30,000
Total Current Liabilities	_____	_____
Long-Term Debt	477,000	339,000
Less Current maturities of long-term debt	−40,000	−40,000
Net Long-Term Debt	$437,000	$299,000
Total Liabilities	_____	_____
Net Worth	_____	_____
Total Liabilities and Net Worth	_____	_____

5. The following table provides the statement of changes in net worth for the Hale Medical Group. Is net worth increasing or decreasing, and how does the change relate to income from operations and nonoperating gains (or losses)?

	For the December 31, 2021	Year Ending December 31, 2022	$ Change	% Change
Net Worth First of Year	$745,000	$1,100,000	_____	_____
Income from operations	345,000	300,000	_____	_____
Investment Income	10,000	−15,000	_____	_____
Net Worth End of Year	$1,100,000	$1,385,000	_____	_____

6. The following table provides the statement of cash flows for the Hale Medical Group. Is cash increasing or decreasing, and how does it relate to operating, financing, and investing activities? What were the three largest sources of cash? What was the largest use of cash?

	For the December 31, 2021	Year Ending December 31, 2022
Operating Activities		
Income from Operations	$345,000	$300,000
Adjustments to reconcile income from operations to net cash flows		
Depreciation	$25,000	$25,000
Changes in asset and liability accounts		
Accounts receivable	$10,000	−$40,000
Inventories	−4,000	−5,000
Prepaid expenses	−2,000	−2,000
Accounts payable	−2,000	5,000
Current maturities of long-term debt	0	0
	_____	_____
Cash Flows from Capital and Related Financing Activities		
Acquisition of equipment	−$50,000	−$20,000
Proceeds from loan for equipment	0	0
Repayment of long-term obligations	−70,000	−138,000
Net Cash Flows from Capital and Related Financing Activities	_____	_____
Cash Flows from Investing Activities		
Interest income received	$10,000	−$15,000

	For the December 31, 2021	Year Ending December 31, 2022
Investments purchased (net)	−30,000	−10,000
Net Cash Flows from Investing Activities	_____	_____
Net Increase (Decrease) in Cash		
Net Increase (Decrease) in Cash	$232,000	$100,000
Cash and Cash Equivalents,		
Beginning of Year	$68,000	$300,000
End of Year	_____	_____

7. Based on your review of the financial statements of the Hale Medical Group, (1) is financial performance improving, (2) are managers doing a good job managing the finance of the organization, and (3) are there any areas of concern that should be investigated?

Notes

1. S. A. Finkler et al., *Essentials of Cost Accounting for Health Care Organizations*, 3rd ed. (Sudbury MA: Jones & Bartlett Publishers, 2007).

2. A. Ellison, "Major Health Systems Report $1B+ Annual Profits," https://www.beckershospitalreview.com/finance/major-health-systems-report-1b-annual-profits.html, accessed April 15, 2021.

CHAPTER 12

Financial Ratios and Operating Indicators, Assessing Financial Performance

PROGRESS NOTES

After completing this chapter, you should be able to:

1. Explain the role of financial ratios in financial management.
2. Calculate and explain the difference between four profitability ratios.
3. Calculate and interpret three liquidity ratios.
4. Calculate and explain the meaning of three capital structure ratios.
5. Calculate and interpret three turnover ratios.
6. Explain how operating indicators are used to examine costs.

Overview: Financial Ratios

Income statements and balance sheets that report multiple years of information can identify whether net income is increasing, stable, or decreasing but shed little insight into what net income should be. Financial ratios and **operating indicators** explore the elements that produce net income. Financial ratios put net income, revenues, and expenses into context by relating them to assets and liabilities as well as exploring liquidity (ability to pay bills), capital structure (use of debt), and asset turnover (productivity).

Operating indicators extend the analysis by relating financial variables to output produced and inputs consumed. A prime goal is to examine the expense per output and its relationship to input costs, efficiency, and utilization. Determining whether managers are producing an appropriate return from the assets they are entrusted with requires comparing organizational performance with appropriate peer institutions.

Ratios are convenient and uniform measures that are widely used in healthcare financial management. Ratio analysis should be conducted as a comparative analysis; in other words, one ratio standing alone with nothing to compare it with does not mean very much. When interpreting ratios, the differences between time periods should be considered and the reasons for such differences should be sought. It is a good practice to compare results with equivalent computations from outside the organization—regional figures from similar institutions would be a good example. Caution and good judgment must always be exercised when working with ratios.

Financial ratios pull together two elements of the financial statements: one as the numerator and one as the denominator. To calculate a ratio, divide the bottom number (the denominator) into the top number (the numerator). Case 32, "Ratios and Operating Indicators," requires the use of financial ratios and operating indicators to assess financial position. We highly recommend that you spend time with this case as it will add depth and background to the contents of this chapter.

In this chapter, we examine profitability, liquidity, capital structure, and **turnover ratios**. **Table 12.1** sets out 13 widely used ratios in healthcare organizations: four profitability, three liquidity, three capital structure, and three turnover ratios.

We will examine the performance of the Westside Clinic for the years 2021 and 2022, **Table 12.2** (i.e., the financial statements introduced in Chapter 11). In Chapter 11, we saw Westside generated $70,000 in net income in 2022. This chapter provides insight into why net income increased over 2021.

Profitability Ratios

Profitability ratios measure the ability of managers to generate more revenue than is spent on resources (i.e., expenses). Nonprofit

Table 12.1 Thirteen Common Financial Ratios

Profitability Ratios	
1. Operating Margin:	Income from Operations
	Total Operating Revenues
2. Total Margin:	Net Income (Revenue and Gains in Excess of Expenses and Losses)
	Total Revenues
3. Return on Assets:	Net Income
	Total Revenues
4. Return on Equity:	Net Income
	Net Worth (fund balance)
Liquidity Ratios	
5. Current Ratio:	Current Assets
	Current Liabilities
6. Days Cash on Hand:	Cash and Cash Equivalents
	(Total Expenses – Depreciation) ÷ Days in Period (365)
7. Days in Accounts Receivable:	Accounts Receivable
	Operating Revenues ÷ Days in Period (365)
Capital Structure Ratios	
8. Times Interest Earned:	Net Income + Interest Expense
	Interest Expense

9. Debt Service Coverage:	Net Income + Interest Expense + Depreciation
	Interest Expense + Current Maturities of Long-Term Debt
10. Equity Financing:	Net Worth (fund balance)
	Total Assets
Turnover Ratios	
11. Total Asset Turnover:	Total Revenue
	Total Assets
12. Current Asset Turnover:	Total Revenue
	Current Assets
13. Fixed Asset Turnover:	Total Revenue
	Fixed Assets

Table 12.2 Westside Clinic Income Statement and Balance Sheet

Income Statement Revenue	For the December 31, 2021	Year Ending December 31, 2022
Net Patient Service Revenue	$1,850,000	$1,950,000
Total Operating Revenue	$1,850,000	$1,950,000
Operating Expenses		
Salaries and wages	$1,215,000	$1,262,000
Fringe benefits	347,000	363,000
Supplies	174,000	200,000
Depreciation	40,000	40,000
Interest	24,000	20,000
Total Operating Expenses	$1,800,000	$1,885,000
Operating Income	$50,000	$65,000
Nonoperating Gains (Losses)		
Interest Income	$2,000	$5,000
Net Nonoperating Gains	$2,000	$5,000
Net Income	$52,000	$70,000
Balance Sheet		
Assets	December 31, 2021	December 31, 2022
Current Assets		
Cash and cash equivalents	$145,000	$190,000

(continues)

Table 12.2 Westside Clinic Income Statement and Balance Sheet   (continued)

Income Statement Revenue	For the December 31, 2021	Year Ending December 31, 2022
Accounts receivable (net)	300,000	310,000
Inventories	20,000	25,000
Prepaid Insurance	3,000	5,000
Total Current Assets	$468,000	$530,000
Property, Plant, and Equipment		
Equipment (net)	$180,000	$190,000
Buildings (net)	300,000	285,000
Land	100,000	100,000
Net Property, Plant, and Equipment	$580,000	$575,000
Investments	32,000	42,000
Total Assets	$1,080,000	$1,147,000
Liabilities		
Current Liabilities		
Current maturities of long-term debt	$48,000	$52,000
Accounts payable and accrued expenses	302,000	310,000
Total Current Liabilities	$350,000	$362,000
Long-Term Debt	430,000	419,000
Less: Current maturities of long-term debt	−48,000	−52,000
Net Long-Term Debt	$382,000	$367,000
Total Liabilities	$732,000	$729,000
Net Worth	$348,000	$418,000
Total Liabilities and Net Worth	$1,080,000	$1,147,000

organizations may not call this result a profit, but the measurement ratios are still called profitability ratios, whether applied to for-profit or nonprofit organizations.

Operating Margin

The **operating margin**, which is generally expressed as a percentage, is operating income (loss) divided by total operating revenues:

$$\frac{\text{Operating Income}}{\text{Total Operating Revenues}} = \frac{\$65,000}{\$1,950,000} = 3.33\%$$

Westside earned 3.33% on every dollar of revenue generated in 2022 (or $3.33 for every $100 of revenue, 3.33% × $100). This is a substantial improvement over 2021 when $2.70 was earned. The improvement was due to management's ability to increase revenue by 5.4% while limiting expense growth to 4.7%.

The operating margin is used for a number of managerial purposes and also sometimes enters into credit analysis (i.e., does the organization earn enough income to ensure its debts can be repaid?). It is so universal that many outside sources are available for comparative purposes. The result of the computation must still be carefully considered because of variables in each period being compared.

Total Margin

The **total margin** is net income divided by total revenues. Total margin measures the ability of managers to generate net income from *all* sources. The numerator is broadened to include nonoperating gains, and the denominator includes non-patient revenues. Westside has zero non-patient revenues, but many nonprofits have substantial nonoperating revenues.

$$\frac{\text{Net Income}}{\text{Total Revenues}} = \frac{\$70,000}{\$1,995,000} = 3.59\%$$

Westside earned $3.59 for every $100 of revenue in 2022. This is a substantial improvement over the prior year when $2.81 was earned. The improvement was largely driven by the increase in the operating margin, but Westside also benefited from an additional $3,000 in interest income (nonoperating gain).

Return on Assets

The **return on assets** (ROA) is net income divided by total assets:

$$\frac{\text{Net Income}}{\text{Total Assets}} = \frac{\$70,000}{\$1,147,000} = 6.10\%$$

Westside is earning $6.10 on every $100 of assets. This is a substantial improvement over the prior year when $4.81 was earned. ROA is a broad measure to assess management's use of assets. A high ROA indicates that management is fully utilizing assets, and a low ROA suggest underutilization of and/or overinvestment in assets. Some analysts use an alternative computation for ROA; they compute this ratio as earnings before interest and taxes (EBIT) divided by total assets.

Return on Equity (ROE)

The **return on equity** (ROE) is net income divided by net worth:

$$\frac{\text{Net Income}}{\text{Net Worth}} = \frac{\$70,000}{\$418,000} = 16.75\%$$

Westside is earning $16.75 on every $100 of equity, a substantial improvement over 2021 when $14.94 was earned. ROE is commonly used to assess management's ability to create wealth for the owners of the organization. **Figure 12.1** demonstrates how figures are taken from the income statement and balance sheet to calculate the profitability ratios for 2022.

Figure 12.2 presents the operating margin, ROA, and ROE for the past four years.

Based on the profitability ratios, we can conclude that management has done a good job generating net income form revenues, assets, and equity. Net income is not only adequate, it has increased over the past four years. We will explore liquidity, capital structure, and turnover ratios to identify how management is producing the reported net income.

Liquidity Ratios

Liquidity ratios reflect the ability of the organization to meet its current obligations. Liquidity ratios measure short-term sufficiency. That is, can the organization pay its obligations when they are due? In other words, does the organization have sufficient cash or assets that can be converted to cash?

Current Ratio

The **current ratio** equals current assets divided by current liabilities. While Westside's balance sheet totals current assets and liabilities, many balance sheets do not, so you may have to add cash and cash equivalents, accounts receivable, inventory, and other current assets to obtain total current assets. For instance, consider this example:

$$\frac{\text{Total Current Assets}}{\text{Total Current Liabilities}} = \frac{\$530,000}{\$362,000} = 1.46$$

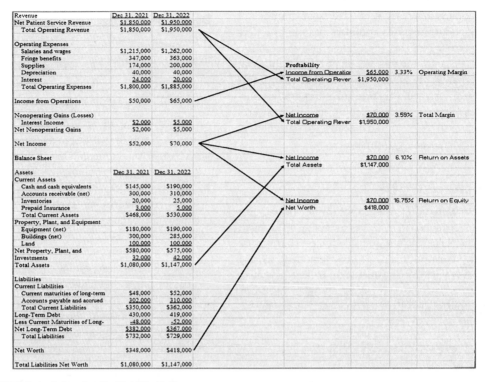

Figure 12.1 Calculating the Profitability Ratios

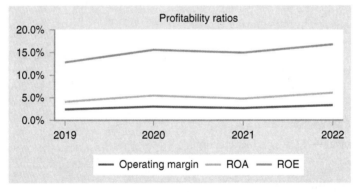

Figure 12.2 Westside Clinic Profitability Ratios

Westside has $1.46 in current assets for every $1.00 in current assets it must pay, so paying short-term obligations should not be a problem. If the ratio were close to 1.00 or below 1.00, the institution may need to liquidate assets or acquire debt to pay its bills.

Days Cash on Hand

Days cash on hand equals unrestricted cash and investments divided by cash operating expenses divided by 365 (i.e., daily cash outlay that does not include depreciation or other expenses that do not require cash payment). Daily cash outlay = (Total Operating Expenses – Depreciation) ÷ 365, ($1,885,000 – 40,000) ÷ 365 = $5,054.79:

$$\frac{\text{Cash and Cash Equivalents}}{\text{Daily Cash Outlay}} = \frac{\$190,000}{\$5,055} = 37.59$$

Based on spending an average of $5,055 per day, Westside could continue to pay its bills for the next 37.59 days with no additional cash inflow. The $45,000 increase in cash and cash equivalents is the primary reason why this ratio increased from 30.07 days in 2021.

Days in Accounts Receivable

Days in accounts receivable equals accounts receivable (net) divided by average daily net patient service revenues. Average daily net patient service revenues is net patient service revenues divided by 365 days (i.e., $1,950,000 ÷ 365 = $5,342.47):

$$\frac{\text{Accounts Receivable (net)}}{\text{Daily Patient Revenue}} = \frac{\$310,000}{\$5,342} = 58.03$$

Based on billing patients an average of $5,342 per day, Westside takes 58.0 days to collect the amounts owed for services provided. Collection is slightly faster than 2021 when it took 59.2 days to collect. Faster collection is desired as money in cash is preferable to accounts receivable and the older a receivable is, the more difficult it becomes to collect. Unpaid bills after 120 days or more often become bad debt. Days in accounts receivable is a common measure of billing and collection performance. There are many regional and national days in accounts receivables benchmarks to compare with your own organization's performance.

Capital Structure Ratios

Liquidity ratios assess an organization's ability to meet its short-term obligations, and **capital structure ratios** expand the focus to include the ability of the organization to pay the annual interest and principal obligations on its long-term debt. Capital structure ratios are also called solvency ratios as they also measure the ratio of assets funded by owners rather than through debt. Overreliance on debt will increase the cost of borrowing funds and in extreme cases may prevent an organization from obtaining additional debt (i.e., creditors do not loan money to those who cannot repay the debt).

Times Interest Earned

Times interest earned measures the ability of an organization to pay its annual interest expense, (Net income + Interest expense) ÷ Interest expense:

$$\frac{\text{Net income} + \text{Interest}}{\text{Interest}} = \frac{\$70,000 + 20,000}{\$20,000} = 4.50$$

Westside has 4.5 times the amount of resources needed to meet its interest obligations. You can see that the predominant factor in this ratio is net income. Profitable organizations will have a ratio greater than 1.00 and should have sufficient resources to meet required interest payments. When an organization loses money, its ratio is less than 1.00, and it may have to sell assets or secure debt to meet its obligations.

Debt Service Coverage Ratio

The **debt service coverage ratio** is net income plus interest, depreciation, and amortization divided by maximum annual debt service (i.e., interest expense plus current maturities of long-term debt):

$$\frac{\text{Net income} + \text{Interest} + \text{Depreciation}}{\text{Interest} + \text{Current maturities of LT Debt}} =$$

$$\frac{\$70,000 + 20,000 + 40,000}{\$20,000 + 52,000} = 1.81$$

Debt service coverage measures the ability of the organization to meet its interest and principal obligations, Westside has $1.81 in resources for every dollar of interest and principal due, an increase from $1.61 in 2021. Lending institutions vary on their requirements for debt service coverage. Lending agreements often have a provision requiring debt service coverage to be at or above a certain figure.

Equity Financing

The **equity financing ratio** is net worth divided by total assets:

$$\frac{\text{Net Worth}}{\text{Total Assets}} = \frac{\$418,000}{\$1,147,000} = 0.36$$

The equity financing ratio measures the percent of total assets financed by owners rather than debt. In this organization, owners supplied 36% of assets versus 64% financed by creditors. In 2021, 32% of assets were financed by owners. The primary driver of the increase in the ratio was the $70,000 net income in 2022. A higher ratio indicating lower reliance on debt is less risky. Organizations with higher equity financing ratios will have lower interest and principal obligations but there is no set standard to assess performance.

Turnover Ratios

Turnover ratios measure the amount of revenue generated from assets (i.e., are managers effectively utilizing assets?). Overinvestment in assets results in less productive (i.e., idle) resources, lower revenues, and higher costs. Similarly, underinvestment may undermine an organization's ability to provide effective care and increase costs.

Total Asset Turnover

Total asset turnover measures how many dollars of revenue are generated for each dollar invested in assets. Total asset turnover is total operating revenue divided by total assets:

$$\frac{\text{Total Operating Revenue}}{\text{Total Assets}} = \frac{\$1,950,000}{\$1,147,000} = 1.70$$

Total asset turnover shows that each dollar of assets generates $1.70 in revenue and was basically equivalent to the $1.71 generated in 2021. Managers' goals should be to maximize the revenue generated per dollar of asset (i.e., ensure assets are fully employed, neither overtaxed nor underemployed).

Current Asset Turnover

Current asset turnover assesses the use of current assets. It is possible that an excess of current assets is offset by underinvestment in fixed assets or vice versa and total asset turnover would appear appropriate despite poor use of assets. Current asset turnover is total operating revenue divided by current assets:

$$\frac{\text{Total Operating Revenue}}{\text{Current Assets}} = \frac{\$1,950,000}{\$530,000} = 3.68$$

The current asset turnover ratio shows that Westside generates $3.68 in revenue for every dollar invested in current assets in 2022. The ratio is significantly lower than the $3.95 generated in 2021 and is due to large increases in cash and cash equivalents and inventory. This ratio should be used as a starting point to determine whether an organization is holding too much or too little in current assets.

Fixed Asset Turnover

Fixed asset turnover assesses the use of long-term assets. Fixed asset turnover is total operating revenue divided by fixed assets, total assets less current assets, $1,147,000 − 530,000 = $617,000:

$$\frac{\text{Total Operating Revenue}}{\text{Fixed Assets}} = \frac{\$1,950,000}{\$617,000} = 3.15$$

The fixed asset turnover ratio shows that Westside generates $3.15 in revenue for every dollar invested in current assets in 2022. The ratio is higher than the $3.02 generated in 2021, suggesting more efficient use of fixed assets. This ratio should be used to determine whether an organization is holding too much or too little in current assets.

Table 12.3 uses arrows to indicate the change in the ratio. In general, higher ratios are desired; the exception is days in accounts receivable, where a lower number of days is desired. Overall, Westside's management has improved performance in 11 of the 13 ratios, the exceptions being no change in total asset turnover and a lower current asset turnover. This concludes the description of profitability, liquidity, capital structure, and turnover ratios.

Operating Indicators

Financial ratios provide an organizational view of performance, and operating indicators relate financial variables to nonfinancial variables to provide senior and department managers with a more organic view of performance. The following benchmarks are taken from Optum360°.[1] Managers often follow expenses on the monthly expense reports and annual income statement. Managers should assess their expenses relative to the output of their organization and department. At the hospital level, an indicator such as total expense per admission provides little guidance for department managers, who need information that relates expenses to the resources used and their output.

Table 12.3 Summary of Westside Clinic Financial Ratios

Profitability	2021	2022	Change
Operating Margin	2.70%	3.33%	↑ improvement
Total Margin	2.81%	3.59%	↑ improvement
ROA	4.81%	6.10%	↑ improvement
ROE	14.94%	16.75%	↑ improvement
Liquidity			
Current Ratio	1.34	1.46	↑ improvement
Days Cash on Hand	30.07	37.59	↑ improvement
Days in Accounts Receivable	59.19	58.03	↓ improvement
Capital Structure			
Times Interest Earned	3.17	4.50	↑ improvement
Debt Service Coverage	1.61	1.81	↑ improvement
Equity Financing	0.32	0.36	↑ lower risk
Turnover			
Total Asset Turnover	1.71	1.70	↔ no change
Current Asset Turnover	3.95	3.68	↓ deterioration
Fixed Asset Turnover	3.02	3.16	↑ improvement

Expense Indicators

Expense indicators relate resource costs to the primary output produced by the department. For example, a head nurse should track RN salaries (other employee salaries or supply expense) per patient day, the director of the clinical lab should track salary or supply expense per lab test (or RVU), and the director of physical therapy should track salary or supply expense per session. In a physician's office, clinic, or emergency department, the physician (other salary, or supply) expense per visit should be tracked. After calculating the resource expense per output, managers should identify the components of cost (i.e., how much is due to the cost of inputs and the use of labor, supplies, equipment, and facilities?). **Table 12.4** presents examples for a nursing unit and physician practice. For a more comprehensive review, see Ross (2018).[2]

Price Indicators

Price indicators examine how much is received for the services provided (outputs) *and* how much is paid for the resources used (inputs). Output price indicators require the revenue received for a service to be divided by the number of outputs produced.

Net price per inpatient discharge = I/P net revenues ÷ Total discharges = $10,154, 25th to 75th percentile range: $7,553 to $14,511

CMI and wage adjusted net price per discharge = I/P net revenues ÷ (total discharges × all patient CMI × wage index) = $6,688, 25th to 75th percentile range: $5,752 to $7,827

Gross price per ambulatory payment classification (APC) = Gross APC revenues ÷ Total APCs = $669, 25th to 75th percentile range: $430 to $1,075

Unit cost indicators examine input prices and costs per discharge by major expense to determine

Table 12.4 Operating Indicators

Nursing Unit		Physician Practice	
Expense Indicator		Expense Indicator	
RN salary (total salary expense)	$800,000	MD salary (total salary expense)	$180,000
Patient days	5,475	Patient visits	4,800
Cost per patient day	$73.06	Cost per patient visit	$37.50
Cost Indicator		Cost Indicator	
RN salary	$800,000	MD salary	$180,000
Total hours paid	21,900	Total hours paid	2,080
Cost per hour	$36.53	Cost per hour	$86.54
Efficiency Indicator		Efficiency Indicator	
Total hours paid	21,900	Total hours paid	2,080
Total patient days	5,475	Total physician visits	4,800
Hours per patient day	4.00	Hours per physician visit	0.43
			(26 min)
Utilization Indicator		Utilization Indicator	
Total patient days	5475	Total physician visits	4,800
Licenced beds	7300	Exam rooms	4.0
Occupancy	75%	Physician visits per room	1,200

which factors, wages, fringe benefits, supplies, depreciation, interest, or other costs (i.e., total cost) for an input divided by number of units purchased.

Salary per FTE = Total salary and wages ÷ Total FTE = $59,380, 25th to 75th percentile range: $52,294 to $67,210, minimum: $50,276 Alabama, maximum: $77,081 Oregon

Pharmaceutical price: Total pharmaceutical expense ÷ total drugs purchased

One reason why the expense per output may be higher than necessary is the organization is paying too much for inputs. When unit cost indicators are higher than expected, the next step is to determine if managers can reduce input prices by better price negotiation and/or use of lower-priced inputs.

Efficiency Indicators

A second reason why the expense per output indicator may indicate costs are higher than necessary is more resources (i.e., variable expenses) are used than necessary. Efficiency indicators require the number of inputs used be divided by output (e.g., hours per patient day; hours per lab test, scan, therapy [lab, radiology, physical therapy]; hours per visit [physicians, clinics, emergency departments]).

Staff hours per discharge = (I/P FTE × 2080) ÷ I/P discharges = 131.1 hours, 25th to 75th percentile range: 101.0 to 194.3 hours

CMI adjusted staff hours per discharge = (I/P FTE × 2080) ÷ (I/P discharges × all patient CMI) = 75.2 hours, 25th to 75th percentile range: 62.9 to 92.8 hours

Outpatient staff hours per visit = (O/P FTE × 2080) ÷ O/P visits, range unavailable

When efficiency indicators are higher than expected, managers should examine the amount of time and/or supplies employees are using to treat patients. Changing processes (i.e., streamlining and eliminating error) is a common way to reduce time and supplies used.

Utilization Indicators

Similar to efficiency indicators, utilization indicators measure the amount of output produced from equipment and facilities (i.e., fixed expenses). Common utilization indicators include occupancy, average length of stay, procedures per surgical suite, scans per machine, and visits per exam or treatment room.

Occupancy = Total patient days ÷ (Licensed beds × 365)

Average length of stay = Total patient days ÷ Total discharges

Procedures per surgical suite = Total surgical procedures ÷ Number of surgical suites

Scans per machine = Total radiological procedures ÷ Number of imaging machines

Patients per exam room = Total patient visits ÷ Total exam rooms

Utilization indicators measure the output produced by a resource. While turnover ratios assess whether managers have over- or underinvested in equipment and facilities, utilization indicators highlight the specific type of investment and hence pinpoint where adjustments, increases or decreases in assets, should be made.

Table 12.4 shows that the head nurse should begin her examination of RN salaries by dividing salary by total patient days, $73.06. Is $73.06 an appropriate expense per output? Let's assume it is high. The next step examines the cost per hour. Is the organization paying an appropriate wage for RNs? We'll assume $36.53 is comparable to other organizations or the prevailing wage in the area. Next, the head nurse assesses the four hours of RN time per patient day. Let's assume other organizations use less time by substituting lower-paid LPNs and/or CNAs. The head nurse may then want to examine how treatment is delivered (i.e., what tasks can be performed by and shifted to other personnel?). Finally, unit occupancy should be calculated. The unit is running at 75% occupancy, so the head nurse should consider if costs could be lowered by increasing utilization. Are inefficiencies created by working at lower output (e.g., operating at minimum staffing guidelines) but insufficient to keep workers fully employed? This discussion is limited; in the real world, providers must also consider intensity (how sick a patient is and how much care [resources] they require and reimbursement indicators (how much is received for the services provided).

Operating indicators explain the components of costs (i.e., if expenses are higher than comparable organizations, what factor(s) account for the higher cost?). Higher-than-necessary cost arises from using more labor or supplies per output, paying more for labor and supplies than other providers, and/or underutilization of equipment and facilities.

WRAP-UP

Summary

Financial ratios put accounting information in context by reporting amounts relative to each other (e.g., net income relative to total assets). This information is essential to evaluating and improving performance. Profitability ratios, operating margin, return on assets, and return on equity should be used to evaluate management. Are managers making decisions and taking actions that increase the net worth of the organization? Answering the question requires understanding an organization's profitability ratios relative to similar organizations and trends. Are ratios higher than other organizations, and are they improving?

After profitability ratios are calculated and especially when the ratios are lower than other organizations and/or deteriorating, managers should investigate liquidity, capital structure, and turnover ratios to identify opportunities for improvement. The liquidity ratios may indicate opportunities in collecting patient revenues or paying liabilities that could increase an organization's cash. Capital structure ratios may indicate opportunities to increase or decrease the use of

debt to reduce financing expenses. Turnover ratios may indicate that assets are not producing sufficient revenues and the organization has overinvested in current and/or fixed assets. Managers should use this information to improve net income.

Operating indicators relate financial data to operational data such as output produced and resources used to illuminate what expenses produce. After identifying the cost per output, managers should be able to explain how the cost of inputs and utilization of labor, supplies, equipment, and facilities contribute to cost and if changes can improve performance.

Key Terms

Current Asset Turnover	Fixed Asset Turnover	Return on Equity
Current Ratio	Liquidity Ratios	Capital Structure Ratios
Days Cash on Hand	Operating Indicators	Total Asset Turnover
Days in Accounts Receivable	Operating Margin	Total Margin
Debt Service Coverage Ratio	Profitability Ratios	Turnover Ratios
Equity Financing Ratio	Return on Assets	

Discussion Questions

1. Explain the role of profitability ratios. Why should net income be assessed relative to operating revenue, assets, and equity?
2. Explain the role of current ratios. Assuming days in accounts receivable are too high, why is this a problem, and what actions should managers take to reduce the number of outstanding days?
3. Explain the role of capital structure ratios. Assuming the equity financing ratio is

higher than similar organizations, what actions should managers take?
4. Explain the role of turnover ratios. Assuming total asset turnover is lower than similar organizations, what actions should managers take to increase the ratio?
5. Explain how operating indicators are used to examine resource use.

Problems

1. The following table provides the income statement and balance sheet for the Hale Medical Group. Complete the ratio

worksheet. Explain the change in the ratios that increased or decreased 20% or more from the prior year.

Revenue	For the December 31, 2021	Year Ending December 31, 2022	Assets	For the December 31, 2021	Year Ending December 31, 2022
Net Patient Service Revenue	$5,000,000	$5,200,000	Current Assets		
Total Operating Revenue	$5,000,000	$5,200,000	Cash and cash equivalents	$300,000	$400,000
			Accounts receivable (net)	450,000	490,000
Operating Expenses			Inventories	35,000	40,000
Salaries and wages	$3,500,000	$3,670,000	Prepaid Insurance	10,000	12,000
Fringe benefits	600,000	660,000	Total Current Assets	$795,000	$942,000
Supplies	500,000	510,000	Property, Plant, & Equipment		
Depreciation	30,000	30,000	Equipment (net)	$200,000	$220,000
Interest	25,000	30,000	Buildings (net)	375,000	350,000
Total Operating Expenses	$4,655,000	$4,900,000	Land	200,000	200,000
			Net Property, Plant, & Equipment	$775,000	$770,000
Income from Operations	$345,000	$300,000	Investments	$32,000	$42,000
			Total Assets	$1,602,000	$1,754,000
Nonoperating Gains (Losses)					
Investment Income	$10,000	–$15,000	**Liabilities**		
Net Nonoperating Gains	$10,000	–$15,000	Current Liabilities		
			Current maturities of long-term debt	$40,000	$40,000
Net Income	$355,000	$285,000	Accounts payable	25,000	30,000
			Total Current Liabilities	65,000	70,000

(continues)

Revenue	For the December 31, 2021	Year Ending December 31, 2022	Assets	For the December 31, 2021	Year Ending December 31, 2022
			Long-Term Debt	477,000	339,000
			Less Current maturities long-term debt	−40,000	−40,000
			Net Long-Term Debt	$437,000	$299,000
			Total Liabilities	$502,000	$369,000
			Net Worth	$1,100,000	$1,385,000
			Total Liabilities and Net Worth	$1,602,000	$1,754,000

Profitability	**Dec. 31, 2021**	**Dec. 31, 2022**
Operating Margin	_____	_____
Total Margin	_____	_____
ROA	_____	_____
ROE	_____	_____
Liquidity		
Current Ratio	_____	_____
Days Cash on Hand	_____	_____
Days in Accounts Receivable	_____	_____
Capital Structure		
Times Interest Earned	_____	_____
Debt Service Coverage	_____	_____
Equity Financing	_____	_____
Turnover		
Total Asset Turnover	_____	_____
Current Asset Turnover	_____	_____
Fixed Asset Turnover	_____	_____

2. The following table provides the income statement and balance sheet for Simpson Community Hospital (amounts in 000s). Complete the ratio worksheet. Explain the change in the ratios that increased or decreased 10% or more from the prior year.

Revenue	For the December 31, 2021	Year Ending December 31, 2022	Assets	For the December 31, 2021	Year Ending December 31, 2022
Net Patient Service Revenue	$95,000	$98,000	Current Assets		
Total Operating Revenue	$95,000	$98,000	Cash and cash equivalents	$5,000	$6,000
			Accounts receivable (net)	18,000	18,500
Operating Expenses			Inventories	12,000	13,000
Salaries and wages	$56,000	$57,900	Prepaid Insurance	2,000	2,100
Fringe benefits	12,000	12,900	Total Current Assets	$37,000	$39,600
Supplies	10,000	10,500	Property, Plant, & Equipment		
Depreciation	5,000	5,100	Equipment (net)	$20,000	$21,000
Interest	2,000	1,900	Buildings (net)	40,000	41,000
Other	6,000	6,300	Land	5,000	5,000
Total Operating Expenses	$91,000	$94,600	Net Property, Plant, & Equip	$65,000	$67,000
			Investments	$4,000	$3,500
Income from Operations	$4,000	$3,400	Total Assets	$106,000	$110,100
Nonoperating Gains (Losses)			**Liabilities**		
Investment Income	$500	$700	Current Liabilities		
Net Nonoperating Gains	$500	$700	Current maturities of LT Debt	$3,000	$3,100
			Accounts payable	5,500	5,300

(continues)

Revenue	For the December 31, 2021	Year Ending December 31, 2022	Assets	For the December 31, 2021	Year Ending December 31, 2022
Net Income	$4,500	$4,100	Total Current Liabilities	$8,500	$8,400
			Long-Term Debt	$50,000	$51,000
			Less Current maturities of long-term debt	−3,000	−3,100
			Net Long-Term Debt	$47,000	$47,900
			Total Liabilities	$55,500	$56,300
			Net Worth	$50,500	$53,800

Profitability			Dec. 31, 2021	Dec. 31, 2022
Operating Margin			_____	_____
Total Margin			_____	_____
ROA			_____	_____
ROE			_____	_____
Liquidity				
Current Ratio			_____	_____
Days Cash on Hand			_____	_____
Days in Accounts Receivable			_____	_____
Capital Structure				
Times Interest Earned			_____	_____
Debt Service Coverage			_____	_____
Equity Financing			_____	_____
Turnover				
Total Asset Turnover			_____	_____
Current Asset Turnover			_____	_____
Fixed Asset Turnover			_____	_____

Notes

1. Optum360°, *2017 Almanac of Hospital Financial and Operating Indicators* (Salt Lake City, UT: Author, 2016).

2. T. K. Ross, *A Comprehensive Guide to Budgeting for Health Care Managers* (Boston: Jones and Bartlett Learning, 2018).

CHAPTER 13

Common Sizing, Trend Analysis, Compound Growth Rates, and Counts Versus Rates

PROGRESS NOTES

After completing this chapter, you should be able to:

1. Describe the role of and use common sizing.
2. Describe the role of and use trend analysis.
3. Calculate and interpret compound growth rates.
4. Explain the difference between counts and rates.
5. Calculate and interpret rates.

Overview: Common Sizing, Trends, Growth Rates, Counts, and Rates

We are constantly warned against comparing apples to oranges, but this advice does not consider that more than 7,000 varieties of apples exist. An apples-to-apples comparison may also be misleading. Life seldom provides a perfect standard to assess performance. Comparing the financial performance of different healthcare providers is complicated due to problems of size, time, location, specialty, goals, and so on. Managers seeking to assess whether their revenues or expenses are appropriate must know how to compare their performance across time and to other organizations to determine when improvement is desirable.

Healthcare managers are often challenged by an absence of information and less-than-perfect reference groups. Even when data for similar organizations can be collected, the time needed to collect data, organize it, and distribute the complied information may be years, so managers are faced with comparing current performance against historical information. In healthcare, differences in location (patient mix, cost of inputs, number of competitors), size (ability to spread fixed costs), and specialty (cost of treatment) can dramatically increase or decrease revenue and expenses for seemingly similar organizations. Building expertise in **common sizing, trend analysis**, calculating **compound growth rates**, and comparing counts and **rates** will allow you to better understand and obtain greater value from the information you receive.

Common Sizing

The process of common sizing puts information on the same relative basis. Generally, common sizing involves converting dollar amounts to percentages. If, for example, total revenue of $200,000 equals 100%, then radiology revenue of $20,000 equals 10% of total revenue. Converting dollars to percentages allows comparative analysis. In other words, comparing the percentages allows a common basis of comparison. Common sizing is sometimes called "**vertical analysis**" because as you will see the computation of the percentages is vertical.

Although such comparisons on the basis of percentages can—and should—be performed on your own organization's data, comparisons can

also be made between or among various organizations. For example, **Table 13.1** shows how common sizing allows a comparison of liabilities for three different hospitals. In each case, the total liabilities equal 100%. Then the current liabilities of hospital 1, for example, are divided by total liabilities to find the proportionate percentage attributable to that line item, $100,000 ÷ $500,000 = 20%, and the long-term liabilities are 80%, $400,000 ÷ $500,000 = 80%. When all the percentages have been computed, add them to make sure they add to 100%. In this case, the sum of current and long-term liabilities equals 100%. If you use a computer, computation of these percentages is available as a spreadsheet function.

Table 13.1 shows the use of liabilities across hospitals. Current liabilities comprise between 12% and 25% of total liabilities, and the average is 20%. **Table 13.2** allows us to assess the use of liabilities across hospitals; for example, long-term debt varies from 75% to 88% of total liabilities, and dividing the difference between the minimum and maximum by the average shows that the variation is only 16.3%.

On the other hand, the use of current liabilities varies dramatically. Current liabilities in hospital 3 are only 12% of total liabilities versus 25% of

Table 13.1 Common Sizing Liabilities Across Hospitals

	Same Year for All Three Hospitals							
	Hospital 1		**Hospital 2**		**Hospital 3**		**Average**	
Current liabilities	$100,000	20%	$500,000	25%	$150,000	12%	$250,000	20%
Long-term debt	400,000	80%	1,500,000	75%	1,100,000	88%	$1,000,000	80%
Total liabilities	$500,000	100%	$2,000,000	100%	$1,250,000	100%	$1,250,000	100%

Table 13.2 Assessing Variance Across Hospitals

	Maximum	**Minimum**	**Range**	**Average**	**Range ÷ Average**
Current liabilities	25%	12%	13%	20%	65.0%
Long-term debt	88%	75%	13%	80%	16.3%

liabilities in hospital 2. Hospital 2 uses more than double the amount of current liabilities, which highlights how current liabilities vary significantly across institutions. Is hospital 3 forgoing the opportunity to use low-cost current liabilities to fund its assets and/or does hospital 2 have cash problems and cannot paid their debts as they are due?

Comparing general services expense across hospitals is more interesting, **Table 13.3**. Once again, the total expense for each hospital is 100%, and the relative percentage for each of the four line items is computed (i.e., hospital 1 dietary expense is 40% of total expense, $320,000 ÷ $800,000). The advantage of comparative analysis is illustrated by the "laundry" line item, where the dollar amounts are $80,000, $300,000, and $90,000 respectively. Yet each of these amounts is 10% of the total expense for the particular hospital, that is, laundry expense is consistent across institutions. The variation in maintenance is more interesting. In hospital 1, maintenance comprises 35% of total cost, whereas in hospital 3, it is only 15%. Is hospital 1 spending too much on maintenance, is hospital 3 spending too little, is spending by both inappropriate, or is spending appropriate in each hospital? Answering this question may require knowing how each hospital categorizes its expenses. For example, are housekeeping duties performed by maintenance in hospital 1, thus accounting for the apparent higher cost?

Table 13.4 allows easy identification of large variances, again pointing out the large differences in maintenance and housekeeping costs between hospitals.

Common sizing is designed to highlight differences in operations (i.e., is an organization spending more to deliver services than other organizations?). Are large differences opportunities for improvement by reducing expenses in areas with high spending and/or increasing expenses in areas with low spending?

Trend Analysis

A vexing question for managers is how fast their expenses should grow from year to year. Expenses should keep pace with inflation (e.g., pharmacy

Table 13.3 Common Sizing Expense Information

General services expense	Hospital 1		Hospital 2		Hospital 3		Average	
	$	%	$	%	$	%	$	%
Dietary	$320,000	40%	$1,260,000	42%	$450,000	50%	$676,667	43%
Maintenance	280,000	35%	990,000	33%	135,000	15%	$468,333	30%
Laundry	80,000	10%	300,000	10%	90,000	10%	$156,667	10%
Housekeeping	120,000	15%	450,000	15%	225,000	25%	$265,000	17%
Total general services expense	$800,000	100%	$3,000,000	100%	$900,000	100%	$1,566,667	100%

Table 13.4 Assessing the Variance in Expenses

General services expense	Maximum	Minimum	Range	Average	Range ÷ Average
Dietary	50%	40%	10%	43.2%	23.2%
Maintenance	35%	15%	20%	29.9%	66.9%
Laundry	10%	10%	0%	10.0%	0.0%
Housekeeping	25%	15%	10%	16.9%	59.1%

expense should increase by 5% when pharmaceutical prices increase 5% to purchase the same amount of drugs). Historically, healthcare input prices have increased faster than general inflation and total expenses also have increased with the volume of patients treated and the severity of their condition. The process of trend analysis compares figures over several time periods. Again, dollar amounts are converted to percentages to obtain a relative basis for purposes of comparison, but now the comparison is across time. If, for example, radiology revenue was $20,000 this period but was only $15,000 for the previous period, the difference between the two is $5,000. The difference of $5,000 is a 33.3% increase because the growth is computed on the earlier of the two years: that is, the base year, $5,000 ÷ $15,000 = 33.3%. Trend analysis is sometimes called "**horizontal analysis**" because the computation of the percentage of difference is horizontal.

An example of horizontal analysis is shown in **Table 13.5**. In this case, the liabilities of hospital

1 for year 1 are compared with its liabilities in year 2. Current liabilities were $60,000 in year 1 and $100,000 in year 2, a difference of $40,000. To arrive at a percentage of difference for comparative purposes, the $40,000 difference is divided by the year 1 base figure of $60,000 to compute the relative differential, $40,000 ÷ $60,000 = 66.7%.

Table 13.5 shows that hospital 1 has increased its liabilities since year 1; the increase is large in long-term liabilities, 17.6%, but the increase in current liabilities is more than three times larger, 66.7%. Financial managers may be choosing to rely on short-term, no-interest loans from vendors, or more ominously, the institution may be unable to secure long-term financing.

Another example of comparative analysis is given in **Table 13.6**. In this case, general service expenses for two years in hospital 1 are compared. The difference between year 1 and 2 for each line item is computed in dollars; then the dollar difference is divided by the year 1 base figure to

Table 13.5 Trend Analysis for Liabilities

	Year 1	% Total	Year 2	% Total	Year-to-Year $ Change	Year-to-Year % Change
Current liabilities	$60,000	15%	$100,000	20%	$40,000	66.7%
Long-term debt	340,000	85%	400,000	80%	60,000	17.6%
Total liabilities	$400,000	100%	$500,000	100%	$100,000	25.0%

Table 13.6 Trend Analysis for Expenses

General services expense	Year 1	% Total	Year 2	% Total	Year-to-Year $ Change	Year-to-Year % Change
Dietary	$290,000	39%	$320,000	40%	$30,000	10.3%
Maintenance	270,000	36%	$280,000	35%	10,000	3.7%
Laundry	76,000	10%	$80,000	10%	4,000	5.3%
Housekeeping	110,000	15%	$120,000	15%	10,000	9.1%
Total general service expense	$746,000	100%	$800,000	100%	$54,000	7.2%

obtain a percentage difference for purposes of comparison. Thus, housekeeping expense in year 1 was $110,000, and in year 2 it was $120,000, a difference of $10,000. The difference amounts to 9.1%, $10,000 ÷ $110,000. The total difference is $54,000 when added down, $30,000 dietary + $10,000 maintenance + $4,000 laundry + $10,000 housekeeping, and average expenses increased by 7.2% over the preceding year. The increase is also $54,000 when added across, $746,000 – $800,000.

The point of calculating year-to year changes is to identify the increase (or decrease) and determine whether it is reasonable and any corrective action is necessary. In this case, dietary and housekeeping should be examined to determine why their expenses increased by 42.9%, 10.3% ÷ 7.1%, and 25.6%, 9.1% ÷ 7.1%, more than the overall increase in general services.

Compound Growth Rates

Financial ratios and operating indicators pointed out the potential pitfalls of drawing conclusions and instituting action based on total expense; one of the largest avoidable financial costs for healthcare providers arises from error. Treatment error often results in lost reimbursement and/or higher expenses. Trend analysis examined the year-to-year change in expenses, but decision-making and action require understanding multiyear changes. Unforeseeable and infrequent events can dramatically increase and decrease volume, revenue, and expenses from one year to the next, so understanding long-run trends often requires calculating multiyear growth rates. **Table 13.7** provides an example of lost reimbursement from readmissions from 2010 through 2021. The problem is Medicare does not pay for unplanned readmissions for the same condition within 30 days of a prior admission and reduces reimbursement to providers with high readmission rates.

Figure 13.1 shows that lost reimbursement has steadily increased over the 12 years, but total dollars lost provides a partial picture of performance.

Focusing on total lost reimbursement, number of readmissions, and lost reimbursement per readmit, one could conclude that readmissions is a growing financial problem. Total lost

Table 13.7 Lost Reimbursement from Unplanned Readmissions

Year	Lost Reimbursement	Readmits	Lost Reimbursement per Readmit
2010	$7,375,000	1,229	$6,001
2011	7,404,000	1,210	6,119
2012	7,747,000	1,241	6,243
2013	7,844,000	1,232	6,367
2014	8,053,000	1,240	6,494
2015	8,314,000	1,255	6,625
2016	8,548,000	1,265	6,757
2017	8,753,000	1,270	6,892
2018	8,900,000	1,266	7,030
2019	9,257,000	1,291	7,170
2020	9,479,000	1,296	7,314
2021	9,765,000	1,309	7,460

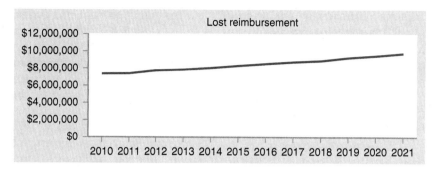

Figure 13.1 Lost Reimbursement from Unplanned Readmissions

reimbursement has grown by $2,390,000 and 34.2% since 2010. Calculating compound growth rates is another way to view the data. The equation to calculate a compound growth rate is:

$$r = (\text{current year} \div \text{base year})^{(1/n)} - 1$$

where n = the number of years between the base and current year

$$r = (\$9,765,000 \div \$7,375,000)^{(1/11)} - 1 = 2.6\%$$

A 2.6% annual increase in lost reimbursement is concerning, but calculating the compound growth rate for readmits and lost reimbursement per readmit provides more insight. The compound growth rate for readmits is 0.6% and 2.0% for lost reimbursement per readmit. The number of readmits has increased by 0.6% per year, but the majority of the loss is due to the higher loss per case (i.e., higher reimbursement per case). Managers should collect data on national readmissions rates before concluding whether the 0.6% annual increase is a major problem, are national readmissions increasing by more or less than 0.6%? Managers should also examine whether the higher loss per case is due to general reimbursement increases over time to account for inflation and/or an increase in readmissions in more complex, higher-reimbursement cases.

Analyzing Operating Data

Comparative analysis is an important tool for managers, and it is worth investing the time to become familiar with both horizontal and vertical analysis. Managers will generally analyze their own organization's data rather than comparing their data against other organizations'. With that fact in mind, we examine 2022 financial performance for the Semmelweis Clinic incorporating common sizing and trend analysis.

Table 13.8 sets out two revenue sources, 13 expenses, and one nonoperating revenue. This is the same as the income statement provided in Chapter 11 with greater detail. Operating revenue in Chapter 11 was rolled up into one line. Table 13.8 divides revenue into physician and therapy services. Likewise, salaries are divided into physician, RN, therapy, and other salaries. Common sizing (vertical analysis) has been performed for the 2021 (prior year) and 2022 (current year), and the percentage results appear in columns 3 and 5. Common sizing shows that physician services account for the largest percent of revenue and physician salaries comprise the largest percent of total expense. Total salaries account for 66.9% of total expenses.

The difference in dollars, labeled "$ Change," appears in column 6 of the analysis. Trend analysis (horizontal analysis) has been performed on each line item, and those percentage items appear in the last column. Trend analysis shows that therapy revenues grew much faster than physician service revenue. Looking ahead toward budgeting, will this rate of increase continue? Medical supplies expense grew at the fastest rate, 19.0%, between 2021 and 2022. The manager should explore whether the growth was appropriate and whether it will continue. The other notable

Table 13.8 Vertical and Horizontal Analysis of 2022 Semmelweis Clinic Operations

Account	December 31, 2021	% Total	December 31, 2022	% Total	$ Change	% Change
Physician services revenues	$1,300,000	70.3%	$1,350,000	69.2%	$50,000	3.8%
Therapy revenue	550,000	29.7%	$600,000	30.8%	50,000	9.1%
Total Operating Revenue	$1,850,000	100.0%	$1,950,000	100.0%	$100,000	5.4%
Physician salaries	$495,000	27.5%	$510,000	27.1%	$15,000	3.0%
RN salaries	283,000	15.7%	$299,520	15.9%	16,520	5.8%
Therapy salaries	208,000	11.6%	$220,000	11.7%	12,000	5.8%
Staff salaries	229,000	12.7%	$232,480	12.3%	3,480	1.5%
Health insurance	116,800	6.5%	$128,000	6.8%	11,200	9.6%
Social security	92,948	5.2%	$96,543	5.1%	3,596	3.9%
Retirement	125,103	7.0%	$125,837	6.7%	735	0.6%
Unemployment	12,150	0.7%	$12,620	0.7%	470	3.9%
Medical supplies	105,000	5.8%	$125,000	6.6%	20,000	19.0%
Office supplies	45,000	2.5%	$50,000	2.7%	5,000	11.1%
Housekeeping supplies	24,000	1.3%	$25,000	1.3%	1,000	4.2%
Depreciation	40,000	2.2%	$40,000	2.1%	.0	0.0%
Interest	24,000	1.3%	$20,000	1.1%	-4,000	-16.7%
Total Operating Expenses	$1,800,000	100.0%	$1,885,000	100.0%	$85,000	4.7%
Interest Income	$2,000	100.0%	$5,000	100.0%	$3,000	150.0%

increase is health insurance, 9.6%, driven by the national (and uncontrollable) trend toward higher health insurance premiums.

Common sizing is designed to focus managers' attention on the largest revenue and expense categories. Likewise, trend analysis is designed to highlight expenses that are increasing faster than inflation or the average for overall expenses. Devoting control efforts on areas to the highest growth rates should yield the greatest benefit to an organization. Comparative analysis is important to managers because it creates a common ground to make judgments for planning, organizing, controlling, and evaluating performance. Comparing the growth rate in expenses should be used extensively when creating a budget, and calculating the difference between actual and budgeted expenses is a primary financial duty of managers and is covered in Chapters 14 and 15.

Counts and Rates

Calculating compound growth rates improved our understanding of lost reimbursement, but calculating rates is another way to view operations.

Data is often reported as the count of events but counts fail to consider the frequency of the event. Rates highlight the number of events (the numerator) relative to potential events (the denominator) (e.g., the number of readmissions relative to total admissions, **Table 13.9**).

Table 13.9 shows that readmissions have increased since 2010, but this conclusion distorts, rather than illuminates, performance. Admissions are increasing 1.1% annually, so, all other things constant, readmissions should increase by a similar amount (i.e., performance is unchanged). Calculating the rate of readmission, readmits ÷ total admissions, shows that the hospital has reduced the rate of readmissions from 6.19% to 5.86% or by 5.3% between 2010 and 2021. A focus on counts, 1,229 in 2010 and 1,309 in 2021, on the other hand, may lead to the conclusion that performance is falling when it is in fact improving.

Figure 13.2 visually demonstrates that the rate of readmissions has fallen while the number of readmissions has increased. Given the variables at play with financial information, it is imperative that managers understand how to assess performance to draw accurate conclusions and initiate effective action when needed.

Table 13.9 Readmissions, Total Admissions, and Readmission Rate

Year	Readmits	Admissions	Rate
2010	1,229	19,856	6.19%
2011	1,210	20,051	6.03%
2012	1,241	20,255	6.13%
2013	1,232	20,610	5.98%
2014	1,240	20,816	5.96%
2015	1,255	21,025	5.97%
2016	1,265	21,359	5.92%
2017	1,270	21,447	5.92%
2018	1,266	21,662	5.84%
2019	1,291	21,843	5.91%
2020	1,296	22,097	5.87%
2021	1,309	22,340	5.86%

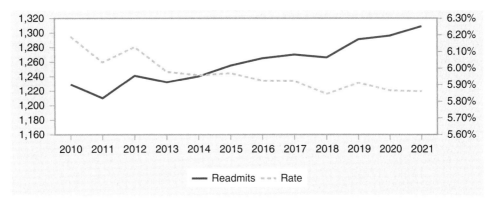

Figure 13.2 Readmits and the Readmission Rate

WRAP-UP

Summary

Hospitals, physician practices, and other healthcare providers vary greatly in size, so obtaining dollar figures to assess expenses is problematic. Common sizing or vertical analysis allows a manager to assess the relative percentage of expenses spent on resources rather than absolute dollars, which should vary with the size of an organization.

In addition to the amount and percent of revenues or expenses spent on resources, a second issue is how rapidly expenses are increasing from year to year. Trend analysis or horizontal analysis allows a manager to assess the dollar and percent growth to identify departments, revenues, and/or expenses that are growing or shrinking relative to the overall organization and assess the appropriateness of the year-to-year changes.

Common sizing and trend analysis provide good information, but managers will gain additional insight by calculating compound growth rates and comparing counts to rates to identify longer-term trends and relationships between variables. Compound growth rates allow managers to calculate multiyear growth rates as unforeseeable events often increase or decrease volume, revenues, and expenses to magnify year-to-year changes and obscure longer trends. Rates allow managers to determine if performance is improving, stable, or deteriorating when the count of events *and* the number of potential events are changing. Managers need the ability to critically assess data to deal with the complexities and challenges of health care.

Key Terms

Common Sizing or Vertical
   Analysis

Compound Growth Rates
   Rates

Trend Analysis or
   Horizontal Analysis

Discussion Questions

1. Explain the purpose of common sizing.
2. Explain the purpose of trend analysis.
3. Explain the difference between simple and compound growth rates.

4. Explain why interpretation of data should consider the number and rate of events.

Problems

1. When considering assets versus liabilities, which hospital has the highest percent of debt (i.e., is the most highly leveraged)?

	Hospital 1	Hospital 2	Hospital 3	Average
Total assets	$1,000,000	$5,000,000	$1,500,000	$7,500,000
Total liabilities	$500,000	$2,000,000	$500,000	$3,000,000
Net worth	$500,000	$3,000,000	$1,000,000	$4,500,000

2. Using the following table, assess the four expenses across four nursing departments. Which departments spend the most on salary and wages _and_ equipment depreciation?

Nursing Expenses	Medical	Surgical	OB	ICU
Salary and wages	$1,000,000	$1,100,000	$600,000	$1,500,000
Supplies	100,000	150,000	75,000	200,000
Equipment depreciation	100,000	200,000	50,000	350,000
Other	200,000	150,000	80,000	200,000
Total expense	$1,400,000	$1,600,000	$805,000	$2,250,000

3. Using the following table, calculate the dollar and percent increase in each expense line on 4 North, a medical unit. What was the average increase in expenses? Which expenses had the highest and lowest year-to-year increase?

4 North Expenses	2021	2022
Salary and wages	$950,000	$1,000,000
Supplies	85,000	100,000
Equipment depreciation	105,000	100,000
Other	195,000	200,000
Total expense	$1,335,000	$1,400,000

4. Using the following table, calculate the compound growth rate for the number of outpatient surgeries, revenue, and overtime expense. Is revenue growing faster than the number of surgeries? Is the use of overtime increasing?

Year	Outpatient Surgeries	Revenue	Overtime
2010	8,556	$3,420,000	$101,000
2011	8,786	3,650,000	111,000
2012	8,921	3,870,000	118,000
2013	9,042	4,190,000	133,000
2014	9,563	4,300,000	141,000
2015	10,126	4,930,000	156,000
2016	10,871	5,230,000	176,000
2017	11,673	5,870,000	185,000
2018	12,899	6,450,000	197,000
2019	13,786	7,010,000	215,000
2020	14,685	7,750,000	246,000
2021	15,447	8,340,000	265,000
2022	15,818	8,500,000	288,000

5. Using the following table, perform a horizontal and vertical analysis of the operations of the Gumbel Family Practice. What is the largest expense, and which expense increased the most from the prior year?

Account	December 31, 2021	December 31, 2022
Revenue		
Physician services	$1,400,000	$1,450,000
Expense		
Admin salaries	$200,000	$210,000
Staff salaries	700,000	735,000
Overtime	50,000	55,000
Fringe benefits	180,000	190,000
Medical supplies	75,000	85,000
Office supplies	10,000	15,000
Depreciation	105,000	100,000
Other	15,000	10,000
Total Expenses	$1,335,000	$1,400,000

6. The following table was obtained from Quality Management and contains the number of surgeries and surgical site infections and births and infant deaths. Calculate the infant mortality rate (IMR). Is the IMR increasing, stable, or decreasing?

Year	Surgeries	Infections	Births	Deaths
2010	8,556	171	3,002	18
2011	8,786	178	2,970	18
2012	8,921	174	2,945	17
2013	9,042	181	2,910	17
2014	9,563	193	2,881	18
2015	10,126	201	2,852	17
2016	10,871	216	2,823	16
2017	11,673	231	2,795	16
2018	12,899	246	2,767	17
2019	13,786	259	2,739	17
2020	14,685	281	2,711	16
2021	15,447	299	2,683	18
2022	15,818	305	2,679	16

PART V

Constructing and Evaluating Budgets

CHAPTER 14

Constructing an Operating Budget

PROGRESS NOTES

After completing this chapter, you should be able to:

1. Explain the goals of budgeting.
2. Describe the steps required to build a budget.
3. Describe the role of forecasting in the budget process.
4. Build an incremental operating budget.
5. Build and restate a flexible budget.

Overview: Operating Budgets

Operating budgets define the goals of the organization and the expected total revenue, expenses, and net income to be earned. The operating budget for a department defines what it should contribute to reach organizational goals and the resources managers will be given to complete the work. Ideally, the budget should provide no more and no fewer resources than are required to produce the projected volume of goods or services at the expected level of quality.

The **master budget** is the compilation of all departments' operating budgets assembled by the finance department to determine whether the organization has sufficient resources to complete the plan. A healthcare provider's mission, values, and objectives should define the patients it will serve and the services it will provide. A department's operating budget will be based on the organization's goals and define the expected activities to be performed, how activities will be completed, and the amount of output it will produce. Budgets are the operating plans of departments and organizations expressed in monetary terms.

Objectives for the Budgeting Process

The American Hospital Association (AHA) provides four primary objectives for the budgeting process:

1. To provide a written expression, in quantitative terms, of a hospital's policies and plans.
2. To provide a basis for the evaluation of financial performance in accordance with a hospital's policies and plans.

3. To provide a useful tool for the control of costs.
4. To create cost awareness throughout the organization.[1]

Operating budgets attempt to quantify the amount of money needed to complete activities in the future. Managers should understand how to construct and use budgets as failure to complete tasks within the budget may have a detrimental impact on patients, the organization, and the manager's career. The adopted budget should provide clear output and financial targets, provide regular feedback on whether goals are being realized, and highlight areas for improvement when goals are not met. The budget should make every employee aware of organizational plans and their role in reaching goals and increase their commitment to making necessary adjustments when goals are not met.

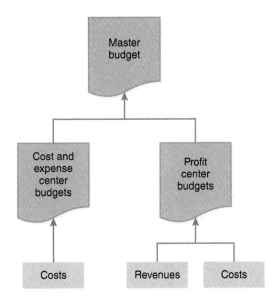

Figure 14.1 Three Common Budget Responsibility Centers

Operating Budgets Versus Capital Expenditure Budgets

Operating budgets generally deal with short-term revenues and the expenses necessary to operate an organization. Operating budgets usually cover the next year, a 12-month period, where expenditures for labor and supplies can be quickly adjusted (i.e., staffing and inventory decisions can often be made on a daily basis). **Capital expenditure budgets** are used to analyze the desirability of acquiring high-cost assets that provide service over multiple years. Multimillion-dollar expenditures for equipment and buildings regularly last five or more years. High-dollar expenditures are not routine decisions, cannot be quickly modified, and, given their impact on an organization, are handled separately from operating expenses. Chapter 19 reviews capital expenditure budgets.

Budget Viewpoints

Responsibility Centers

In a responsibility center, the manager has the authority over and is accountable for a particular set of activities and outcomes. In the context of operating budgets, there are three common types of responsibility centers: cost, expense, and profit centers. As shown in **Figure 14.1**, managers in cost and expense centers are responsible for controlling costs. Managers in profit centers are responsible for costs and revenues. Thus, we expect that operating budgets for cost and expense centers will have only costs, while a profit center budget should contain revenues and costs.

Budget Basics: A Review

Direct Versus Allocated Budget Costs

In a small organization like a physician practice, all costs are direct costs, and the budget preparer must account for all costs in their budget. That is, the budget preparer must estimate the expense for all resources expected to be used. In a large organization like a hospital, the managers of the emergency department, nursing units, and ancillary services must prepare a budget for the resources they control. Expenses that will be allocated generally are not budgeted, that is, the expenses incurred in other areas such as patient accounting, housekeeping, and security are not part of patient care departments' budgets. Finance compiles all department budgets, patient care and support areas, into the master budget that reports total planned expenses and revenues for the organization. The purpose of the master budget is to ensure the budget is workable (i.e., the organization will have sufficient resources to complete the plan and continue operating if the plan is followed). When expenses exceed revenue and threaten the goals or existence of the organization, the department budgets will be returned to department managers to increase revenue and/or reduce expenses until a financially feasible budget is established. Your role as a budget preparer is to estimate the expenses needed in a future fiscal period and the amount of revenues your department will generate when you manage a profit center.

Fixed Versus Variable Costs

The resources you control can be categorized as fixed or variable. You will recall that fixed costs do not change in total when workload increases or decreases. Variable costs, however, rise or fall in proportion to a rise or fall in output. In healthcare organizations, output or volume generally means the number of patient days (inpatient services), number of procedures (outpatient services), or prescriptions filled (pharmacy services). **Figure 14.2** illustrates the difference between fixed and variable costs. The distinction between them is a critical component to the construction of budgets.

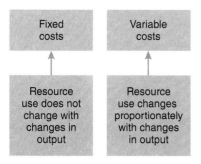

Figure 14.2 Fixed Versus Variable Costs

Building an Operating Budget: Preparation

Preparation is the first step in building an operating budget. It is often difficult for managers to allow adequate time for budget preparation because this effort is in addition to their daily responsibilities. Understanding the steps in preparing a budget assists in predicting how much time will be required.

Construction Stages

Operating budget construction stages include the following:

- Planning
- Gathering information
- Preparing input
- Constructing and submitting a preliminary budget
- Making required revisions to preliminary budget
- Submitting final budget

Input includes both assumptions and calculations; required revisions to the draft version would occur after upper-level management has reviewed the draft. Additional revisions will typically be required after the preliminary budget has been presented. The preliminary budget almost never becomes the final version without some revision.

Construction Elements

What will your budget look like? Will it follow guidelines from last year, or will it take on a new form? What will be expected of you, the manager? Understanding the budget construction elements will help you create a budget that is a useful tool.

As part of the preparation process, you should determine the following:

- Format to be used
- Budget scope
- Available resources
- Levels of review
- Time frame

As to format, will templates be available for use? If so, will they be required? As to budget scope, will your budget be an input to a larger budget to be combined and consolidated with other areas at a later stage (e.g., the human resource budget may be composed of the VP office plus the recruitment, training and development, and compensation review budgets)? If this is so, you may lose some of your line items as you do not control the final budget. Necessary resources made available to you could include, for example, special data processing runs or extra staff assistance to locate required information. The levels of review, along with how many revisions of the budget will be required, depend upon the structure and expectations of the particular healthcare organization. Many organizations start the budget process six months before the start of the budget year to ensure adequate time for creation, revision, and approval of budgets.

Budget Information Sources

Three primary sources of operating budget information are illustrated in **Figure 14.3**. They include the operating revenue forecast and the staffing plan or forecast along with actual or budgeted operating expenses. As Figure 14.1 illustrated earlier in this chapter, the manager who is responsible for both costs and revenues would require the revenue forecast. If, however, the manager is responsible only for costs, the revenue forecast would not be part of his or her responsibility.

When the preliminary operating budget is under construction, the capacity-level checkpoints should also be taken into consideration. This step may be undertaken at a different level and thus may not be your own responsibility.

Budget Assumptions and Computations

Building a budget means making a series of assumptions and choices. The budget process should begin with a review of strategy and objectives. The first choice is where the data come from. That is, when forecasting revenues, salaries, and other expenses, what is the starting point? Typically, the data come from current year actual revenues and expenses. In some cases, managers may elect to use current year budgeted revenues and expenses or the last full year of data. In this chapter, we will use current year actual revenues and expenses.

The challenge when using current year actual revenues and expenses is the budget process begins prior to the completion of the current year so managers will not know what total revenues and expenses will be for the entire year. Managers thus need to know how to annualize partial-year

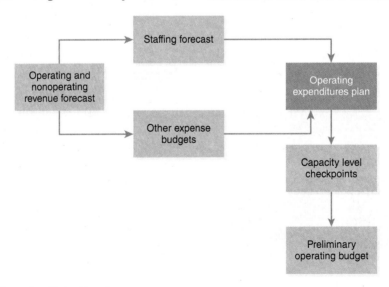

Figure 14.3 Operating Budget Inputs

expenses. **Table 14.1** reports the actual expenses for the first six months of 2023 for the Semmelweis Clinic that employs three physicians and 13 other employees. The actual year-to-date (YTD) expenses are converted to a 12-month basis, or annualized, as shown in the fourth column of Table 14.1.

These computations were performed on a computer spreadsheet; however, the calculation is as follows. Using physician salaries as an example, $262,500 was spent during the first six months, or an average of $43,750 is spent per month. To obtain an estimate for the entire year, $43,750 is multiplied by 12 months (i.e., $43,750 × 12 = $525,000). A second means to annualize expenses multiplies YTD amounts by 12 divided by the number of YTD months—in this case, $262,500 × (12 ÷ 6). Both methods produce the same estimate. This method is used in Table 14.1. The annualized 12-month figure

provides a starting point and comparison for the next year's budget. In the absence of major changes annualized 2023 year-to-date actual should be similar to 2022 actual revenues and expenses.

Basing budget estimates on annualized revenues and expenses assumes little or no change in volume. Given a growing, aging, and/or mobile population, healthcare providers should consider whether their patient loads will increase or decrease. Forecasting workload is a critical part of building a budget as providers expecting higher (lower) volume should expect higher (lower) revenues and expenses.

Forecasts

The goal of forecasting is to define the expected amount of work to be performed in the budget year as revenues and expenses should be related

Table 14.1 Annualizing Semmelweis Clinic's YTD Revenues and Expenses

Account	Actual December 31, 2022	YTD Budget June 30, 2023	YTD Actual June 30, 2023	Annual Factor	Annualized YTD Actual
Physician services revenues	$1,345,000	$693,000	$687,500	12/6	$1,375,000
Therapy revenue	$569,000	293,000	312,500	12/6	625,000
Total Operating Revenue	$1,914,000	$986,000	$1,000,000		$2,000,000
Physician salaries	$510,000	$263,000	$262,500	12/6	$525,000
RN salaries	292,000	150,000	156,500	12/6	313,000
Therapy salaries	214,000	110,000	115,000	12/6	230,000
Staff salaries	236,000	122,000	122,000	12/6	244,000
Health insurance	128,000	66,000	67,000	12/6	134,000
Social security	95,778	49,343	50,184	12/6	100,368
Retirement	62,600	32,250	32,800	12/6	65,600
Unemployment	12,520	6,450	6,500	12/6	13,000
Medical supplies	108,200	56,000	68,000	12/6	136,000
Office supplies	46,400	24,000	25,500	12/6	51,000
Housekeeping supplies	24,700	12,700	12,750	12/6	25,500
Depreciation	40,000	20,600	21,000	12/6	42,000
Interest	22,000	11,300	9,750	12/6	19,500
Total Operating Expenses	$1,792,198	$923,643	$949,484		$1,898,968

to the amount of work performed. It is pretty simple today to create "what if" scenarios on the computer, but the important thing for managers to remember is that assumptions directly affect the results of forecasts.

Forecasts are based on assumptions that are expected to exist and actions that are expected to occur. Operating budget forecasts are relatively short term and should be based on realistic assumptions that we expect to exist along with actions that we can reasonably expect to occur.

Forecasting Approaches

The approach to producing a forecast usually involves three different sources of information and forecast assumptions:

- The first level derives from the personnel who are directly involved in the department or unit. They know the operation and can provide important ground-level detail such as use of department services and prices of inputs.
- The second level comes from statistical information, including trend analysis. Databases can provide information on patient volume (admissions and visits) by service and payer, use of services and expenses, and reimbursement and nonoperating revenues, and there is a skill to selecting relevant information for forecasting purposes.
- The third level represents executive-level judgment that is typically applied to a preliminary rough draft of the forecast. For example, adjusting volume upward or downward due to the anticipated future impact of local competition would most likely be an executive-level judgment.

The amount and type of information that is readily available greatly affects the forecast difficulty. Templates and standardized worksheets may also greatly influence the final forecast results.

Common Types of Forecasts in Healthcare Organizations

The three most common types of forecasts found in most healthcare organizations include revenue forecasts, staffing forecasts, and operating expense forecasts. This section discusses all three forecasts.

Revenue Forecasts

A prime input into the operating budget is the revenue forecast as it often sets the upper limit on expenses (i.e., an organization's goals and planned expenses should be limited by its expected revenue). The revenue forecast thus estimates how much the organization will earn from patient services and nonoperating sources over the budget year. Longer-range multiyear forecasts are useful for executive decision-making regarding the future of the organization. **Figure 14.4** illustrates a multiyear forecast; in the real world, the revenue forecast would be the product of an output forecast and the prices expected for the services.

The graph shows low growth from 2020 through 2022 followed by higher expected growth in the upcoming budget years through 2027 as the practice adds services and patients. Revenue growth in 2028 is expected to slow as the practice reaches capacity and growth is limited to increases in reimbursement. A single-year forecast is generally for the coming year and is thus a short-range forecast. Reliable forecasts of revenue are a vital part of the organization's planning process and are an input into the operating budget. **Figure 14.5** illustrates a short-range forecast. Note that the graph in Figure 14.2 could report data by month instead of by quarter as shown.

The revenue forecast may assist managers in assembling their staffing and expense budgets. For example, revenues (and patient volume) are projected to be low in April and December, which could encourage managers to schedule vacations in those months and avoid scheduled time off in the high-demand months of March and November.

Revenue Forecast Assumptions
Utilization Assumptions

In health care, significant changes in utilization patterns can occur that need to be taken into account in the manager's forecast assumptions.

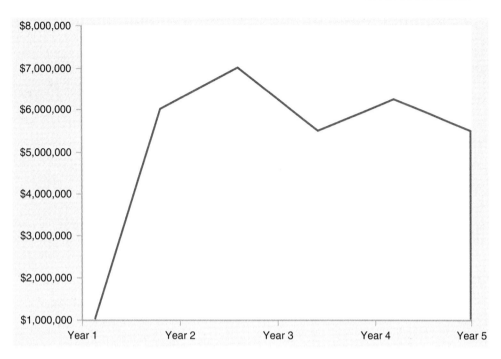

Figure 14.4 Five-Year Operating Revenue Forecast

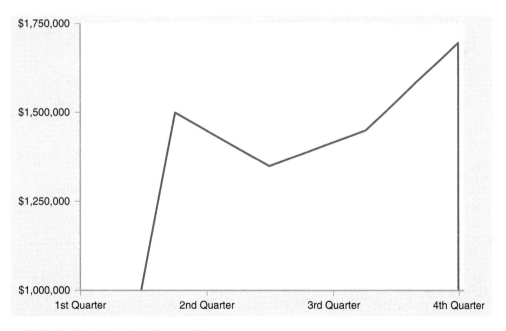

Figure 14.5 One-Year Operating Revenue Forecast

The inexorable shift to shorter lengths of stay for hospital inpatients over the past decade and the continuing growth in outpatient services are examples of basic shifts in utilization patterns.

Patient Mix Assumptions

It is also important to specify the anticipated patient mix for each service. Patient mix means the number or percent of patients whose services are paid by Medicare, Medicaid, private insurance, and self-pay. When payers are thus identified, this information allows the appropriate payments to be associated with the service utilization assumptions.

Contractual Allowance Assumptions

The forecasted utilization of a service (or its volume) is multiplied by reimbursement for each payer or charges for self-pay patients to arrive at total expected operating revenue. A word of warning, however: Revenue forecasted at "gross charges" is not a valid figure. Virtually all payers—Medicare, Medicaid, and private insurers—pay a stipulated amount for a particular service that is vastly lower than charges. Optum360° calculated that the average hospital receives 31 cents for every $1.00 billed.[2] The reimbursement each payer pays for the same service varies, so forecasters must calculate the contractual allowance and expected net revenue for each major payer. To calculate expected net revenue, the forecaster must identify the following:

- *Gross charge*: Amount for a service as shown on the claim form; a uniform charge generally greater than most expected payments received for the service.
- *Allowed charge*: Net amount that the particular payer's contract or participation agreement will recognize, or "allow," for a certain service.
- Multiply the expected number of services for each major payer by the allowed charge to obtain total expected revenue and add the totals for each payer.
- *Contractual allowance*: The difference between the gross charge and the allowed charge is recorded as a reduction of the gross charge within the accounting system.

It should also be noted that part of the payer's allowed charge is generally due from the patient as their deductible or copayment and the remaining portion of the allowed charge is due from the payer.

Trend Analysis Assumptions

One of the basic purposes of performing trend analysis is to compare data between or among years to determine how volume and reimbursement have changed over time. When trends are found (e.g., patient volume has grown by 1% per year), it makes sense to incorporate the trend into the forecast. If volume has averaged a 1% increase over the past five years, that should be the starting point, but managers should consider whether changes in population, the number of competitors, and/or the addition or subtraction of services should warrant a higher or lower rate of growth.

Labor and Expense Forecast Assumptions

Table 14.2 reports the expected number of paid hours by position at the Semmelweis Clinic in the unit. There may not be enough detail in this report to forecast labor requirements because it does not indicate, among other things, hours by type of staff and/or staff level. Sufficient information at the proper level of detail is essential in creating a budget.

Computations

Computations should be supported by their assumptions and should be replicable; that is, another individual should be able to reproduce your computations when using the same assumptions. Computations must also be comparable; that is, the same type of computation must be used by each unit or department. Thus, when the departmental budgets are combined, they will all be stated on the same basis.

An example of computations that must be comparable is contained in **Figure 14.6**. Recall the information provided in Chapter 9 on the

Table 14.2 Semmelweis Clinic Expected Paid Hours for Fiscal 2023

Position	FTE	Regular Hours	Overtime Hours	Total Hours
Physician	3	6,240	0	6,240
Register Nurse	4	8,320	520	8,840
Therapist	4	8,320	206	8,526
Support Staff	5	10,400	360	10,760
Total	16	33,280	1,086	34,366

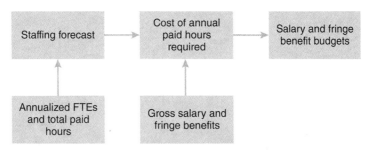

Figure 14.6 Calculating Salaries and Fringe Benefits in the Operating Budget

preparation of a staffing forecast, now an input to the operating budget. Costs must be attached to the staffing forecast for budget purposes. As shown in Figure 14.6, the forecast should first contain annual FTEs and total paid days required.

When cost is attached to the cost of annual paid days required, that cost should include gross salaries and fringe benefit costs (**Table 14.3**).

The fringe benefit expense equals the sum of annualized health insurance, Social Security, retirement, and unemployment insurance in Table 14.1. In multidepartment organizations, all departments must define fringe benefits in the same way to ensure the resulting master budget's staffing dollars will be computed on a comparable basis.

Finalize and Implement the Budget

The final budget must be approved by the practice owner or senior management and the

Table 14.3 Using Scheduled Hours, Wage Rates, and Fringe Benefits Rates to Calculate 2023 Annualized Salaries and Fringe Benefits

Position	Hourly Wage w/OT	Hourly Fringe Benefit	% FB to Wage		2023 Annualized Salary	2023 Annualized Fringe Benefits
Physician	$84.13	$15.50	18.4%		$525,000	$96,739
Register Nurse	$34.40	$8.62	26.6%		$313,000	$76,196
Therapist	$26.65	$7.61	29.3%		$230,000	$64,874
Support Staff	$22.30	$6.99	32.4%		$244,000	$75,159
Total	$37.58	$9.11	25.0%		$1,312,000	$312,968

board of directors in large organizations. Preliminary budgets may require multiple reviews and revisions before an acceptable final budget is reached. The final step is then to implement the new budget. It is important to explain the contents to all involved personnel. It may also be necessary to provide training for new report formats or similar issues.

Building an Operating Budget

Two types of budgets will be constructed: an **incremental budget** and a **flexible budget**. Incremental budgets are based on forecasted output, often last year's output adjusted for anticipated increases or decreases in volume. Incremental budgets do not change if actual budget year output differs from the forecast. Incremental budgets are easy to prepare and should be used when output is predictable. Flexible budgets create a preliminary budget based on forecasted output and are restated (or flexed) at the end of a budget period when actual output is known. The final flexible budget provides more resources to managers whose areas are providing more services (i.e., when departments serve more patients than expected their expenses should be higher) and reduces the budget in departments that produce lower output than forecasted.

Incremental Budgets

Incremental budgets should be used when managers expect little change between the current year and the budget year. In many cases, an incremental budget assumes the same volume of patients and the same production methods. The only change is an expected price increase for services provided and resources due to inflation.

An incremental (also known as a fixed or static) budget is based on a single level of output (e.g., a nursing unit is funded to deliver 5,475 patient days of care, an emergency department or physician practice for 15,000 visits, or a clinical lab for 1,000,000 tests). After an incremental budget has been approved and finalized, expenses are not adjusted. Managers' performance is measured by how far actual expenses differ from budget projections (e.g., are actual expenses less than, equal to, or greater than the budget?). The budget is an agreement between a manager and their superior that a specified amount of work will be produced with the budgeted resources. Producing the work while meeting the budget is expected, completing the work and spending less than budgeted is superior performance, and failing to complete the work and/or exceeding the budget is unsatisfactory.

The computation of a budget variance only requires one calculation:

$$\text{Actual Expenses} - \text{Budget Expense} = \text{Budget Variance}$$

The basic thing to understand is that incremental budgeted expense never changes even when actual volume differs from forecasted volume. We will use patient days as an example of volume or output. Assume the budget anticipated 5,475 patient days during the year, 75% occupancy for a 20-bed unit. Revenue and expenses were budgeted based on the expected 5,475 patient days. At the end of the year, the unit provided care for 6,205 patient days, 85% occupancy, but the budgeted revenues and expenses still reflect the original forecast of 5,475 patient days. Obviously, an increase of 730 patient days will require more resources and the department will overrun its expense budget for the year. On the positive side, the department's revenue should also increase with the higher-than-expected occupancy.

On the other hand, assume only 4,745 patient days are delivered, 65% occupancy, or 86.7% of forecasted output. An incremental budget will provide too many resources for the work provided. Given the reduction in patient days, hospital revenues may be 13.3% lower, and we should expect a comparable reduction in expenses.

Incremental budgets are used to plan what resources will be needed to produce the forecasted output and determine if the organization has sufficient money to purchase the resources. When utilized in this way, these budget figures represent a goal for the budget period. **Table 14.4** illustrates this concept. The table shows 100 procedures that were performed and the corresponding revenue and expenses. Column 3 documents the current expenses per procedure and column 4 the budget year assumptions. No change in procedures is expected, average reimbursement is expected to increase 2.6%, and expenses from 5.0% for supplies to 0.0% for depreciation. Based on these assumptions, net income is expected to be $3,500 in the budget period, a slight decline from the current year.

When expected net income is less than budgeted, Table 14.4 should be used to determine the cause (i.e., were procedures or net revenue per procedure lower than expected and/or were salary, supply, other, or depreciation expenses higher than expected?). Incremental budgets should be used when output can be predicted accurately. In cases where department output cannot be predicted, a flexible budget should be used that will increase budgets when more work is performed than expected and reduce budgets when less work is performed.

Flexible Budgets

A flexible budget creates a preliminary budget for revenues and expenses based on forecasted output and adjusts the final budget based on actual output at the end of the budget period. A flexible budget is restated or flexed to the actual level of output achieved during the budget period.[3] Flexible budgeting recognizes that producing an accurate output forecast is difficult and managers should not be expected to hold expenses to a budget that underestimated actual output and the resources needed to meet that output. Similarly, managers should not expect to receive the budgeted level of resources when actual output is less than forecasted.

Flexible budgets became important in health care when payment based on diagnosis-related groups (DRGs) was established in hospitals in the 1980s. Formerly Medicare reimbursed hospitals on the basis of cost rather than output for inpatient care. Medicare cost reimbursement assured hospitals that they would recoup their costs even if they overran the budget. Under DRG reimbursement, hospitals receive a flat fee for inpatient care, and managers must work to minimize expenses, if

Table 14.4 Incremental Budget: Establishing a Plan and a Goal

	Current Year	Current Per Procedure	Incremental Budget Assumptions	Budget Per Procedure	Incremental Budget
Procedures Performed	100		No Change, 100		100
Average Reimbursement	$195	$195	2.6% increase	$200	$200
Net Revenue Expenses	$19,500	$195.00		$200.00	$20,000
Salaries	$9,615	$96.15	4.0% increase	$100.00	$10,000
Supplies	3,810	$38.10	5.0% increase	40.00	4,000
Other	980	$9.80	2.0% increase	10.00	1,000
Depreciation	1,500	$15.00	No change	15.00	1,500
Total Expense	$15,905	$159.05		$165.00	$16,500
Net Income	$3,595	$35.95		$35.00	$3,500

not keep expenses under the fixed payment. Constructing a flexible budget requires more time and effort than building an incremental budget. An incremental budget projects expenses at a single level of output, whereas the restated flexible budget calculates what expenses should have been if output had been accurately forecasted.[4]

Flexible budgets can readily be used to review the prior performance of the unit, department, and organization. **Table 14.5** illustrates this concept. The table shows a forecasted volume of 100 and 110 actual procedures performed during the budget period, along with the per-procedure assumptions for revenues and variable expense plus the total fixed expenses that accompany these procedures.

Table 14.5 shows net income should increase by 14.3% if the budget assumptions hold. A 10% increase in volume and revenue should be accompanied by a 9.1% increase in total expenses as depreciation expense does not change. The flexible budget thus allows managers to evaluate performance. An increase in net income of more than 14.1% would indicate superior management of resources. On the other hand, an increase of less than 14.1% may indicate the need to review revenues and expenses to determine if improvements are needed.

Building an Incremental Budget

The examples in Tables 14.4 and 14.5 illustrate the essential differences in incremental and flexible budgets. In the real world, a budget preparer must work with more detail to build a budget. Most notably, the budget preparer will have to create a budget for each expense line item (e.g., salaries may be budgeted by job classification rather than total salaries). There are four major steps required to build an incremental (static) budget (**Box 14.1**).[5] First, determine an expenditure base; this is what was spent or budgeted in prior periods and should be used as the starting point for the following year's budget. Preparations for the following year's budget generally begin midway through the current operating year, thus creating three choices for the budget base: current YTD expenditures, the current full-year budget, or the last full-year expenditures.

Table 14.4 uses YTD actual as the starting point, and since only six months have been completed in the current year, revenues and expenses are annualized to determine what total spending for the year may be. **Annualization** requires multiplying YTD revenues and expenses by 12 months divided by the number of months reported. In this case, physician salaries for the

Table 14.5 Flexible Budget: Reviewing Performance

	Flexible Budget Assumptions	Preliminary Budget	Final, Restated Budget	% Change
# Procedures Performed	100 procedures	100	110	10.0%
Net Revenue	$200 per procedure	$20,000	$22,000	10.0%
Expenses				
Salaries	$100 per procedure	$10,000	$11,000	10.0%
Supplies	$40 per procedure	4,000	4,400	10.0%
Other	$10 per procedure	1,000	1,100	10.0%
Depreciation	$1,500 fixed cost	1,500	1,500	0.0%
Total Expense		$16,500	$18,000	9.1%
Net Income		$3,500	$4,000	14.3%

Box 14.1 **The Incremental Budgeting Process**

1. Identify the expenditure base.
2. Identify inflation factors and timing.
3. Multiply the expenditure base and the inflation factor and sum for all line items.
4. Modify for expected changes in output, production processes, and regulatory mandates.

year should be $525,000, $262,500 × (12 ÷ 6), if current spending levels continue.

The second step determines the appropriate rate to increase line item expenditures (i.e., how will hourly wages and the price of supplies and other expenses increase in the next year?). The prices of different resources used in the production process are unlikely to increase at the same rate. As you see in Table 14.4, salaries are expected to increase by 3%; the **inflation factor** is 1.03, 1.00 + 0.03. Medical supplies are expected to increase by 6%, office supplies by 2%, and so on.

The third step is the easiest: multiply the expenditure base (step 1) by the expected change in prices for each budget line (step 2). Annualized physician salaries for 2023 are $525,000, and if wages increase by 3%, $540,750, $525,000 × 1.03, should be budgeted for 2024. After multiplying each line item, the products are totaled for all budget lines (**Table 14.6**).

The third step produces a budget assuming only output and input prices have changed, while the

Table 14.6 Incremental Budget for Semmelweis Clinic

Account	YTD June 30, 2023	Annualized	Inflation Factor	2024 Budget
Physician services revenues	$687,500	$1,375,000	1.04	$1,430,000
Therapy revenue	312,500	625,000	1.04	650,000
Total Operating Revenue	$1,000,000	$2,000,000	1.04	$2,080,000
Physician salaries	$262,500	$525,000	1.03	$540,750
RN salaries	156,500	313,000	1.03	322,390
Therapy salaries	115,000	230,000	1.03	236,900
Staff salaries	122,000	244,000	1.03	251,320
Health insurance	67,000	134,000	1.10	147,400
Social security	50,500	101,000	1.03	104,030
Retirement	66,000	132,000	1.03	135,960
Unemployment	6,500	13,000	1.03	13,390
Medical supplies	68,000	136,000	1.06	144,160
Office supplies	25,500	51,000	1.02	52,020
Housekeeping supplies	12,750	25,500	1.02	26,010
Depreciation	21,000	42,000	1.00	42,000
Interest	9,750	19,500	1.00	19,500
Total Operating Expenses	$983,000	$1,966,000	1.036	$2,035,830
Interest Income	$2,750	$5,500	1.00	$5,500
Net Income	$19,750	$39,500	1.257	$49,670

fourth step recognizes that other factors may change: It will be extremely rare that an organization or department will do everything in the future exactly as it did in the past and outputs and inputs will simply cost more. Adjustments should be made for changes in the quantity or quality of output produced or changes in production processes or regulatory mandates that may affect expenses. The manager should review the budget before submission to ensure it will provide adequate resources to complete work; in other words, in the absence of major changes (step 4), the budget should be comparable to past revenues and expenses. The term *incremental* alludes to the fact that prior revenues and expenses are increased (incremented) each year for expected price increases.

Building a Flexible Budget

An incremental budget is appropriate when output is predictable from year to year; however, when output fluctuates and cannot be accurately predicted, an incremental budget may provide too many or too few resources for the actual output produced. A flexible budget avoids this problem by reestimating revenues and expenses based on actual output rather than forecasted output at the end of the budget period. Creating a flexible budget requires eight (or nine when restating the budget for actual output is included) steps beginning with forecasting budget year output (**Box 14.2**).[6]

Step 1 defines the output that will be produced and the expected number of individual services. The Semmelweis Clinic provides two major services— physician and therapy visits—and the practice manager expects a modest increase in both in 2024. The 2024 forecast calls for 15,606 physician visits and 9,600 therapy visits (**Table 14.7**). Step 2 defines how work will be completed, what resources are required, and whether more or fewer of the resources will be needed if output increases or decreases. Physician and staff salaries are a fixed cost and do not change with output. RN salaries are a variable cost based on total physician visits (V_{MD}), and therapist salaries are based on total therapy visits (V_{TH}). Medical and office supplies are based on total visits (V_{Total}).

Step 3 then identifies how much more of variable resources will be required for every one unit increase in output. For example, RN time

---

Box 14.2 The Flexible Budgeting Process

1. Define the output measure and estimate the budget year output.
2. Identify how work will be performed and what inputs will be required.
3. Develop productivity standards (input per output) for variable costs.
4. Translate productivity standards into cost standards (dollars per output).
5. Inflate cost standards for expected price increases to produce budget standards.
6. Multiply the budget standards by estimated output to obtain budget allocations.
7. Develop budget allocations for fixed costs (administrative salaries, health insurance, rent, etc.) using the incremental budgeting process (select an expenditure base, identify the inflation factor, and multiply the base by the inflation factor).
8. Modify for expected changes in output quality, production processes, regulatory mandates and so on to get a preliminary budget.
9. At the end of the fiscal period, recalculate variable costs by multiplying budget standards by actual output to get a final budget.

Data from Ross, T. K. (2018). *A comprehensive guide to budgeting for health care managers.* Jones and Bartlett Learning; Ross, T. K. (2021). *Practical budgeting for health care, a concise guide.* Jones and Bartlett Learning.

---

is determined by the number of physician visits delivered (i.e., how many minutes of RN time are needed to treat each patient and then multiplied by the hourly wage). Step 3 was not used in this example. Instead, a **cost standard** was developed, step 4, based on total RN salaries and total patient visits in the expenditure base. Total RN salaries were $156,000 for the first six months of 2023, and divided by 7,650 physician visits over the same time period, average RN salaries per physician visit is $20.46. Likewise, medical supplies were calculated to be $5.48 per visits, $68,000 ÷ 12,400 total visits.

Step 5 inflates the expenditure base cost standard to a **budget standard** (i.e., the expected expense per visit in the budget year). Assuming RN wages are expected to increase by 3%, the budgeted expense per physician visit should be $21.07, $20.46 × 1.03. The price of medical supplies are expected to increase by 6% in 2024, so the

Table 14.7 Flexible Budget for Semmelweis Clinic

Output	June 30, 2023					Budget Forecast
Physician visits (V_{MD})	7,650					15,606
Therapy visits (V_{TH})	4,750					9,600
Total Visits (V_{Total})	12,400					25,206

Account (line item)	June 30, 2023	F, V, %	Cost Std	Inflation Factor	Budget Std	Preliminary 2024 Flexible Budget
Physician services revenues	$687,500	V	$89.87	1.04	$93.46	$1,458,600
Therapy revenue	312,500	V	65.79	1.04	68.42	656,842
Total Operating Revenue	$1,000,000					$2,115,442
Physician salaries	$262,500	F	$525,000	1.03	$540,750	$540,750
RN salaries	156,500	V_{MD}	20.46	1.03	21.07	328,838
Therapy salaries	115,000	V_{Th}	24.21	1.03	24.94	239,394
Staff salaries	122,000	F	244,000	1.03	251,320	251,320
Health insurance	67,000	F	134,000	1.10	147,400	147,400
Social security	50,500	%	7.65%			115,339
Retirement	66,000	%	10.00%			136,030
Unemployment	6,500	%	1.00%			13,603
Medical supplies	68,000	V_{Tot}	5.48	1.06	5.81	146,520
Office supplies	25,500	V_{Tot}	2.06	1.02	2.10	52,872
Housekeeping supplies	12,750	F	25,500	1.02	26,010	26,010
Depreciation	21,000	F	42,000	1.00	42,000	42,000
Interest	9,750	F	19,500	1.00	19,500	19,500
Total Operating Expenses	$983,000					$2,059,575
Interest Income	$2,750					$5,500
Net Income	$19,750					$61,367

budgeted cost for medical supplies will be $5.81, $5.48 × 1.06. Step 6 multiplies the budget standard by forecasted output. For RN salaries, it is $21.07 × 15,606 physician visits = $328,838. Note that RN salaries should increase or decrease by $21.07 for every visit over or under 15,606 physician visits. The total expense for medical supplies is expected to be $146,520, $5.81 × 25,206 total visits.

Step 7 calculates the budget allocation for fixed resources such as physician salaries, health insurance, and housekeeping supplies, which should not change with changes in output, and uses the incremental budgeting process introduced previously. Managers select an expenditure base; annualize partial-year data when used, to obtain a 12-month estimate; identify an inflation factor; and multiply the annualized expense by the inflation factor to determine the budget for each fixed line item. Budgeted physician salaries will be the annualized 2023 salaries multiplied by expected 3% wage increase. The only factor that should affect outlays for fixed resources is changes in input prices.

The final step in constructing the preliminary flexible budget is the same as in incremental budgeting: Managers should modify their budgets for new work processes or regulations that add steps, introduce new expenses, or expand the time required to complete present tasks.

Restating the Flexible Budget

Managers will only know the number of outputs produced *after* the end of the budget period. After actual output is known, the flexible budget is restated or flexed to provide the amount of resources needed for actual output. All variable expenses and the expenses based on variable expenses, such as

Social Security, payroll tax, retirement, and unemployment, are increased when more output is produced than forecasted or reduced when forecasted output exceeds actual output.

Table 14.8 shows that physician visits were lower than forecasted and therapy visits were higher than forecasted, so physician revenue is less than the preliminary budget and therapy revenue is higher. The net effect is a $21,197 reduction from planned revenue. Expenses for all fixed costs are unchanged, while the drop in physician visits reduced the need for RN hours and their salary and the increase in therapy visits increased the need for therapists and their salary. The other major reduction was in medical supplies; the lower number of total visits reduced medical and office supply expenses.

The net impact of the change in output is net income *should* decline by $15,073, 24.6%, emphasizing that a 1.0% reduction in revenue combined with a 0.3% reduction in expenses has a large negative effect on net income. Managers

Table 14.8 Final, Restated Budget for Semmelweis Clinic

Output	Actual	Budget	Difference	% Difference
Physician visits	15,306	15,606	−300	−1.9%
Therapy visits	9,700	9,600	100	1.0%
Total visits	24,006	24,206	−200	−1.0%

Account (line item)	Restated 2024 Flexible Budget	Preliminary 2024 Flexible Budget	$ Difference	% Difference
Physician services revenues	$1,430,561	$1,458,600	−$28,039	−1.9%
Therapy revenue	663,684	656,842	6,842	1.0%
Total Operating Revenue	$2,094,245	$2,115,442	−$21,197	−1.0%
Physician salaries	$540,750	$540,750	$0	0.0%
RN salaries	322,516	328,838	−6,321	−1.9%
Therapy salaries	241,887	239,394	2,494	1.0%
Staff salaries	251,320	251,320	0	0.0%
Health insurance	147,400	147,400	0	0.0%
Social security	115,046	115,339	−293	−0.3%
Retirement	135,647	136,030	−383	−0.3%

Account (line item)	Restated 2024 Flexible Budget	Preliminary 2024 Flexible Budget	$ Difference	% Difference
Unemployment	13,565	13,603	−38	−0.3%
Medical supplies	145,357	146,520	−1,163	−0.8%
Office supplies	52,452	52,872	−420	−0.8%
Housekeeping supplies	26,010	26,010	0	0.0%
Depreciation	42,000	42,000	0	0.0%
Interest	19,500	19,500	0	0.0%
Total Operating Expenses	$2,053,452	$2,059,575	−$6,124	−0.3%
Interest Income	$5,500	$5,500	$0	0.0%
Net Income	$46,293	$61,367	−$15,073	−24.6%

that understand the relationship between output, revenue, and expenses should monitor output and pricing on a monthly basis to prevent year-end surprises.

Incremental and flexible budgets are designed to create an operating plan that specifies a set of outputs and the resources needed to produce the output. Actual performance should be compared to the budget to assess performance. Did managers and employees produce higher or lower net income than anticipated, and if so, were the causes of the increase or decrease controllable?

There is no one right way to prepare an operating budget. The budget construction depends on factors such as the organizational structure, the reporting system, the manager's scope of responsibility and controllable costs, variability of output, and so on. When output and revenue are stable and predictable, incremental budgets provide an equitable budget and are easy to prepare. Flexible budgets should be used when output and revenue are not stable and predictable to ensure managers receive more resources when output increases and vice versa. Flexible budgets are more difficult to prepare, but managers who understand the flexible budgeting process will gain greater insight into their department's operations and finances. **Exhibit 14.1** sets out a series of questions and steps to undertake when building a budget.

Exhibit 14.1 Checklist for Building a Budget

1. What is the proposed output (volume) for the new budget period?
2. What is the appropriate inflow (revenues) and outflow (cost of services delivered) relationship?
3. What will the appropriate dollar cost be? (Note: This question requires a series of assumptions about the nature of the operation for the new budget period.)
   3a. Forecast service-related workload.
   3b. Forecast non-service-related workload.
   3c. Forecast special project workload if applicable.
   3d. Coordinate assumptions for proportionate share of interdepartmental projects.
4. Does the organization have sufficient resources to meet planned expenses?
5. Will this budget accomplish the appropriate managerial objectives such as meeting the community's need for care and financial return for the organization?

It is also important to note that the budget for operations is usually part of an overall, or comprehensive, financial budget. Responsibility for the comprehensive financial budget always rests with upper-level financial officers of the organization and is beyond the scope of this chapter.

Budget Review

The questions discussed in constructing a budget also serve to evaluate an existing budget. Issues of valid and replicable assumptions and comparability are especially essential. Comparative analysis is an important skill to for managers, as discussed in Chapter 13. **Exhibit 14.2** sets out a series of questions and steps to undertake when reviewing and evaluating a budget.

Exhibit 14.2 Checklist for Reviewing a Budget

---

1. Is this budget incremental (not adjusted for volume) or flexible (adjusted for volume during the year)?
2. Are expenses designated as fixed or variable?
3. Is the budget for a defined unit of authority?
4. Are the line items within the budget (i.e., the expenses and revenues, if applicable) controllable by the manager?
5. Is the format of the budget comparable with that of previous periods so that several reports over time can be compared if so desired?
6. Are the actual and budget amounts for the same period?
7. Are YTD amounts annualized?
8. Are the line-item calculations correct including the dollar differences and percentage changes?
9. Is the budget request reasonable compared to the expenditure base and expected output? The total amount should be approximately similar, neither too high or low, unless major changes are anticipated.

WRAP-UP

Summary

The job of a budget is to set goals and estimate needed resources for the next fiscal period and provide managers with information to assess budget year performance. The critical element in a budget is the level of output expected as it should determine operating revenues and expenses. Managers should be able to assess past trends in output, expenses, and sometimes revenue as the starting point for forecasting output, expenses, and revenue.

Two primary budget processes were reviewed. The first, incremental budgeting, depends primarily on identifying prior actual or budgeted expenses, an expenditure base, and increasing these amounts for expected price increases in the budget year. Any major changes in output are then incorporated into expense estimates.

The second method, flexible budgeting, recognizes that accurately forecasting output may be difficult, so a preliminary budget is created based on forecasted output, and the final budget is adjusted after the close of the budget period for actual output to increase the budget for departments producing higher than forecasted output and reduce resources to departments producing lower output. Flexible budgets eliminate output as a cause of budget variances so managers can focus on other issues that result in spending more or less than the budget. Chapter 15 demonstrates how managers should examine budget variances to gain greater control over the financial performance of their departments.

Key Terms

Annualization
Budget Standard
Capital Expenditure Budget
Cost Standard

Flexible (preliminary and final) Budget
Incremental (static or fixed) Budget

Inflation Factor
Master Budget
Operating Budget

Discussion Questions

1. Explain the goals of budgeting.
2. Describe the steps required to build a budget.
3. Explain the role of forecasting in budgeting.

4. Describe the difference between an incremental and flexible operating budget and when each should be used.
5. Explain the difference between the preliminary and final, restated flexible budgets.

Problems

1. Using the following table, create an incremental budget for the pediatric nursing unit at Codman Medical Center based on 2022 year-to-date actual expenses assuming no change in output. Finance has stipulated that the inflation factors for 2023 should be 3% for wages and fringe benefits, 5% for supplies, and 2% for all other expenses.

has stipulated the inflation factors for 2023 should be 3% for wages and fringe benefits, 5% for supplies, and 2% for all other expenses. (2) Fiscal year 2023 has ended, and the unit provided 97,339 patient days. Restate the budget for actual output to create the budget to which the unit manager should be accountable. (3) Assume actual expenses for fiscal

Expense	2021 Actual	2022 YTD Actual	2022 YTD Budget	2023 Budget
Salaries and Wages-V	$376,700	$200,200	$194,000	_____
Fringe Benefits-V	131,700	69,200	68,000	_____
Supplies-V	200,600	111,000	109,000	_____
Depreciation-F	57,400	25,000	24,000	_____
Interest-F	17,800	8,400	9,000	_____
Other-V	187,400	99,300	100,000	_____
Total Expenses	$971,600	$513,100	$504,000	_____
Patient days	95,000	47,700	47,200	96,400

2. Using the table in Problem 14–1, (1) create a flexible budget for the pediatric nursing unit based on year-to-date actual expenses and patient days with 96,400 forecasted patient days for 2023. Finance

year 2023 totaled $1,092,456. Did the manager do a good job managing the budget?

3. The Fleming Medical Group has had a modest net income recently, and the

	2021	2022 YTD Actual	2022 YTD Budget	Budget 2023
Revenue	$4,885,987	$2,964,750	$2,950,000	_____
Operating expenses				
Physician salaries	$960,000	$585,306	$576,800	_____
Nursing staff salaries	1,380,000	857,157	829,150	_____
Mgt and clerical salaries	780,000	466,971	468,650	_____
FICA	238,680	143,397	143,407	_____
Health Insurance	390,000	238,760	234,325	_____
Retirement	124,800	76,763	74,984	_____
Unemployment	31,200	18,323	18,746	_____
Medications	148,152	91,687	89,015	_____
Medical instruments	102,792	64,287	61,761	_____
Bandages, gauze...	57,468	34,140	34,529	_____
Gloves, gowns...	40,416	24,476	24,283	_____
Sterile wipes	26,820	15,780	16,114	_____
Office supplies	115,200	69,388	69,216	_____
Cleaning supplies	39,048	23,103	23,461	_____
Rent	144,000	89,251	86,520	_____
Maintenance	13,764	11,245	8,270	_____
Electricity	10,788	6,684	6,482	_____
Gas	18,504	11,215	11,118	_____
Water and Sewage	6,756	4,225	4,059	_____
Telephone	3,228	2,004	1,939	_____
Housekeeping	36,000	21,694	21,630	_____
Travel/meetings/meals	7,908	4,744	4,751	_____
Prof. insurance	22,380	15,669	13,447	_____
CME	29,856	17,994	17,938	_____
Other expenses	57,732	35,955	34,687	_____
	$4,785,492	$2,930,218	$2,875,282	_____
Total Visits	51,986	30,331	30,672	52,560

first six months of 2022 indicate that their profit margin may be less than 2% if current performance continues. The owners want to put greater emphasis on budgeting to improve financial performance. Using the following table, create an incremental budget for the practice based on 2022 year-to-date actual expenses and a 4% inflation factor for each line item. What are the total budget, projected net income, and profit margin?

4. One of the owners of the Fleming Medical Group recently attended a conference on medical practice management, learned of flexible budgeting, and believes it can help the practice better manage its revenues and expenses. Using the table in Problem 14–3, create a flexible budget based on 2022 year-to-date actual expenses and visits, a 4% inflation factor for each line item, and 52,560 forecasted patient visits in 2023. What are the total budget, projected net income, and profit margin? Did net income and profit margin increase from the incremental budget prepared in Problem 14–3?

Notes

1. W. O. Cleverly, *Essentials of Health Care Finance*, 4th ed. (Gaithersburg, MD: Aspen Publishers, Inc., 1997).
2. Optum360°, *2017 Almanac of Hospital Financial and Operating Indicators* (Salt Lake City, UT: Author, 2016).
3. C. Horngren et al., *Cost Accounting: A Managerial Emphasis*, 9th ed. (Englewood Cliffs, NJ: Prentice Hall, 1998), 228.
4. J. R. Pearson et al., "The Flexible Budget Process—A Tool for Cost Containment," *American Journal of Clinical Pathology*, 84, no. 2 (1985): 202–208.
5. T. K. Ross, *A Comprehensive Guide to Budgeting for Health Care Managers* (Burlington, MA: Jones and Bartlett Learning, 2018); T. K. Ross, *Practical Budgeting for Health Care, A Concise Guide* (Burlington, MA: Jones and Bartlett Learning, 2021).
6. Ibid.

CHAPTER 15

Variance Analysis and Sensitivity Analysis

PROGRESS NOTES

After completing this chapter, you should be able to:

1. Explain the role of variance analysis.
2. Explain the four ways managers can compare the financial performance of their areas of responsibility.
3. Calculate and interpret budget variances.
4. Explain the purpose of sensitivity analysis and describe how it is performed.
5. Calculate a contribution margin and break-even output.

Overview: Variance Analysis

The operating budget defines the expected amount of work and how much should be spent to accomplish the work during the budget year. **Variance analysis** examines differences between the amount spent and the amount budgeted. Variance analysis may be the most important financial skill a manager should master, as failing to deliver the required work within budget may spell the end of a manager's career. Multiple unanticipated factors may arise that will increase or decrease expenses, and determining whether budget overruns arise from controllable or uncontrollable factors may be crucial to how a manager is evaluated. The ability to quantify why more money was spent than budgeted is also critical to improving performance. While noncontrollable factors cannot be altered, managers should act promptly when controllable variances arise to minimize year-end variances (i.e., a controllable factor that arises in March should be acted on in April so budget overruns do not continue through the end of the year).

A variance is the difference between the amount spent and the amount budgeted. One reason that actual spending will exceed the budget is producing higher output. (In a flexible budget, the final, restated budget would be increased for higher output and thus no variance would arise.) The second reason is each output costs more to produce than expected (i.e., the actual cost per output exceeded the amount budgeted [the standard] due to an increase in the price of resources and/or the amount of resources used).

Comparative Budget Review

Managers need to know how to effectively review financial data to determine the appropriateness of their expenses. Review typically involves comparing actual and budgeted expenses so managers must first understand how the budget was constructed. In general, the operating expense budget under review will have a column for actual expenditures, a column for budgeted expenditures, a column for the dollar difference between actual and budget, and the percent difference (i.e., the dollar difference divided by the budget). Each line item will have a horizontal analysis (discussed in Chapter 13) that measures the amount of the difference against the budget. Sometimes the actual expense column and the budget column will have a vertical analysis of percentages showing the percent of total expense that each line item accounts for. (This is also discussed in Chapter 13.)

Table 15.1 illustrates the operating expense budget configuration just described. Note that the "Budget Variance $" column has positive and negative amounts. The negative amounts indicate that the department spent less than its budget (e.g., dietary had an actual expense of $400,000 against a budget of $405,000, resulting in a $5,000 budget savings). The next line is maintenance, which exceeded its budget, so the difference is positive. The maintenance budget was $270,000, and actual expenses were $290,000, so the department was $20,000 over budget. Negative amounts are good (under budget) and positive amounts are

bad (over budget) in expenses. In revenues, negative amounts are bad (under budget) and positive amounts are good (over budget).

Table 15.1 illustrates a comparison of actual expenses versus budgeted expenses. This format reflects both dollars and percentages, as is most common. Table 15.1 shows the grand totals for each department (dietary, maintenance, etc.) contained in the general services expense for the hospital. There is, of course, a detailed budget for each of these departments that adds up to the totals shown in Table 15.1. For example, all the detailed expenses of the laundry department—labor, supplies, and so on—are contained in a supporting detailed budget whose total actual expenses amount to $50,000 and whose total budgeted expenses amount to $45,000.

Department managers are responsible for analyzing and managing the detailed budgets of their own departments. Division managers are responsible for analyzing and controlling the budgets of their subordinate departments, and the chief financial officer (CFO) may be responsible for making a comparative analysis of the overall operations of the organization. This comparative analysis at a higher level will condense each department's details into a departmental grand total, as shown in Table 15.1, for convenience and clarity in review.

The CFO may also convert this comparative data into charts or graphs in order to "tell the story" in a more visual manner. For example, the total general service expense in Table 15.1 can be readily converted into a graph. **Figure 15.1** illustrates such a graph.

Table 15.1 Comparative Analysis of General Services Budgeted and Actual Expense

General Services Expense	2023 Actual	% GS Expense	2023 Budget	% GS Expense	Budget Variance $	Budget Variance %
Dietary	$400,000	43%	$405,000	45%	–$5,000	–1.2%
Maintenance	290,000	32%	270,000	30%	$20,000	7.4%
Laundry	50,000	5%	45,000	5%	$5,000	11.1%
Housekeeping	180,000	20%	175,000	20%	$5,000	2.9%
Total GS Expense	$920,000	100%	$895,000	100%	$25,000	2.8%

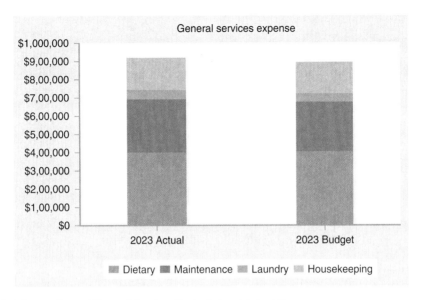

Figure 15.1 A Comparison of General Services Budgeted and Actual Expenses

Compare Current Actual Expenses to Prior Periods in Own Organization

Trend analysis compares current actual expenses to expenses incurred in prior periods in the same organization. For example, consider that maintenance is over budget by $20,000 for the current year. The director of maintenance and the vice president of support services, the director's superior, should compare past financial performance (i.e., year-to-year or current YTD performance versus prior year performance over the same time period as well as the trend over multiple years). **Figure 15.2** displays annual maintenance expense for the past five years. The question that should be addressed is "Is the 2023 maintenance expense appropriate?" The large increase in the 2023 expense may be due to maintenance that should have been performed in prior years being completed in 2023 or because severe weather resulted in unplanned damage to equipment or buildings. Another explanation is an increase due to poor management. The next two graphs attempt to determine the cause of the increase.

Compare to Industry Standards

It often makes little sense to compare the total expenses or revenues of one organization to another. The primary problem is differences in size (i.e., the number of licensed beds and patients served). A 200-bed hospital should not be compared against a 500-bed institution as the larger organization should have revenues and expenses 250% larger than the smaller one. Likewise, differences in mission, location, type of patients served, accounting methods, and so on should also be considered when comparing financial performance. **Figure 15.3** reports the maintenance cost per bed for Codman Medical Center and the industry average to provide a more valid comparison (i.e., is Codman spending a similar amount per bed compared to the industry?).

Maintenance costs are often related to the average age of the facility (i.e., older facilities require more maintenance and managers should determine if their assets are newer or older than the industry average *before* judging the appropriateness of the expense and management performance). Healthcare organizations are particularly

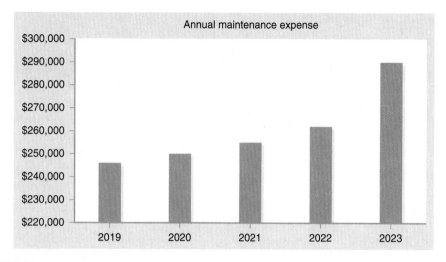

Figure 15.2 Maintenance Expense, 2019–2023

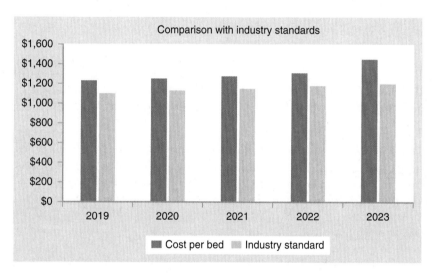

Figure 15.3 A Comparison of Maintenance Cost per Bed with Industry Standards

well suited to use industry standards because both the federal and state governments release a wealth of public information and statistics regarding the provision of health care. Chapter 16 will explore benchmarking (i.e., what are appropriate and desirable performance targets?).

Compare to Similar Organizations

Figure 15.3 showed that the maintenance cost per bed at Codman exceeds industry standards and

that the difference between the hospital and the standard almost doubled between 2022 and 2023. A more appropriate measure may be obtained by comparing Codman to similar organizations. For example, an eastern teaching hospital should not compare itself against a midwestern community hospital as the cost of living is more expensive on the East Coast and teaching hospitals have higher investments in equipment and facilities that increase their costs. In this case, the eastern teaching hospital may have a higher-than-average cost per bed but be spending less than comparable

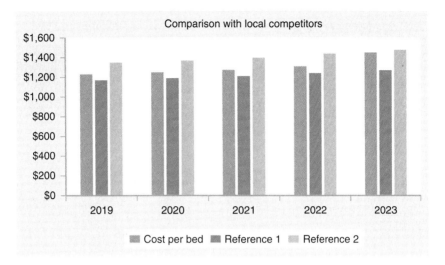

Figure 15.4 Comparison of Maintenance Cost per Bed with Local Competitors

institutions. On the other hand, a community hospital's cost may be excessive, but when compared to high-cost organizations, it may appear reasonable. Figure 15.4 compares the maintenance cost per bed to other community hospitals in the same city.

Figure 15.4 shows that Codman's maintenance costs were between the highest- and lowest-cost competitors from 2019 through 2022. In 2023, its costs were similar to the high-cost competitor. Managers should identify the cause of the recent increase. Is it aging equipment and facilities (noncontrollable) or poor management (controllable)?

Starting the Budget Review

The first step in determining the appropriateness of actual expenses is to collect information and understand (or calculate) dollar and percent differences between actual and budgeted expenses. Dollar and percent differences are required as large expense items may have large dollar differences that are small percent differences. Small changes should be expected due to the large number of factors that can change actual spending and the difficulty creating a precise budget. On the other

hand, small expense items may have relatively small dollar variances that are large percent differences relative to expected expenses. **Table 15.2** provides financial information for Codman Medical Center's Operating Room and Recovery Room.

Checklist Questions and Answers for the Comparative Budget Review

1. Q. Are the actual and budget amounts reported for the same period?
   A. The actual and budget amounts are for the same period.
2. Q. Are the actual and budget amounts for the month, year-to-date, and/or complete year?
   A. The amounts are for the entire year, October 1, 2022, through September 30, 2023.
3. Q. Is this budget incremental (not adjusted for volume) or flexible (adjusted for volume) during the year?
   A. This budget is incremental, so increases (decreases) in surgical volume should explain some if not all of the variation in actual expenses.

Table 15.2 Codman Medical Center Operating Room and Recovery Room Budgets
For the Fiscal Year October 1, 2022, to September 30, 2023

Operating Room					
Account #	Expense	Actual	Budget	$ Variance	% Variance
1010-020	RN Salaries	$470,640	$459,710	$10,930	2.4%
1010-030	LPN Salaries	44,685	41,234	3,451	8.4%
1010-040	Other Nursing Salaries	68,390	56,937	11,453	20.1%
1010-200	OR Supplies-Req.	54,350	57,162	(2,812)	−4.9%
1010-220	Supplies-Direct Purchase	3,833	3,540	293	8.3%
1010-221	Instruments	50,727	52,310	(1,583)	−3.0%
1010-245	Uniform Expense	628	410	218	53.2%
1010-605	Periodicals and Books	670	750	(80)	−10.7%
1010-610	Employee Education	4,720	4,192	528	12.6%
1010-620	Maintenance	6,387	5,940	447	7.5%
1010-730	Purchased Maintenance	9,366	8,550	816	9.5%
1010-740	Purchased Service	864	864	0	0.0%
	Total Expense	$715,260	$691,599	$23,661	3.4%
Recovery Room					
Account #	Expense	Actual	Budget	$ Variance	% Variance
1012-020	RN Salaries	$173,527	$174,807	($1,280)	−0.7%
1012-040	Other Nursing Salaries	26,155	21,617	4,538	21.0%
1012-200	Recovery Room Supplies	10,114	12,375	(2,261)	−18.3%
1012-213	Minor Equipment	422	422	0	0.0%
1012-220	Supplies-Direct Purchase	482	295	187	63.4%
1012-610	Employee Education	125	63	62	98.4%
1012-620	Maintenance	1,037	758	279	36.8%
1012-730	Purchased Maintenance	438	310	128	41.3%
	Total Expense	$212,300	$210,647	$1,653	0.8%

4. Q. Is the budget for a defined unit of authority?
   A. The budgets are for two interrelated units of authority: the operating and recovery rooms, which fall under the aegis of the Department of Surgery.
5. Q. Is the format of the budget comparable with that of previous periods so that several reports over time can be compared if so desired?
   A. The format is comparable. One can compare fiscal year 2023 with past years. Year-to-year comparisons of individual expenses codes may be invalid if codes have been added or deleted.
6. Q. How are the "percent variance" figures calculated?
   A. Using Account #1010-020, Operating Room RN Nursing Salaries, the variance of $10,930 is divided by the budgeted amount of $459,710, resulting in a +2.4% variance. The less commonly used method would divide $10,930 by the actual amount of $470,640, resulting in a +2.3% variance.
7. Q. What are the largest dollar and percent differences, and are the line items controllable by the manager?
   A. The largest dollar and percent differences are in 1010-040, Other Nursing Salaries, $11,453 and 20.1% over budget. Whether this variance or other variances are controllable by the manager requires additional information that we will explore in the next section.

Budget Variances

We'll begin our examination of the potential causes and controllability of variances by focusing on a single expense. Assume a physician practice employs one physical therapist who is paid $35.00 per hour and is scheduled for 2,080 hours per year. The budgeted salary expense is $72,800. At the end of the year, the physician, the practice owner, is reviewing expenses and notes that the therapist was paid $79,100. The total variance is $6,300 over budget or 8.7% over budget, $6,300 ÷ $72,800 (**Table 15.3**). The

Table 15.3 Operating Statistics

	Expense	Hours	Visits
Actual	$79,100	2,200	2,276
Budget	$72,800	2,080	2,080
Variance	$6,300	120	196
% Variance	5.8%	8.7%	9.4%

higher-than-expected cost is concerning, but the physician needs the information that variance analysis provides before concluding if action is necessary and what action should be taken. The physician, and managers in general, should not jump to the conclusion that employee salary or other expenses must be reduced when they are over budget.

Table 15.3 indicates that the cause of the budget overage may be due to higher-than-expected visits. The purpose of variance analysis is to determine if differences between actual and budget expenses are appropriate.

Volume Variance

The first variance we should examine is the **volume variance**. The volume variance is the portion of the total variance caused by a difference between the actual and budgeted output and is calculated as the difference between actual and budgeted output multiplied by the budgeted cost per output, (actual output − budgeted output) × (budgeted cost ÷ budgeted output). The therapist was budgeted to provide 2,080 sessions (60 minutes each) over the course of the year. During the year she was paid for 2,200 hours and provided 2,276 therapy sessions, 120 hours and 196 sessions more than budgeted. The volume variance is: (2,276 − 2,080) × ($72,800 ÷ 2,080) or 196 × $35 = $6,860 The practice should have paid the therapist more based on the higher-than-expected output. The volume variance calculates what the budget should have been (i.e., the increase or decrease in the budget if actual workload had been known in advance).[1]

Cost Variance

The **cost variance** is the difference between the actual and budgeted cost per output and arises due to differences between the expected and actual use of inputs and the budgeted and actual price of inputs. The cost variance is calculated as ((actual cost ÷ actual output) – (budgeted cost ÷ budgeted output)) × actual output. The cost variance is (($79,100 ÷ 2,276) – ($72,800 ÷ 2,080)) × 2,276 actual visits. The actual cost per session was $34.75 versus a budgeted cost of $35.00. The practice saved $0.25 per session for a total savings of –$560. Note that the sum of the volume and cost variances equals the total variance, $6,860 – 560 = $6,300.

Efficiency Variance

A cost variance can arise from using more of a resource than budgeted or paying more for the resource than budgeted. The efficiency (also known as a quantity or use) variance is the portion of the cost variance that is caused by a difference between the actual and budgeted quantity of input needed per output. The **efficiency variance** is calculated as the difference between the actual and budgeted quantity of inputs used per output multiplied by the actual output level and the budgeted unit price. The budgeted therapist time per session was 60 minutes. An unfavorable efficiency variance arises when sessions take more than 60 minutes. Increases in the quantity of inputs used could be due to the need to provide more services for sicker patients requiring more care (i.e., an intensity variance, and vice versa). Readers seeking more information on intensity variances should see Ross (2018) or Ross (2021).[2] On the other hand, if visits are completed in less than 60 minutes, a favorable efficiency variance arises, and the therapist may be able to see more patients in an eight-hour day.

The efficiency variance for the practice is ((2,276 hours ÷ 2,200 sessions) – (2,080 hours ÷ 2,080 sessions)) × 2,276 sessions × $35 or the actual time per session equals 0.9667 hours (58 minutes) versus a budgeted time of one hour (60 minutes). The cost savings due to faster completion of work is 0.0333 hours per session (or 2 minutes) multiplied by the budgeted cost of

$35.00 per hour; thus $1.17, was saved per session or –$2,660 was saved in total.

Price Variance

The second factor accounting for a cost variance is a price or rate variance. A **price variance** is the portion of the cost variance caused by a difference between the actual and budgeted price of an input and is calculated as the difference between the actual and budgeted input price multiplied by the actual quantity of labor or supplies used per unit of output. The price variance is ((actual expense ÷ actual input units) – (budgeted expense ÷ budgeted input units)) × actual input units.

The practice's price variance is (($79,100 ÷ 2,200 paid hours) – ($72,800 ÷ 2,080 budgeted hours)) × 2,200 paid hours. The practice paid the therapist $35.95 per hour due to overtime, time and a half for every hour over 2,080, versus a budgeted rate of $35.00. Paying $0.95 more per hour across 2,200 paid hours increased the salary expense by $2,100. Note that the sum of the efficiency and price variance equals the cost variance, –$2,660 + $2,100 = –$560. **Table 15.4** summarizes this example.

In this case, the physician should be happy as the therapist is working more efficiently (taking less time per session), providing more sessions, and generating more revenue for the practice. As long as the additional revenue generated by the therapist exceeds the $35.95 labor expense plus the cost of any supplies needed to provide the additional therapy sessions, the practice benefits from going over budget.

Two-Variance and Three-Variance Analysis

Variance analysis can be performed as a two- or three-variance analysis. The two-variance analysis calculates **volume and cost (or revenue) variance** as compared with budgeted costs. The three-variance analysis calculates **volume, efficiency, and price variances** (Figure 15.5).

Another complexity in variance analysis that contributes to confusion is all three variable cost

Table 15.4 Variance Calculations

	Actual	Budget	Difference	Budgeted Wage	Variance	
Volume	(2276 –	2080) =	196 ×	$35.00 =	$6,860	
	Actual	Budget	Difference	Actual Visits	Variance	
Cost	($34.76 –	$35.00) =	–$0.24 ×	2276 =	–$560	
Total Variance					$6,300	
	Actual	Standard	Difference	Actual Visits	Budgeted Wage	Variance
Efficiency	(0.9667 –	1.0000) =	–0.0333 ×	2276 ×	$35.00 =	–$2,660
	58 minutes	60 minutes	–2 minutes	($1.17)		
	Actual	Standard	Difference	Actual Hours		
Price	($35.95 –	$35.00) =	$0.95 ×	2200 =		$2,100
Cost Variance						–$560

Elements of two-variance analysis	Elements of three-variance analysis
1. Volume (output) variance 2. Cost or revenue variance	1. Volume (output) variance 2. Efficiency (or use) variance 3. Price (or rate) variance

Figure 15.5 Elements of Variance Analysis

elements—that is, direct labor, direct materials, and variable overhead—can have a price variance and an efficiency variance computed, but the variance is not described by the same names. **Exhibit 15.1** sets out the different names. Even though the names differ, the calculation for all three is the same. Note that variance analysis is primarily a matter of input–output analysis. The inputs represent actual quantities of direct labor, direct materials, and variable overhead used. The outputs represent the services or products delivered for the applicable time period expressed in terms of standard hours for labor and standard quantity for materials. In other words, the

Exhibit 15.1 Different Names for Materials, Labor, and Overhead Variances

Price Variance = Materials Price Variance [for direct materials]
Price Variance = Labor Rate Variance [for direct labor]
Price Variance = Overhead Spending Variance [for variable overhead]

standard hours or standard quantity equates to what should have been used (the budget standard) rather than what was actually used. This is an important point to remember.

Cost and Volume Variance Analysis: Curie Imaging Center

The financial report for the Curie Imaging Center is given in **Table 15.5**. As shown, the budgeted number of imaging tests was 1,000, while the actual number performed was 1,100. An increase in volume is favorable. The budgeted revenue per test was $400, $400,000 ÷ 1,000 tests, while actual revenue was $438,000 for 1,100 tests or $398.18 per test, an unfavorable variance of $1.82 per test. The net revenue variance, $38,000, $438,000 – $400,000, is favorable.

The salaries and benefits expense line item exceeded the budget by an unfavorable balance of $20,000. Likewise, the supply expense line item exceeded budget by an unfavorable balance of $15,000, insurance was $500 more than budgeted, and actual depreciation equaled budgeted depreciation. The total expense variance is an unfavorable $30,500. The operating income variance, $7,500, is favorable, the net difference between the $38,000 favorable revenue variance and the $30,500 unfavorable total expense variance.

Calculating a cost variance—we will call it a revenue variance as it examines revenue rather than an expense—indicates the center received $1.82 less per test than expected, (($438,000 ÷ 1100 tests) – ($400,000 ÷ 1000 budgeted tests)) × 1100 actual tests, for a revenue loss of $2,000 (**Table 15.6**). The negative price variance may be due to patients or third parties paying less than expected (i.e., higher-than-expected contractual discount or bad debt and/or an increase in low reimbursement or charity patients). Calculating the volume variance for revenue indicates that revenue should have increased by $40,000, (1,100 tests – 1,000 tests) × $400.

Actual salaries increased $20,000, so the cost variance shows the labor cost per test increased $4.55 over the budget, (($170,000 ÷ 1,100 tests) – ($150,000 ÷ 1,000 budgeted tests)) × 1,100 actual tests, ($154.55 – $150.00) × 1,100, increasing salary and benefits by $5,000. The increase in the labor cost per test may arise from paying higher-than-expected wages and/or benefits and/or radiology technicians taking more time to complete tests. Calculating the volume variance for salaries and benefits indicates that salaries should have increased by $15,000, (1,100 tests – 1,000 tests) × ($150,000 ÷ 1,000 budgeted tests). The sum of the cost, $5,000, and volume, $15,000, variances equals the total variance, $20,000.

Table 15.5 Operating Data for the Curie Imaging Center

Curie Imaging Center	Actual	Budget	Variance	Favorable/ Unfavorable
Imaging Tests Performed	1,100	1,000	100	Favorable
Net Revenue	$438,000	$400,000	$38,000	Favorable
Expenses				
Salaries and Benefits	$170,000	$150,000	$20,000	Unfavorable
Supplies	35,000	25,000	10,000	Unfavorable
Insurance	15,500	15,000	500	Unfavorable
Depreciation	150,000	150,000	0	
Total Expense	$370,500	$340,000	$30,500	Unfavorable
Operating Income	$67,500	$60,000	$7,500	Favorable

Table 15.6 Variance Calculations for the Curie Imaging Center

Variance	Act. Price	Bud. Price	Difference	Act. Volume	$ Variance
Revenue Price	$398.18	$400.00	–$1.82	1,100	–$2,000
	Act. Volume	**Bud. Volume**	**Difference**	**Bud. Price**	
Revenue Volume	1,100	1,000	100	$400	<u>$40,000</u>
Total					$38,000
	Act. Cost	**Bud. Cost**	**Difference**	**Act. Volume**	
Salaries Cost	$154.55	$150.00	$4.55	1,100	$5,000
	Act. Volume	**Bud. Volume**	**Difference**	**Bud. Cost**	
Salaries Volume	1,100	1,000	100	$150	<u>$15,000</u>
Total					$20,000
	Act. Cost	**Bud. Cost**	**Difference**	**Act. Volume**	
Supplies Cost	$31.82	$25.00	$6.82	1,100	$7,500
	Act. Volume	**Bud. Volume**	**Difference**	**Bud. Cost**	
Supplies Volume	1,100	1,000	100	$25	<u>$2,500</u>
Total					$10,000

Actual supply expense increased $10,000, so the cost variance shows the supply cost per test increased $6.82 over the budget, (($35,000 ÷ 1,100 tests) – ($25,000 ÷ 1,000 tests)) × 1,100 actual tests, ($31.82 – $25.00) × 1,100 = $7,500. The $6.82 increase in the supply cost per test could be due to higher-than-budgeted supply prices and/or higher-than-expected supply usage per test. Calculating the volume variance for supplies indicates that supplies should have increased by $2,500, (1,100 tests – 1,000 tests) × ($25,000 ÷ 1,000 budgeted tests). Again, the sum of the cost and volume variances equals the total variance for supplies.

The increase in insurance cost should be attributed entirely to an unanticipated increase in the insurance premium since insurance is a fixed cost that does not change with increases or decreases in output. Depreciation is a fixed cost and had no variance, so there is no need to calculate cost or volume variances.

Price, Efficiency, and Volume Variance Analysis: Semmelweis Clinic

A three-variance example is provided in **Table 15.7** that presents the financial report by line item for six months of operations at the Semmelweis Clinic. Budgeted revenue was calculated at $90.00 per visit for physician services and $65.00 for therapy. Physicians are paid a fixed salary independent of hours worked or visits provided. RN salaries are considered a variable cost that changes with physician visits, and therapist salaries are a variable cost based on therapy visits. Medical and office supplies are variable costs that change with total visits. Fringe benefits, Social Security, retirement, and unemployment are based on a percent of total physician, RN, therapist, and staff salaries. All other costs are consider fixed.

Table 15.7 Six-Month Operating Results for Semmelweis Clinic

Output	Actual June 30, 2023	Budget June 30, 2023	Variance	% Variance	
Physician visits	7,650	7,700	−50	−0.6%	
Therapy visits	4,800	4,700	100	2.1%	
Total Visits	12,450	12,400	50	0.4%	
Account (Line item)					F,V,%
Physician services revenues	$687,500	$693,000	−$5,500	−0.8%	V
Therapy revenue	312,500	305,500	7,000	2.3%	V
Total Operating Revenue	$1,000,000	$998,500	$1,500	0.2%	
Expenses					
Physician salaries	$262,500	$265,000	−$2,500	−0.9%	F
RN salaries	156,500	149,000	7,500	5.0%	V_{MD}
Therapy salaries	115,000	114,000	1,000	0.9%	V_{TH}
Staff salaries	122,000	125,000	−3,000	−2.4%	F
Health insurance	67,000	67,000	0	0.0%	F
Social security	50,500	49,955	546	1.1%	%
Retirement	66,000	65,300	700	1.1%	%
Unemployment	6,500	6,530	−30	−0.5%	%
Medical supplies	68,000	62,000	6,000	9.7%	V_{Total}
Office supplies	25,500	25,000	500	2.0%	V_{Total}
Housekeeping supplies	12,750	12,800	−50	−0.4%	F
Depreciation	21,000	21,000	0	0.0%	F
Interest	9,750	9,750	0	0.0%	F
Total Operating Expenses	$983,000	$972,335	$10,666	1.1%	

Semmelweis is over budget on total visits, revenue, and expenses, and the net effect of these differences is a $9,166 reduction in anticipated net income—that is, the increase in revenue, $1,500, was less than the increase in expenses, $10,666. Due to the lower-than-expected income, the clinic manager must determine why expenses increased more than seven times faster than revenues.

Variance analysis will be performed for line items more than $5,000 over budget (highlighted in Table 15.7), which include RN salaries and medical supplies. RN salaries should vary with the number of physician visits, so with actual visits being less than budgeted, RN salary expense should fall by $19.35 per visit, $149,000 ÷ 7,700. The volume variance indicates RN salary expense should have declined by $968 due to lower-than-expected output, (7,650 actual visits − budgeted 7,700 visits) × $19.35. Given RN salaries were $7,500 higher than budgeted, the cost variance must be positive. The cost variance is $8,468, (($156,500 ÷ 7,650 actual visits) − ($149,000 ÷ 7,700 budgeted visits)) × 7,650 actual visits or ($20.46 − $19.55) × 7,650.

RN salaries increased because the cost per actual visit was $0.91, $20.46 − $19.55, higher than expected. The cost variance is primarily due to the $9,599 price variance, (($156,000 ÷ 4,200) − ($149,000 ÷ 4,260)) × 4,200 hours. RNs were paid $2.29 more per hour than budgeted. The increase in RN wage was partially offset by RNs using less time per visit. The efficiency variance is −$1,131, ((4,200 ÷ 7,650) − (4,260 ÷ 7,700) × $34.98 budgeted hourly wage × 7,650 physician visits. Determining the cause of the higher hourly wage, the price variance, and lower time per visit, the efficiency variance, requires more investigation. The sum of the volume and cost variance equals the total variance, −$968 + $8,468 = $7,500.

Medical supplies is the other line item more than $5,000 over budget and was expected to vary with total visits rather than physician visits. Total visits increased due to the increase in therapy visits, so we should expect medical supply expenses to increase. The volume variance indicates that medical supplies should have increased by $250 due to higher-than-expected output, (12,450 actual visits − 12,400 budgeted visits) × ($62,000 ÷ 12,400 budgeted visits) or 50 additional, unbudgeted visits at a cost of $5.00 each. The increase was more than expected, so the cost variance again is positive. The cost variance is $5,750, (($68,000 ÷ 12,450 actual visits) − ($65,300 ÷ 12,400 budgeted visits)) × 12,450 actual visits or ($5.46 − $5.00) × 12,450. Medical supply expense increased primarily due to paying $0.46 more per visit than expected.

Medical supply costs increased because the cost per supply was $0.31, ($5.31 − $5.00), higher than expected. The price variance was $4,000, (($68,000 ÷ 12,450) − ($149,000 ÷ 4,260)) × 12,800 supply units. In addition, more supplies were used per visit,. The efficiency variance is $1,750, ((12,800 ÷ 12,450) − (12,400 ÷ 12,400) × $5.00 budgeted supply cost × 12,450 total patient visits. Determining the cause of the higher per-unit supply cost, the price variance, and higher amount of supplies used per visit, the

efficiency variance, requires more investigation. Again, the sum of the volume and cost variances equals the total variance.

Two additional line items will be examined to flesh out the role of variance analysis. The first is physician salaries. Physicians are a fixed cost in that the doctors are paid a salary independent of hours worked. Physician salaries were under budget by $2,500. The volume variance indicates that had they been paid on visits they would have earned $1,721 less due to the lower number of visits, (7,650 actual visits − 7,700 budgeted visits) × ($265,000 ÷ 7,700 budgeted visits) or −50 × $34.42. That is, physicians were budgeted to receive an average of $34.42 per visit, but they delivered 50 fewer visits. The cost variance shows that physicians were paid only $34.31 per visit, $262,500 ÷ 7,650 actual visits, rather than the $34.42 expected in the budget, reducing their actual salaries by $779.

The last line item we will examine is therapist salaries. Therapy visits are higher than expected, and they were paid $1,000 more than budgeted. The volume variance indicates that therapist salaries should have increased by $2,426 due to providing 100 more visits than expected, (4,800 actual visits − 4,700 budgeted visits) × ($114,000 ÷ 4,700 budgeted visits) or $24.26 per visit. The increase was less than expected. The actual variance was only $1,000, so the cost variance must be negative. The cost variance is −$968, (($115,000 ÷ 4,800 actual visits) − ($114,000 ÷ 4700 budgeted visits)) × 4,800 actual visits or ($23.96 − $24.26) × 4,800. Saving $0.30 per visit reduced therapist salaries by $1,426. Again, the manager must determine if the $0.30 savings per visit is due to paying therapists a lower hourly wage or therapists taking less time per visit. **Table 15.8** summarizes the variance analysis for the four line items examined.

The totals in Table 15.8 show that the primary cause of spending more for RN salaries and medical supplies is wages and supply cost (cost per input) was higher than budgeted. Efficiency (inputs per visit) and volume (visits) accounted for a small percent of the total variance.

Variance analysis does not tell us the cause of budget variance but rather guides us to potential causes (i.e., is overspending the budget due to higher output, higher resource prices, using more

Table 15.8 **Variance Analysis Summary for Semmelweis Clinic**

Line Item	Price	Efficiency	Volume	Total
Physician salaries	−$2,500	$1,721	−$1,721	−$2,500
RN salaries	9,599	−1,131	−968	7,500
Therapy salaries	−213	−1,213	2,426	1,000
Medical supplies	4,000	1,750	250	6,000
Total	$10,886	$1,127	−$13	$12,000

resources per output, or a combination of all three?). Variance analysis is a powerful tool that all managers should master. All managers are evaluated on their ability to manage a budget. When their area(s) go over budget, they must (or should) identify and take corrective action on controllable factors and quantify the increase in costs due to noncontrollable factors such as volume increases, increases in market prices for resources, and/or sicker patients requiring more labor and/or supplies.

In closing, when should variances be investigated? Revenues and expenses will fluctuate within some type of normal range, and being over budget one month may be offset by being under budget in a subsequent month. The trick is to separate normal randomness from those factors requiring correction. The manager would be well advised to calculate the cost and benefit of performing a variance analysis before commencing the analysis. In many cases, variances are not investigated unless they exceed a dollar threshold (e.g., more than $5,000 over budget) and/or a percent threshold (more than 10% over budget).

Sensitivity Analysis Overview

Sensitivity analysis is a "what if" proposition (i.e., what may happen to net income if major assumptions change or predicted events do not occur). The "what if" feature allows managers to plan for a variety of possibilities in different scenarios.

Forecasts should be subjected to sensitivity analysis. As previously defined, a forecast is a view of the organization's future. The future cannot be predicted with absolute precision, so forecasts will contain a degree of uncertainty. "What if" analysis is important to managers' decision-making; for example, "*What* will the radiology department's operating income be *if* the department's revenue is 10% greater than expected?" or "*What* will the radiology department's operating income be *if* the department's revenue is 10% less than expected?"

A common form of sensitivity analysis computes three levels of a variable such as a revenue forecast: the most likely, the planned outcome; a best case (high revenue); and a worst case (low revenue). A chart illustrating the three potential outcomes for revenue appears in Figure 15.5.

Sensitivity Analysis Tools

Managers' tools involving sensitivity analysis that are described in this section include most likely, best- and worst-case scenarios, the **contribution margin** and the contribution income statement; and finding the breakeven point using the contribution margin method.

Contribution Margin and the Contribution Income Statement

The contribution income statement specifically identifies the contribution margin within the income statement format. You will recall that the contribution margin is the difference between revenue and variable costs. The remaining difference is available to cover fixed costs and increase operating income after fixed costs are paid.

For example, assume 100 units are sold at $50 each for a total of $5,000 revenue. Further, assume variable costs amount to $30 per unit. One hundred units have been sold, so variable costs amount to $3,000 (100 times $30 per unit = $3,000). The contribution margin equals $2,000 ($5,000 revenue less $3,000 variable costs). For a further discussion of the contribution margin, refer to Chapter 8 on cost behavior and break-even analysis. Now further assume that fixed costs in this example amount to $1,200. Therefore, the operating income will amount to $800 ($2,000 contribution margin less $1,200 equals $800). **Table 15.9** provides the worst-case, most likely, and best-case assumptions and the projected contribution margin and net income using the most likely assumptions for price, variable cost, and fixed cost while varying output.

If worst-case output occurs, assuming price, variable cost, and fixed costs meet the most likely assumptions, the organization will break even—contribution margin equals fixed cost. If best-case output is achieved, the organization will earn $1,400. You can see that sensitivity analysis allows an analyst to alter one or more variables to determine the effect on net income.

Break-Even Point Using the Contribution Margin Method

You will recall that the break-even point is the point at which operating revenues and costs equal each other and operating income is zero. A graph method illustrates the break-even point (which was previously discussed in Chapter 8, "Cost Behavior and Break-Even Analysis"). In this sensitivity analysis section, we will describe another method to determine the break-even point. It is called the "contribution margin method." The advantage of this method is its transparency. The manager can easily explain his or her results because the computations can be easily seen and understood.

It is understood that operating income is zero at the break-even point. It follows, then, that the number of units at the break-even point can be computed. The formula is

$$\text{Break-Even Number of Units} = \frac{\text{Fixed Costs}}{\text{Contribution margin per Unit}}$$

To compute the contribution margin per unit, subtract the variable costs per unit from the sales price per unit. In the target operating income formula inputs as previously described, the sales price per unit

Table 15.9 Sensitivity Analysis

Assumptions	Worst Case	Most Likely	Best Case
Output	70	100	130
Price	$45	$50	$55
Variable Cost	$35	$30	$25
Fixed Cost	$1,500	$1,200	$1,000
	Worst Case	Most Likely	Best Case
Output	60	100	130
Revenue	$3,000	$5,000	$6,500
Variable Cost	$1,800	$3,000	$3,900
Contribution Margin	$1,200	$2,000	$2,600
Fixed Cost	$1,200	$1,200	$1,200
Net Income	$0	$800	$1,400

Table 15.10 Proving the Break-Even Output

Break-Even Output	60	
Revenue	$3,000	($50 × 60 units)
Variable Cost	$1,800	($30 × 60 units)
Contribution Margin	$1,200	
Fixed Cost	$1,200	
Net Income	$0	

was $50, the variable costs per unit were $30, and the contribution margin per unit is $20, $50 − $30. Given fixed costs of $1,200, break-even output is

$$\text{Break-even output} = \frac{\$1,200}{(\$50-30)} = \frac{\$1,200}{\$20} = \$60$$

Table 15.10 shows an income statement to prove this formula's results. Creating an income statement is a great way to check your conclusion and catch math errors.

Managers may feel even more confident in pursuing this project as the break-even output, 60, is lower than the worse-case output prediction, 70, developed earlier. Furthermore, Table 15.9 highlights that even if output is at its expected minimum, the organization will still break even. Sensitivity analysis is designed to assess the risk surrounding an investment. In this case, the manager should be confident that this investment will not lose money, should earn $800, and could earn $1,400 if favorable conditions occur.

WRAP-UP

Summary

Variance analysis is designed to examine differences between actual and budgeted expenses to improve operations. Variance analysis allows managers to determine if actual expenses exceed the budget due to higher output (volume variance) or higher cost per output (cost variance). When managers know the quantity of resources used, they can break the cost variance into the amount due to increases or decreases in resource prices (price variance) and changes in the amount of resources used (efficiency variances). Managers should be able to identify expense increases due to controllable and uncontrollable factors and take effective action to minimize the financial impact of controllable factors.

Sensitivity analysis is designed to assess the degree of risk in a financial investment. The expected return on a financial investment is based on assumptions about output, revenue, and expenses. Sensitivity analysis allows a manager to assess the return based on different assumptions (i.e., will the investment be worthwhile if output and revenues are lower than expected and expenses are higher?). Break-even analysis asks how much actual output can fall below expected output before an organization will not recover its investment. Sensitivity analysis is a useful and flexible tool for planning purposes. It is used again in Chapter 19, "Constructing a Capital Budget."

Key Terms

Contribution Margin
Cost and Volume
 (Two-Variance)
Cost Variance

Efficiency Variance
Price, Efficiency, and Volume
 (Three-Variance)
Price Variance

Variance Analysis
Volume Variance

Discussion Questions

1. Explain the role of variance analysis.
2. Explain the four ways managers can compare the financial performance of their areas of responsibility.
3. Explain what volume, cost, price, and efficiency variances measure.
4. Explain the role of sensitivity analysis and describe how it is performed.
5. Explain how a contribution margin and break-even output are calculated.

Problems

1. Using the following table, calculate the volume and cost variances for the pediatric nursing unit at Codman Medical Center. Is the overage due primarily to volume or cost increases? Salaries account for $6,200 of the total variance of $9,100. Explain why salaries and benefits cost $6,200 more than budgeted.

Expense	2022 YTD Actual	2022 YTD Budget	$ Difference	% Difference
Salaries and Wages	$175,200	$169,000	$6,200	3.7%
Fringe Benefits	69,200	68,000	1,200	1.8%
Supplies	126,000	124,000	2,000	1.6%
Depreciation	25,000	24,000	1,000	4.2%
Interest	8,400	9,000	−600	−6.7%
Other	109,300	110,000	−700	−0.6%
Total Expenses	$513,100	$504,000	$9,100	1.8%
Patient Days	47,700	47,200	500	1.1%

2. Using the following table, calculate the volume, price, and efficiency variances for salaries and wages, fringe benefits, and supplies for the pediatric nursing unit at Codman Medical Center. The efficiency variance for salaries and wages and fringe benefits should be based on paid hours. The efficiency variance for supplies should be based on supply units. Explain each variance for salaries and benefits and supplies so others can understand why these two line items accounted for $8,200 of the total $9,200 variance.

Expense	2022 YTD Actual	2022 YTD Budget	$ Difference	% Difference
Salaries and wages	$175,200	$169,000	$6,200	3.7%
Fringe benefits	69,200	68,000	1,200	1.8%
Supplies	126,000	124,000	2,000	1.6%
Depreciation	25,000	24,000	1,000	4.2%

(continues)

Expense	2022 YTD Actual	2022 YTD Budget	$ Difference	% Difference
Interest	8,400	9,000	−600	−6.7%
Other	109,300	110,000	−700	−0.6%
Total Expenses	$513,100	$504,000	$9,100	1.8%
Patient Days	47,700	47,200	500	1.1%
Paid Hours	5,078	4,829	249	5.2%
Supply Units	66,303	68,440	(2,137)	−3.1%

3. The Fleming Medical Group financial results are under budget for the first six months of 2022. Using the following table, calculate the volume, revenue, and cost variances for all variances greater than $5,000. What is the primary cause of the negative $40,186 net income variance? Explain the major cause behind the $54,936 increase in expenses.

Description	YTD 2022 Actual	YTD 2022 Budget	$ Difference	% Difference
Revenue	$2,964,750	$2,950,000	$14,750	0.5%
Operating Expenses				
Physician salaries	$585,306	$576,800	$8,506	1.5%
Nursing salaries	857,157	829,150	28,007	3.4%
Mgt and clerical salaries	466,971	468,650	(1,679)	−0.4%
FICA	143,397	143,407	(10)	0.0%
Health insurance	238,760	234,325	4,435	1.9%
Retirement	76,763	74,984	1,779	2.4%
Unemployment	18,323	18,746	(423)	−2.3%
Medications	91,687	89,015	2,672	3.0%
Medical instruments	64,287	61,761	2,526	4.1%
Bandages, gauze...	34,140	34,529	(389)	−1.1%
Gloves, gowns...	24,476	24,283	193	0.8%
Sterile wipes	15,780	16,114	(334)	−2.1%
Office supplies	69,388	69,216	172	0.2%

Description	YTD 2022 Actual	YTD 2022 Budget	$ Difference	% Difference
Cleaning supplies	23,103	23,461	(358)	–1.5%
Rent	89,251	86,520	2,731	3.2%
Maintenance	11,245	8,270	2,975	36.0%
Electricity	6,684	6,482	202	3.1%
Gas	11,215	11,118	97	0.9%
Water and sewage	4,225	4,059	166	4.1%
Telephone	2,004	1,939	65	3.4%
Housekeeping	21,694	21,630	64	0.3%
Travel/meetings/meals	4,744	4,751	(7)	–0.1%
Prof insurance	15,669	13,447	2,222	16.5%
CME	17,994	17,938	56	0.3%
Other expenses	35,955	34,687	1,268	3.7%
	$2,930,218	$2,875,282	$54,936	1.9%
Net income	$34,532	$74,718	($40,186)	–53.8%
Profit margin	1.16%	2.53%		
Output	**Actual**	**Budget**	**Difference**	**% Difference**
Visits	15,451	15,408	43	0.3%

4. Using the following table, calculate the volume, price, and efficiency variances for all variances greater than $5,000 in the Fleming Medical Group. The efficiency variance for salaries should be based on paid hours. The efficiency variance for medications should be based on medications dispensed. Explain each variance for physician and nursing salaries so others can understand why these two line items accounted for $36,513 of the total $54,936 total expense variance.

Description	YTD 2022 Actual	YTD 2022 Budget	$ Difference	% Difference
Revenue	$2,964,750	$2,950,000	$14,750	0.5%
Expenses				
Physician salaries	$585,306	$576,800	$8,506	1.5%
Nursing salaries	857,157	829,150	$28,007	3.4%
Mgt and clerical salaries	466,971	468,650	($1,679)	–0.4%

(continues)

Description	YTD 2022 Actual	YTD 2022 Budget	$ Difference	% Difference
FICA	143,397	143,407	($10)	0.0%
Health insurance	238,760	234,325	$4,435	1.9%
Retirement	76,763	74,984	$1,779	2.4%
Unemployment	18,323	18,746	($423)	−2.3%
Medications	91,687	89,015	$2,672	3.0%
Medical instruments	64,287	61,761	$2,526	4.1%
Bandages, gauze...	34,140	34,529	($389)	−1.1%
Gloves, gowns...	24,476	24,283	$193	0.8%
Sterile wipes	15,780	16,114	($334)	−2.1%
Office supplies	69,388	69,216	$172	0.2%
Cleaning supplies	23,103	23,461	($358)	−1.5%
Rent	89,251	86,520	$2,731	3.2%
Maintenance	11,245	8,270	$2,975	36.0%
Electricity	6,684	6,482	$202	3.1%
Gas	11,215	11,118	$97	0.9%
Water and sewage	4,225	4,059	$166	4.1%
Telephone	2,004	1,939	$65	3.4%
Housekeeping	21,694	21,630	$64	0.3%
Travel/meetings/ meals	4,744	4,751	($7)	−0.1%
Prof Insurance	15,669	13,447	$2,222	16.5%
CME	17,994	17,938	$56	0.3%
Other expenses	35,955	34,687	$1,268	3.7%
	$2,930,218	$2,875,282	$54,936	1.9%
Net income	$34,532	$74,718	($40,186)	−53.8%
Profit margin	1.16%	2.53%	−1.37%	−54.0%
Output	**Actual**	**Budget**	**Difference**	**% Difference**
Visits	15,451	15,408	43	0.3%
Inputs used	**Actual**	**Budget**	**Difference**	**% Difference**
Physician hours	6,240	6,240	0	0.0%
Nursing hours	34,611	33,280	1,331	4.0%

Description	YTD 2022 Actual	YTD 2022 Budget	$ Difference	% Difference
Mgt and clerical hours	11,200	11,440	−240	−2.1%
Medications dispensed	17,464	17,803	−339	−1.9%

Notes

1. S. A. Finkler, "Flexible Budget Variance Analysis Extended to Patient Acuity and DRGs," *Health Care Management Review*, 10, no. 4 (1985): 21–34.
2. T. K. Ross, *A Comprehensive Guide to Budgeting for Health Care Managers* (Burlington, MA: Jones and Bartlett Learning, 2018); T. K. Ross, *Practical Budgeting for Health Care, A Concise Guide* (Burlington, MA: Jones and Bartlett Learning, 2021).

CHAPTER 16

Benchmarking, Estimates, and Measurement Tools

PROGRESS NOTES

After completing this chapter, you should be able to:

1. Explain the reasons for using estimates.
2. Explain the purpose of benchmarking.
3. Describe the idea behind the Pareto rule.
4. Describe how quartiles are computed and how they should be used for management.

Overview: Assessing Performance

Life seldom provides a perfect standard to assess performance. Comparing the financial performance of different healthcare providers reveals the problems of size, location, specialty, goals, and so on. Similarly, assessing times for runners should consider a host of factors. The world record for running a mile is 3 minutes and 43 seconds. This standard is only appropriate for comparing the run times for professional male runners between the ages of 20 and 29. Excellence for older and younger nonprofessional males and females should be judged against longer completion times.

Improving future financial performance requires understanding existing performance. Managers must estimate the amount of output that may be sold, the prices that will be received

for the product, and the amount and price of resources needed to produce the output to construct a budget. Understanding the range in performance is vital. Has the organization performed in the top half of the industry, at the average, or in the bottom half on output, reimbursement, and costs, *and* is performance expected to improve, stay the same, or deteriorate? **Estimates** are also needed to construct financial statements—for example, determining the allowance for bad debt.

Estimates may be of the following:

- Amount
- Value
- Size

The first question should be "Is it capable of being estimated?" Relying on estimates for input to reports, financial statements, forecasts, budgets, internal monthly statements, and so on means sacrificing some degree of accuracy.

Common Uses of Estimates

Using estimates often involves trade-offs, such as gaining a quick answer that is less accurate. Four common reasons for using estimates are described here.

Timeliness Considerations

Deadlines may dictate the use of estimates because there is insufficient time to develop more accurate figures. Some managers call these "quick and dirty" results. The quick and dirty estimates may then be followed at a later date by a more detailed report.

Benefit and Cost Considerations

Situations arise where an estimate is adequate. The manager may decide upon using estimates instead of proceeding with a more formal forecasting process. After assessing the effort and time involved to gather and prepare a forecast, the manager may make a cost–benefit decision; is the cost of forecasting greater than or equal to the benefit of the more precise information, or will estimates adequately serve the purpose?

Lack of Data

Estimates must be used when there is no or not enough information available to prepare a full forecast. For example, how many units can be sold of a new service or to a previously unserved group of patients? There is no choice but to estimate.

Internal Monthly Statements

Estimates are commonly used to prepare short-term financial statements. For example, the monthly statements that managers receive often contain a number of estimates derived from various ratios and percentages. These estimates will probably have a historical basis because they are typically based on the organization's prior years' operating history. Thus, if bad debts for the past two years averaged 2%, the monthly statements for the current year may estimate bad debts at the same 2%.

Estimating the Economic Impact of Adding a New Specialty to a Physician Practice

Estimates can be extremely general, total revenue and expenses, or they can reflect considerable judgment, revenue and expense by line item that have been well thought out. **Figure 16.1** illustrates an example of a general estimate and its subsequent impact.

In this case, we have a four-doctor physician practice in which the doctors must decide whether to bring another doctor, a pulmonary specialist, into the practice. The county population and average income have grown faster than the country as a whole, and the local hospital has just expanded. The doctors determine there is a sufficient demand within this growing area to support the services of a pulmonary specialist. They believe adding a pulmonary specialist would benefit their patients by providing more services

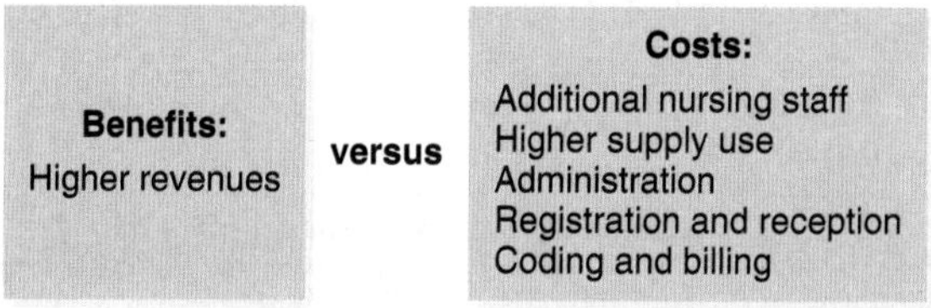

Benefits:
Higher revenues

versus

Costs:
Additional nursing staff
Higher supply use
Administration
Registration and reception
Coding and billing

Figure 16.1 Estimated Economic Impact of a New Pulmonary Specialist in a Physician Practice

at a single location but want to be confident that the addition will improve the financial performance of the practice.

One morning, the senior doctor asks the practice manager to estimate the expense involved in adding a pulmonary specialist to the practice. He wants the report for their four o'clock meeting that afternoon. They must make a decision quickly because the desired specialist has received another offer.

The practice manager is trying to close the books for the month but makes time to produce an estimate. The doctors already know the amount that the specialist wants as a guaranteed salary for the first year, and they have already projected the revenue that should be produced in the first year. The practice has an empty office available that was acquired in the initial lease for purposes of future expansion. The practice manager needs to estimate the impact on basic practice operational costs. His "quick and dirty" estimate is in two parts.

Part 1: Add one half-time RN for direct support and assume existing nursing staff can take up any slack and $30,000 for medical supplies.

Part 2: Assume an overall 10% increase in practice administration operating costs. He has no specific basis for the 10% estimate but knows that labor is the greatest part of practice administration costs. As a result of his "back of the envelope" calculation, he thinks that administrative staff is not overworked at present and can handle tasks imposed by an additional physician. Since he does not think adding any administrative staff is needed, he feels that an overall 10% increase for administrative expenses of the practice is adequate.

Three months after the pulmonary specialist has joined the practice, the senior doctor meets with the practice manager to discuss the financial performance to date. Operational costs to absorb the new specialist have far exceeded the original estimate. The doctors want an explanation from the practice manager for their meeting the next afternoon.

The practice manager realizes that his estimate did not allow for startup costs. He composes a memo explaining that the administrative expenses were impacted by startup costs such as coder training for the new pulmonary codes, the consultants'

fees for the new super-bill setup in the office software, training about pulmonary services for the medical records transcriptionist, and training for the office biller regarding the new codes. He also notes that the front office problems arising from increased patient intake had been underestimated. While explaining the lower-than-expected performance for the first three months is important, the office manager should provide the outlook for the next quarter including expectations for patient visits, reimbursement, and expenses and the resolution of front office, coding, and billing problems.

Other Estimates

Other commonly used computations are actually estimates including bad debt, interest rates, malpractice costs, and so on. The weighted average inventory method is a good example (see Chapter 10). Weighted average cost is determined by dividing the cost of goods available for sale by the number of units available. The resulting average cost of inventory is in fact an estimate.

Importance of a Variety of Performance Measures

A variety of **performance measures** must be in place if operations are to be effectively managed. Generally, a broad variety of such measures are available, and different organizations tend to lean toward using one type over another. Generally speaking, a wider variety of performance measures are evident in organizations that have adopted a total quality approach. The acronym SQTCM typifies the wider perspective, S = safety, Q = quality, T = timeliness, C = cost, and M = morale (employee). Managers should develop one or more measures to monitor their performance in each area. One healthcare organization, for example, may rely heavily on one type of measure, whereas another organization may rely on a different measurement profile. Given that this is a finance text, we will focus on cost measures, but issues of patient and employee satisfaction should not be ignored, as failure in these areas will undermine an organization's competitiveness.

Adjusted Performance Measures Over Time

We have previously discussed how tracking measures over time is necessary to evaluate the use of money. The example in **Figure 16.2** combines a financial measure, the cost per discharge, with an acuity measure. **Case mix adjustment** refers to adjusting measures for the acuity level of the patient (i.e., the number of complications or comorbidities a patient has). Medicare inpatient reimbursement increases with the acuity of the patient as it has been shown that the level of resources required to provide care for patients increases with the acuity level. The vertical axis reports cost per discharge, and the horizontal axis tracks performance over five years. Two measures are plotted: The first is cost unadjusted for case mix, and the second adjusts for case mix. Unadjusted cost rises over the five-year period, while the case mix adjusted cost flattens out over time.

Figure 16.2 shows that the cost per discharge is rising over time, but the increase was driven by the higher level of care needed by patients. After adjusting for patient acuity, the cost of treatment has increased by less than 1% per year.

Benchmarking

Benchmarking is or should be the continuous process of measuring products, services, and activities against industry averages or best-in-class performance. Best-in-class performance may be found inside or outside an organization's industry (e.g., a hospital seeking to improve its food or housekeeping services may look to the food service or hotel industries for performance measures). Benchmarks are used to measure performance gaps.

There are three types of benchmarks:

1. A financial variable reported in an accounting system
2. A financial variable not reported in an accounting system
3. A nonfinancial variable

How to Benchmark

Benchmarking involves the identification of processes producing superior outcomes and adapting these processes for use in your organization. The benchmarking method is predicated on the assumption that a superior, if not an exemplary, process similar to the process being examined

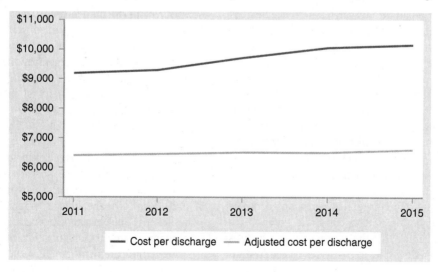

Figure 16.2 Cost per Discharge and Case Mix Adjusted Discharge

can be identified and examined to improve performance. Benchmarking can be accomplished in one of several ways, including (1) studying the methods and end results of your prime competitors, (2) examining the analogous process of noncompetitors with a world-class reputation, and (3) analyzing processes within your own organization or health system that are worthy of being emulated. In any of these three cases, the necessary analysis will rely on one or both of the following methods: parametric analysis or process analysis. In parametric analysis, the characteristics or attributes of similar services or products are examined. In process analysis, the process that serves

as a standard for comparison is examined in detail to learn how and why it performs the way it does. Benchmarking is used to identify opportunities for improvement (i.e., information about the way things should or possibly could be).

Benchmarking in Health Care

Financial benchmarking compares financial measures among groups. One of the most common types of comparison is industry averages, as seen in **Table 16.1**. Optum360° compiled the data in Table 16.1 and also provides more specific benchmarks

Table 16.1 Financial Ratio and Operating Indicator Hospital Benchmarks

Financial Ratios	Median	25th	75th
Total Margin	4.4%	–0.2%	9.7%
Operating Margin	3.8%	–0.8%	9.1%
Return on Equity (ROE)	8.4%	1.2%	18.0%
Return on Assets (ROA)	4.5%	–0.1%	10.4%
Days in Accounts Receivable	56.1	46.8	70.5
Equity Financing	57.5%	35.2%	79.2%
Times Interest Earned	4.7	0.9	13.1
Total Asset Turnover	1.2	0.8	1.7
Current Asset Turnover	3.7	2.4	5.1
Fixed Asset Turnover	2.7	1.9	4.3
Operating Indicators	**Median**	**25th**	**75th**
Occupancy	55.3%	39.0%	68.4%
Discharges per Bed	33.0	17.4	47.5
Adjusted ALOS	2.7	2.4	3.0
Medicare % Discharges	40.3%	30.0%	52.9%
Medicaid % Discharges	5.7%	1.9%	12.9%
Outpatient Revenue %	58.4%	44.2%	71.5%
Salaries per Adjusted Discharge	$2,382	$1,982	$2,866
FTE's per Occupied Bed	3.7	3.2	4.3
Salaries as % of Total Expense	39.8%	34.6%	44.7%
Deductible Ratio	62.7%	48.8%	72.0%

based on location (region of the country and urban or rural), number of beds, ownership status, and teaching programs so managers can compare their organization with a more relevant peer group.[1] The computation of ratios included in this report was discussed in Chapter 12. The computation of **quartiles**, the thresholds for organizations operating in the top and bottom 25% of their industry, is described later in this chapter.

Statistical benchmarking is a related method of benchmarking. In this case, the statistics of utilization and service delivery (i.e., operating indicators on which inflow and outflow are based) are compared with those of certain other hospitals.

Examining operating margin and total asset turnover leads to an interesting conclusion. Operating margin averages 3.8%, but 25% of hospitals earn –0.8% or less (i.e., more than 25% of hospitals lose money). Twenty-five percent of hospitals earn 9.1% or more, and thus the high margins of successful organizations offset the losses of organizations in the bottom 25% to produce the 3.8% average. Total asset turnover indicates that the difference in profitability may be related to revenue, as the top 25% produce $1.70 of revenue for every $1.00 in assets versus $0.80 of revenue in the bottom quartile (i.e., organizations in the top 25th percentile earned more than twice as much revenue per dollar of investment in assets than organizations in the 75th percentile).

The difference in profitability may also be related to costs and patient mix. The percent of admissions reimbursed by Medicaid is dramatically different between the top and bottom quartiles. While the average is 5.7% of admission, Hospitals in the top quartile serves 12.9% or more Medicaid patients, while the bottom quartile services 1.9% or less. A high percent of Medicaid patients reduces average reimbursement and thus operating margins. Salaries per adjusted discharge are at least 44.6%, $2,866 ÷ $1,982, higher for hospitals in the 75th percentile, probably those with negative operating margins, than for those in the 25th percentile, who may be earning 9.1% or more. While patient mix may be uncontrollable, managers should strive to hold down costs and maximize revenue to ensure the financial viability of their organizations.

In summary, benchmarking is a comparative method that assists in evaluating an organization's performance. Objective measures (i.e., performance gaps) are often required to motivate employees to elevate their performance and achieve better outcomes.

Compare to Industry Standards

The CFO of Codman Medical Center wants to assess his organization's operating margin. Codman has an operating margin of 3.8%, equal to the national average. However, he knows that 25% of hospitals earn over 9.1% and that other factors should be considered such as whether a hospital is located in an urban area and affiliated with a health system. **Figure 16.3** supplies some relevant benchmarks.

If Codman is located in an urban area and affiliated with health system, the CFO may conclude that financial performance should be improved as Codman's operating margin is 28.2%, –1.5% ÷ 5.2%, lower than the average for system affiliated hospitals. Likewise, its operating margin is 17.0%, –0.8% ÷ 4.5%, below the average for urban hospitals. If Codman is an independent, rural hospital, its operating margin is 71.7%, 1.6% ÷ 2.2%, above the average for non-system hospitals and 39.8%, 1.1% ÷ 2.7%, above the average for rural hospitals. The point is managers must choose an appropriate peer group for comparison. If Codman is an independent, rural hospital, improving performance may be difficult if it wants to remain independent. On the other hand, managers should identify and correct the factor(s) leading to low performance if Codman is an urban hospital and part of health system. The first step toward better performance is establishing credible benchmarks so employees understand the financial strengths and weaknesses of their organization.

Healthcare organizations are particularly well suited to use industry standards because both the federal and state governments release a wealth of public information and statistics regarding the provision of health care.

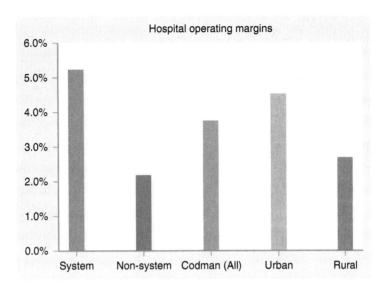

Figure 16.3 Codman's Operating Margin Compared with Industry Benchmarks

Measurement Tools

Pareto Analysis

Creating benchmarks, especially in an organization committed to continuous quality improvement, ultimately leads managers to explore how to improve one or more steps in a process. **Pareto analysis** is an analytical tool that employs the Pareto principle and helps in this exploration. Vilfredo Pareto was a 19th-century economist who was a pioneer in applying mathematics to economic theory. The Pareto principle states that 80% of events arise from 20% the potential causes, thus the "80/20 Rule." For example, 80% of the medication errors in a hospital may involve 20% of the medications dispensed.

The usual way to display a Pareto analysis is through the construction of a Pareto diagram. A Pareto diagram displays the important causes of variation, as reflected in data collected on the causes of such variation. **Table 16.2** provides data on the number of inpatient claim denials for Codman Medical Center. **Figure 16.4** presents inpatient claim denials in a Pareto diagram and reinforces the idea behind the Pareto analysis that the majority of

Table 16.2 Inpatient Claim Denials

Problem	Denied Claims	% of Denials
Diagnosis or procedure code error	162	41.6%
Not medically necessary	114	29.3%
Lack of preauthorization	65	16.7%
Submitted after deadline	19	4.9%
Out of network provider	8	2.1%
Other	21	5.4%
Total	389	100.0%

claim denials are due to a small number of identifiable causes (i.e., diagnosis and procedure code errors and lack of medical necessity).

The CFO of Codman Medical Center believes the billing and collection department is inefficient—or, to be more specific, that the process

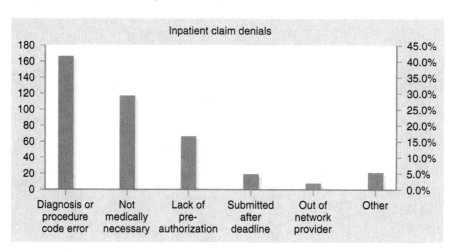

Figure 16.4 Pareto Analysis of Billing Department Data

is probably inefficient. Based on Figure 16.4, some of the inefficiency is due to billing personnel spending too much time on unproductive work (i.e., rebilling claims). The Pareto diagram indicates that the major causes of denied claims may lie outside the billing and collection area. Improvement may require coordination with medical records and registration areas to reduce the top two causes for denied claims. Resubmitting denied bills is an inefficient and nonproductive activity and also delays payment for services.

Constructing a Pareto diagram is straightforward. The first step is to prepare a table that shows the activities recorded, the number of times the activities were observed, and the percentage of the total number of times represented by each count. In Figure 16.4, the total number of times inpatient claims were denied was 389. The number of times that inpatient claims were denied for diagnostic or procedure code errors was 162. Thus, diagnostic or procedure code errors account for 41.6%, 162 ÷ 389, of inpatient billing problems. Similar calculations complete the table.

The Pareto diagram has two vertical axes, the left one corresponding to the number of denied claims column in the table and the right one corresponding to the percent of denials. On the

horizontal axis, the reasons for denial are listed, creating bases of equal length for the rectangles shown in the diagram. The activities are listed in decreasing order of occurrence (i.e., the most frequently observed activity lies on the left extreme of the diagram and the least frequently observed activity on the right extreme). The heights of the rectangles show the frequencies of the activities.

Adding the denials for diagnostic and procedure code errors and lack of medical necessity shows these two problems account for 71.0% of denied claims, not quite the 80% suggested by the Pareto rule. Pareto analysis highlights the substantial improvement that can be realized if these two problems can be reduced.

Pareto charts highlight the activities requiring priority attention—the "vital few"— on the left of the diagram. Pareto diagrams are often constructed before and after improvement efforts for comparative purposes. When the improvements are effective, the height of the bars, if not the order of the bars, will change.

Many authorities recommend that Pareto analysis take the costs of the activities into account (i.e., instead of the number of denied claims, the horizontal axis would measure the total cost of denied claims). The concern is that a commonly occurring problem may nevertheless cost less than a relatively rare but disastrous problem. Also, before basing a Pareto analysis on frequencies, as this example does, the analyst needs to decide that the seriousness of the problem is roughly proportional to the frequency. If seriousness fails to satisfy this criterion, then activities should be measured in some other way.

Quartile Computation

Reporting data by quartiles is an effective way to show ranges of either financial or statistical results. Quartiles divide events into four classes, each of which contains one-quarter of the whole. Each of the four classes is a quartile. Quartile computation is not very complicated, although several steps are involved. We can use occupancy in Table 16.1 to illustrate the computation of quartile data. We see from the first line that 500 hospitals were used for benchmarking. The median, 55.3%, means half of hospitals have an occupancy rate above 55.3% and half lower. The median is easy to identify—when hospitals are sorted from highest to lowest occupancy, the median is the midpoint. Percentages are then arrayed; in this case, cutoffs were then arranged into three groups. The percentages that were between 0% and 25% are designated

as the low-quartile group, those between 25 and 75% are designated as the mid-quartile groups, and those between 75% and 100% are designated as the upper-quartile group.

The average (also known as the arithmetic mean) of each quartile group is then presented in this report. Thus, occupancy for the upper-quartile group is 68.4% or more, 55.3% to 68.4% for the second quartile, 39.0% to 55.3% for the third quartile, and 39.3% or lower for the low-quartile group. Quartiles supply greater information than averages. Managers can only determine if performance is above or below average when only an average is available. Quartiles allow managers to determine if performance is in the top or bottom 25%. Deciles, which separate performance by 10%, supply greater information and indicate the degree of potential improvement. For example, if your hospital's operating margin is 14.7% or more, it is in the top 10% in profitability' conversely, the bottom 10% loses 5.9% or more. The managers at Codman thus know if they want to perform in the top 25% of the industry, they must increase their operating margin from 3.8% to 9.1%. If their goal is to perform in the top 10%, they must increase it to 14.7%.

WRAP-UP

Summary

Estimates are widely used in finance to assess performance when timely information is more important than accurate information or when data are unavailable. Managers also use estimates to assess the financial risk associated with new undertakings.

After performance measures are collected or estimated, managers require benchmarks to assess how their department or organization is performing. Use of industry averages provides a starting point to determine if performance is above or below average, but managers should seek more appropriate benchmarks—that is, performance should be judged against similar organizations when this information is available. Managers should master Pareto analysis to identify the factors that comprise the largest number of events and quartiles to determine how far above (or below) average an organization performs.

Key Terms

Benchmarking
Case Mix Adjustment

Estimates
Pareto Analysis

Performance Measures
Quartiles

Discussion Questions

1. Explain the reasons for using estimates.
2. Explain the purpose of financial benchmarking.

3. Describe the idea behind the Pareto rule.
4. Describe how quartiles are computed and how they should be used for management.

Problems

1. Given the following table, assess Mercy Hospital against the benchmarks for urban teaching hospitals. Explain Mercy Hospital's strengths and weaknesses in profitability, liquidity, capital structure, and turnover.

Profitability	Mercy Hospital	Median	25th	75th
Total Margin	4.7%	4.4%	−0.2%	9.7%
Operating Margin	4.2%	3.8%	−0.8%	9.1%
ROA	4.2%	4.5%	1.2%	18.0%
ROE	8.9%	8.4%	−0.1%	10.4%
Liquidity				
Days in AR	69.2	56.1	46.8	70.5
Capital Structure				
Times Interest Earned	3.25	4.7	0.9	13.1
Equity Financing	47.6%	57.5%	35.2%	79.2%
Turnover				
Total Asset Turnover	0.90	1.2	0.8	1.7
Current Asset Turnover	2.57	3.7	2.4	5.1
Fixed Asset Turnover	1.38	2.7	1.9	4.3

2. Given the following table, assess Redwood Hospital against the benchmarks for community hospitals. Explain Redwood Hospital's strengths and weaknesses in profitability, liquidity, capital structure, and turnover.

Profitability	Redwood Hospital	Median	25th	75th
Total Margin	3.4%	4.4%	−5.0%	8.7%
Operating Margin	2.3%	3.8%	−1.1%	7.5%
ROA	3.0%	4.5%	0.1%	9.0%
ROE	5.6%	8.4%	−0.2%	16.8%
Liquidity				
Days in AR	55.9	59.5	42.5	72.4
Capital Structure				
Times Interest Earned	2.75	3.70	0.10	10.90
Equity Financing	55.8%	51.8%	37.6%	75.8%
Turnover				
Total Asset Turnover	1.1	1.1	0.9	1.8
Current Asset Turnover	2.4	3.4	2.5	4.6
Fixed Asset Turnover	1.8	2.6	1.8	3.9

3. Given the following table, assess Mercy Hospital against the benchmarks for urban teaching hospitals, and so on. Explain Mercy Hospital's strengths and weaknesses in occupancy, payer mix, service mix, and labor use. Identify two areas you would recommend for improvement and explain why these two areas should be given priority.

Operating Indicators	Mercy Hospital	Median	25th	75th
Occupancy	64.3%	55.3%	39.0%	68.4%
Discharges per Bed	37.2	33.0	17.4	47.5
Adjusted ALOS	2.8	2.7	2.4	3.0

(continues)

Operating Indicators	Mercy Hospital	Median	25th	75th
Medicare % Discharges	44.9%	40.3%	30.0%	52.9%
Medicaid % Discharges	5.2%	5.7%	1.9%	12.9%
Outpatient Revenue %	62.3%	58.4%	44.2%	71.5%
Salaries per Adjusted Discharge	$2,696	$2,382	$1,982	$2,866
FTEs per Occupied Bed	3.6	3.7	3.2	4.3
Salaries as % of Total Expense	42.70%	39.8%	34.6%	44.7%
Deductible Ratio	63.10%	62.7%	48.8%	72.0%

4. Given the following table, assess Redwood Hospital against the benchmarks for community hospitals. Explain Redwood Hospital's strengths and weaknesses in occupancy, payer mix, service mix, and labor use. Identify two areas you would recommend for improvement and explain why these two areas should be given priority.

Operating Indicators	Redwood Hospital	Median	25th	75th
Occupancy	52.4%	51.3%	35.8%	64.7%
Discharges per Bed	31.5	31.0	15.6	45.7
Adjusted ALOS	3.2	2.8	2.3	3.1
Medicare % Discharges	44.8%	42.3%	33.1%	55.1%
Medicaid % Discharges	6.1%	5.5%	2.0%	10.7%
Outpatient Revenue %	55.9%	56.1%	45.8%	70.8%
Salaries per Adjusted Discharge	$2,235	$32,158	$1,945	$2,766
FTEs per Occupied Bed	3.8	3.7	3.1	4.4
Salaries as % of Total Expense	44.6%	42.5%	36.9%	42.7%

5. Given the following table, create a Pareto chart reporting the major diagnostic categories (MDCs) with the highest inpatient revenue first (on the left) to the lowest revenue last (on the right). What percent of revenue is generated by the top 20% of MDCs?

MDC	Revenue
Blood and blood-forming organs	$1,668,475
Injury and poisoning	$1,803,197
Musculoskeletal system	$14,137,767
Infectious and parasitic	$3,458,147
Perinatal conditions	$3,923,030
Mental	$9,369,685
Digestive system	$15,841,269
Endocrine, nutritional, etc.	$5,432,203
Nervous system	$14,092,523
Circulatory system	$43,579,068
Genitourinary system	$11,149,038
Neoplasms	$23,082,428
Respiratory system	$19,367,421
Total Revenue	$206,904,250

6. Given the following table, create a Pareto chart reporting the insurers with the highest revenue first (on the left) to the lowest revenue last (on the right). What percent of revenue is generated by the top 20% of insurers?

Insurer	Revenue
Aetna	$6,200,000
Anthem	8,000,000
Blue Cross Blue Shield	6,000,000
Cigna	7,500,000
Humana	12,500,000
UnitedHealth Group	11,000,000
WellCare	4,000,000
Other (13 plans)	9,800,000
Total Revenue	$65,000,000

Note

1. Optum360°, *2017 Almanac of Hospital Financial and Operating Indicators* (Salt Lake City, UT: Author, 2016).

CHAPTER 17

Using Lean Six Sigma to Improve Financial Performance

PROGRESS NOTES

After completing this chapter, you should be able to:

1. Explain the objectives and method of Lean Six Sigma.
2. Describe the eight wastes.
3. Explain the five pillars of Lean Six Sigma.
4. Describe the Define, Measure, Analyze, Improve, and Control (DMAIC) methodology.
5. Describe the evolution from point kaizen, kaizen events, and kaizen systems.

Overview: Lean Six Sigma

Prior chapters have discussed measuring financial performance and what constitutes superior performance. Reaching higher performance requires a clear method that can be and is followed to completion. Identifying that your organization has higher costs (or lower outcomes) than other organizations is easy; determining why costs are higher requires insight given the amount of resources involved in producing healthcare services, and reducing costs requires determination to carry on to success. **Lean Six Sigma** provides insight and a method to pursue improvement.

Lean Six Sigma has two distinct and interrelated parts. Lean seeks to reduce waste in production systems by visually examining processes to improve performance and increase efficiency. The goal of Lean Six Sigma has been stated as cutting cost, errors, time, and space requirements in half three times, $50\% \times 50\% \times 50\% = 12.5\%$, or a total reduction of 87.5%. Research indicates that medication errors in hospitals may occur once in every 10 opportunities. Reducing the error rate from 10% to 1.25% may seem to be an impossible task, but history shows that improvements of this magnitude have been achieved. Infant mortality rates and deaths due to anesthesia have fallen by more than 87.5% in the past 70 years, and Henry

Ford cut the time to produce a car by 87.4% by instituting the assembly line.

Six Sigma is a statistical approach to reduce defects. Improving outcomes requires continuous monitoring of performance to know when outcomes are no longer meeting customer requirements, technical standards, and/or prior performance. Statistical process control (SPC) developed by Walter Shewhart in 1924 summarized historical performance for the output of a production system and established an acceptable range of variation based on past performance. When output stays within the established range, typically plus or minus three standard deviations from the average, no action is required. When output goes outside the acceptable range, workers should investigate the cause of the deviation and determine whether correction is required. SPC was designed to be used by frontline workers (who may have no statistical training) to ensure consistent output by identifying unacceptable variation and enabling them to make rapid corrections before deficiencies reach customers. Six Sigma builds on SPC and aims for 3.4 defects or less per million opportunities.

The Eight Wastes

Reducing excessive costs is easier when waste is understood and can be identified; the **eight wastes** highlight common problems in production processes that increase costs. The first waste is defects, errors that require work to be corrected or previous work to be scrapped and redone. The cost of defects is obvious; rework requires additional labor, supplies, and equipment to correct problems and satisfy customers. Scrapping previous work and starting over doubles the amount of labor, supplies, and equipment required and their cost to produce a single output. The second waste is time waste or idleness (i.e., employees or customers waiting for the next step in a process). The cost of idle employees is unproductive time multiplied by the hourly wage (e.g., the cost of 5 idle minutes per hour for an employee earning $60,000 a year is $2.40 per hour, $19.23 per day, and $4,615 over 48 weeks per year). The cost

of customer waiting is more subtle. How many customers are lost to other organizations due to long wait times? Are employees engaged in value-adding work, non-value-adding work, or idle; how long do patients spend to obtain care; and how much of that time is spent waiting? Idleness is easy to observe yet the total cost of time waste is rarely quantified, and thus little effort is taken to reduce it.

Overproduction is the creation of goods and services before they are needed. When output is not needed or desired, customers may be unwilling to purchase the product at any price, resulting in the complete loss of all invested costs or the producer having to sell the product at a price that does not fully cover costs. When output is produced before it is wanted or needed by customers and can be stored, it can be placed into inventory, producing additional costs. The fourth waste is excessive inventory, the acquisition and storage of material not immediately needed. Excessive inventory covers raw materials, work in process, and finished goods. Excessive inventory increases costs in three ways. The first is handling and storage costs. Space must be provided to store materials and staff employed to move and safeguard it. The second set of costs deals with spoilage or obsolescence. Will the material go bad, be damaged, or will customers no longer want the product after a certain time? The third cost is theft or shrinkage (i.e., the difference between actual inventory and reported inventory). Japanese producers minimize inventory costs using just-in-time processes where inventory is minimized and suppliers are expected to deliver new materials as production exhausts current stocks. Just-in-time inventory systems, in addition to the costs named previously, reduce the average inventory investment cost, the outlay to purchase materials, and allow any mismatch between the supplies received and the requirements of a production process to be quickly identified and rectified as supplies quickly move into production processes rather than being placed in storage for days, weeks, or months before being used.

The next three wastes focus on how work is done. The first looks at excessive motion. Do employees walk unnecessary distances to complete work, and/or once at the work site, are tools and materials within reach? Eliminating excessive motion seeks to minimize unnecessary movement by people (i.e., walking and reaching take time that could be used to create goods and services). The sixth waste, excessive transportation, examines unnecessary movements of materials and products. The goal is to minimize distances traveled by moving all supplies or equipment needed to complete work from inventory to the work site one time. Workers should not have to return to storage areas to obtain additional materials to complete work or restock unused supplies to inventory. Employees should know the amount of material they will require to complete tasks and transport no more or less material than they need to complete their jobs. Additionally, frequently used items should be stored close to where work is performed to minimize worker movement, whereas infrequently used items should be stored in more distant locations or offsite. The seventh waste, unneeded processing, explores whether more work or higher-quality work is performed than required by the customer. In health care, unneeded processing includes excessive lab tests or image studies that may be driven by defensive medicine concerns. Physicians seeking to avoid malpractice litigation order more medical services than necessary to minimize the probability of being accused of overlooking something or failing to do enough.

The final waste, underutilized talent, may be the most difficult to observe. Are managers underutilizing employee's skills and knowledge? People have different skill sets and are paid different wages. Managers should assign work to ensure each individual's skills are fully employed. More demanding tasks should be performed by more highly skilled workers, and any lower-skill duties they are performing should be delegated to lower-paid workers capable of performing the job. More subtle are the questions of whether employee improvement ideas are being fully examined and implemented and/or whether employees are leaving for better jobs. Workers generally have the best understanding of their work and know

what improvements are possible. Incorporating workers' ideas not only makes the most of their talents but also increases their commitment to the work as it increases their ownership of processes. The Japanese again offer an easy means to fully integrate employees into a production system via stop-the-line authority, or **jidoka**. There is no clearer sign of employee empowerment than to give them the authority to stop production when they identify problems. Finally, high staff turnover provides a clear indicator of employee dissatisfaction with their role in the organization. The eight wastes form an invaluable tool focused on employee attention on the types of actions that increase costs; recognizing these costs will motivate improvement.

The Five Principles of Lean Six Sigma

Identifying waste is the first step; the more challenging step is reducing waste. Lean Six Sigma pursues waste reduction by focusing employee attention on **value**, value streams, **flow**, **pull**, and **perfection**. Value focuses on product features that enhance patient satisfaction encompassing the total product experience. Patients evaluate the value of care based on the goods and services delivered, service (i.e., how goods or services are delivered), timeliness, the environment where goods or services are received, involvement in the treatment process (i.e., are patients active participants in developing their care plan?), and price. Managers must ensure that each of these six elements meets the expectations of customers to maximize their satisfaction.

Employees should spend the majority of their time producing goods and services that customers want. When employees spend large amounts of time on work that is not valued by customers, work should be restructured. The value stream is every step taken to design, produce, and deliver a product. The value stream is not what is supposed to happen but what really happens. The goal of **value stream mapping** is to document every step and determine if current activities increase, reduce, or have no impact on customer value.

Value-adding activities should then be enhanced, and activities that reduce or have no impact on value should be eliminated.

After examining the activities performed and determining whether they increase customer value and should be retained, flow focuses on how activities work together. Does the production process work continuously toward the desired goal without wasted time or motion? Healthcare managers should ensure an efficient flow of patients, family members, providers, medications, supplies, machinery, and information in their organization. Patient flow begins when care is sought, encompassing appointment making, registration, transfer to room, movement to and from testing and treatment areas, discharge, and follow-up. Long waits at any point undermine patient satisfaction. Similarly, long walks from parking areas and the inability to locate a family member's room (i.e., poor signage) reduce visitor satisfaction. Poor flows of providers, medications, supplies, and information within an organization (i.e., poorly integrated processes) delay decision-making and action, waste employee time, misuse supplies and equipment, and undermine patient outcomes. Finally, providers should follow up after care is delivered to determine how patients are faring after discharge. This not only ensures that providers know outcomes but also demonstrates continuing concern for the patient. Poor patient, provider, medication, supply, machinery, and information flows have a direct and negative impact on cost. The more disjointed the process, the higher the cost of care.

Pull seeks to ensure that nothing is produced until needed by customers. Pull in health care should ensure that tests are run, pharmaceuticals are delivered, and food is prepared when patients need or want these services. Providers should not be running tests, preparing medications or meals when staff has the time as their efforts and any required supplies will be wasted if the work is not subsequently needed. Perfection seeks to identify defects in processes to retrain employees and/or redesign systems to ensure that errors are not repeated. The goal is to do it right the first time. Tests and procedures that must be redone because they were not done right the first time not only increase costs but inconvenience patients and possibly subject them to pain and bodily harm. By focusing on what is produced, how it is produced, and outcomes, employees can identify where improvements can be made. The next step is designing and implementing change.

Define, Measure, Analyze, Improve, and Control (DMAIC)

Most organizations have long histories of failed improvement initiatives. Good ideas are seldom sufficient to change established processes. Change requires a compelling reason, a plan, and the tenacity to follow it through. **Define, Measure, Analyze, Improve, and Control (DMAIC)** provides a structured process for identifying opportunities and implementing improvements (**Table 17.1**).[1] Improvement often falters when there is no clear path forward. While completing every step in a DMAIC process will not guarantee success, it will reduce the probability of failure due to overlooking critical factors.

Define begins the process by identifying areas of concern or opportunity. Areas for improvement may be suggested by patients, frontline employees, finance, or quality management. Given an abundance of opportunities, managers must identify the projects that offer the greatest benefit to the organization. Once a project is selected, a compelling business case must made (what is at stake if improvement does not occur) and communicated to all stakeholders who will be affected by changes and an improvement team assembled with people who have the ability to motivate others and/or skills to complete improvement projects. Charles Kettering, head of research for GM, said, "A problem well-stated is half-solved." Obviously little can be accomplished when members of an improvement team are pursuing different problems and goals. The final step develops a data collection plan specifying how performance should be measured.

The second stage, *Measure*, adds detail to the chosen project. Measure collects data to document

Table 17.1 The DMAIC Process

Define	1. Identify improvement project and stakeholders
	2. Assemble performance improvement team
	3. Develop project charter
	4. Create project plan
	5. Create voice of the customer and voice of the process data collection plan
Measure	6. Measure voice of the customer
	7. Measure voice of the process
	8. Benchmark and assess capability
	9. Define cost of poor quality and expected benefit
Analyze	10. Identify potential causes of lower-than-desired performance
	11. Test causes of lower-than-desired performance and identify root causes
	12. Determine process capability
Improve	13. Identify and select improvements
	14. Perform cost–benefit analysis
	15. Design future state
	16. Establish performance targets
	17. Obtain approval to implement, train, and implement
Control	18. Measure and report results
	19. Manage change
	20. Identify replication opportunities
	21. Embed continuous improvement across the organization

what customers want (voice of the customer) and how a system is performing (voice of the process). After data are collected, the improvement team must determine if the system meets customer expectations. When gaps exist between customer expectations and system performance, the team should assess the importance of the deficiencies. Is the problem as great as originally believed, and will improvement produce the expected benefit?

When a gap must be rectified, *Analyze* seeks to identify the most important factors preventing superior performance (i.e., is the gap due to deficiencies in performance of workers, the materials or equipment used, how the current treatment process is structured, or environmental factors?).

After identifying potential factors, Analyze uses small-scale tests to alter one variable at a time while holding others constant to determine how much improvement may be achieved if the variable is altered. Sequential testing of factors thus allows the improvement team to identify the factors that could produce the greatest improvement.

Improve identifies the potential solutions that could be implemented and whether the benefit of improvement is likely to exceed the cost of change. Common problems arise from poor design of products or services; failure to remove or reduce obstacles to performance; poor training of employees (do they use the most effective and efficient methods to complete work?); lack of measurement and/or feedback (are best methods followed?); incoming material problems; equipment that is unsuitable for the work, incorrectly calibrated, or out of order; multiple input streams with variation; and nonoptimal working conditions due to noise, lighting, vibration, dirt, temperature, humidity, ventilation, and so on.

When the expected benefits of improvement exceed their cost, the improvement team develops one or more presentations to secure organizational support for change. A high-level report emphasizing the expected benefits and costs should be created for senior managers to obtain their approval and funding for necessary changes. A more detailed report identifying proposed changes in processes should be created for production employees to alert them to how the change may affect their work and obtain their input. After a project has been greenlighted, the team develops training materials for employees and assists in implementing new procedures.

The process should not end with implementation. The team should collect post-implementation data to evaluate the effectiveness of the new procedures. *Control* follows one of two paths. When the expected improvements are achieved, Control seeks to maintain improvements through continuous reporting of outcomes and reducing opportunities for failure. (As seen in other chapters, run charts are highly effective means of conveying change over time.) The next step evaluates whether the improvement can be introduced in other areas with similar processes. Replication should not simply impose the same changes in other areas but should recognize differences and modify improvements for new areas.

The second path when the expected benefit does not occur requires the improvement team to review prior steps to determine whether the improvements were appropriate. Was the correct cause identified and/or were improvements properly implemented? The team must decide whether additional effort is warranted on the current project or work should move to other projects that offer greater benefit to the organization. The ultimate goal of Lean Six Sigma is to encourage every employee to embrace change and continually pursue improvements that will increase customer and/or employee satisfaction and improve financial performance.

Assume the cost per CMI adjusted discharge or patient visit is believed to be excessive. Define creates a high-level value stream map identifying major functions (clearly defines the parameters of the project, the point where the work begins and ends), the stakeholders, and key performance metrics so the process to be improved and improvement goals are clear to the team. Measure should define the extent of the problem. How high are costs, by how much do costs exceed the costs of similar providers, and where do the excess costs arise in the production process? A detailed value stream map is then developed to identify how work is performed (i.e., where costs are incurred to eliminate non-value-adding steps, improve inefficient work processes, and/or reduce defects), and what level of performance is possible (industry average, top 25%, or best-in-class). The final step in the Measure stage quantifies the cost of nonoptimal performance to determine how much benefit the organization may obtain from improvement. If the cost per surgical discharge in MDC 5 is $7,200 and the industry average is $6,609, a hospital could potentially save $591 per discharge. A hospital with 1,200 annual surgical discharges could save $709,200 per year by meeting the industry average. The business case should demonstrate what the organization can do with this additional income. In a struggling hospital, $709,200 may determine whether it survives.

Analyze attempts to identify the major cause(s) of the high cost and whether they are controllable. Obviously, the cost per discharge varies by body system and treatment choices. Certain MDCs will have costs above and below the industry average. In this example, Define identified a subset—MDC 5, diseases of the circulatory system—where a targeted group of stakeholders can be identified and a value stream can be mapped for specific types of care (i.e., DRGs). Let's assume the high cost has been identified in the surgical DRGs. We can then examine the cost of surgery, the cost of nursing care, and the cost of ancillary services. Is the time spent in surgery excessive, or is it the cost of surgical inputs (i.e., labor, supplies, and/or facilities)? Similar analysis must look at the LOS, nursing staff levels, and wage rates, numbers of lab tests, images, and so on ordered, and ancillary staffing levels and wages.

After identifying potential controllable causes, the improvement team should alter each cause while holding other factors constant to assess the effect on the desired goal. If time in the OR is excessive, can the surgical process be streamlined to complete cases faster? If labor costs are too high, can staffing be reduced and/ or lower-cost employees utilized to perform lower-skill functions? Can the price of surgical supplies be lowered by better contracting and/ or elimination of less frequently used items on the surgical cart? After testing each controllable cause, the team should determine the level of performance possible (i.e., process capability). For example, when surgical processes can be streamlined or unnecessary tests and procedures can be reduced, how much can the cost per CMI adjusted discharge be reduced?

The testing of causes of suboptimal performance in the Analyze stage documents what could be accomplished; Improve identifies how these changes can be incorporated into the production process by focusing on a small number of caregivers. Improve should identify how the small-scale test can be enlarged to encompass all caregivers and calculate the cost of implementing each alternative, including the resistance of those affected by the desired changes. Ultimately, Improve determines whether changes should be pursued; will an improvement increase revenue or reduce cost by more than the cost of implementing change? When the expected benefits of a project exceed its costs and a project is greenlighted by senior managers, Improve creates a new value stream map to define how future work should be performed, establishes performance targets, trains employees, and assists in implementation.

The final stage in the DMAIC process, Control, evaluates the results of implemented improvements. Did the cost of surgical DRGs with MDC 5 fall by the expected amount, and were the costs of change greater than expected?

If the expected cost savings are not realized, the team must determine whether additional changes are needed. When expectations are met, Control seeks to institute systems to ensure improvements are sustained over time. Sustaining improvements requires continuous reporting of outcomes to demonstrate to employees that maintaining improvements remains a priority and alert them when performance falls and corrections are needed. In addition, new safeguards, mistake proofing, audits, and so on should be introduced to reduce opportunities for error and ensure that new procedures are followed. The final two steps in the Control stage assess whether improvements can be replicated in other areas and seek to ensure that improvement becomes an integral part of operations (i.e., what areas should be explored to achieve further improvements?).

Getting Started and Documenting Achievement

You've seen that the DMAIC process involves multiple steps and many stakeholders. The number of steps should not be an impediment to getting started. **Kaizen**, continuous improvement, can begin with small projects that one or two people can complete in a day. Point kaizen is discrete, independent, and opportunistic problem solving. The 30-30-30 exercise emphasizes how anyone can start an improvement effort.[2] 30-30-30 requires 30 minutes of observation of a process with a goal of identifying 30 problems or opportunities. The final 30 holds that the observer should then take 30 minutes to select and resolve one problem or implement one improvement.

A point kaizen project could be reorganizing a storage area or workspace using 5S. The goal in reorganizing a storage area is to reduce the time needed to locate supplies and reduce the chance of retrieving a wrong item. The first step is to examine input use:—which items are used most frequently and which are rarely used. Sort, the first S, moves infrequently used items to another area (of course balancing the cost of infrequent retrieval against the time gained from removing clutter). After infrequent items are relocated, the next step, set-in-place, designs and establishes places for regularly used items. The most frequently used items should be placed at eye level and within easy reach. Lightweight, lesser-used items should be located on higher shelves and heavier items placed on lower shelves. The third step, shine, requires ensuring that the area is clean and items are visible.

Standardization is the next step. In a storage area, there must be a procedure for indicating reorder and restocking needs. Lean Six Sigma relies on **Kanban**, a two-bin inventory system where emptying of a bin indicates the need for reordering. Everyone assessing supplies should know the procedure and alert the responsible party or place the empty bin in the appropriate location for replenishment, and/or the stock person must monitor bins. Once the standardized inventory system is established, identifying the location for empty bins and the reorder quantity, it must be sustained, the final S by monitoring, until the desired behavior becomes habitual. Point kaizen may be undertaken without a defined set of steps to demonstrate that anyone can initiate improvement and then use their success to pursue bigger and more impactful changes.

A kaizen event is a targeted focus on a process and how to improve it versus the opportunistic approach pursued in point kaizen. Kaizen events often require multiple days and should be guided by a defined set of steps, although 21 steps as recommended here may not be necessary. A kaizen event begins by defining the issues and mapping a process, what steps are taken, who performs each step, what they produce, how the steps work together, what the output is, and setting goals. A kaizen event is wider ranging than point kaizen, where one person can observe, redesign, and implement change. In a kaizen event, all parties must be represented, their knowledge and input secured to design new workflows, and their buy-in obtained to implement changes. A single person could redesign a paper medical record storage system, but redesigning the medical record system would require input from all users, doctors, nurses, file technicians, and so on. All participants must be included as any change may affect when

files are pulled, where they will be placed for use, where they will be placed after use, and when the files will be refiled. The effectiveness and efficiency of any change will depend upon how solutions are identified, tested, implemented, and sustained, all of which require full participation by affected parties. As the scope of the kaizen event increases, encompassing more people, processes, and time, the 21-step process should be used to ensure that critical activities are not overlooked.

Kaizen systems signal organizational transformation. Continuous improvement has become a way of life or philosophy. This could be door-to-door, where changes not only impact operating room or medical record processes but encompass everything from initial appointment making, reception, the nurse taking vital signs, the physician interaction, and discharge. In multisite organizations, kaizen systems would strive to produce consistency across sites (i.e., when best practice is identified that maximizes patient satisfaction and/or medical outcome or minimizes cost, it becomes standard practice across sites). At its fullest potential, a kaizen system synchronizes performance across organizations—that is, a hospital may seek closer integration with admitting physician offices and home health services. Pre-admission, in-house, and post-discharge services are synchronized. As discussed earlier, kaizen systems would also focus on medical supplies. Inventory levels should be reduced by developing relationships with suppliers that ensure that supplies arrive when needed.

The Path from Problem Solving to Continuous Improvement

Figure 17.1 documents the desired evolution of Lean Six Sigma in an organization. At adoption, point kaizen methods are used for discrete problem solving. Employees lack knowledge and experience and use Lean Six Sigma for small projects that have limited impact on processes and outcomes. When successful, employees gain confidence and skills and begin to see wider applicability for Lean Six Sigma tools. At the second level,

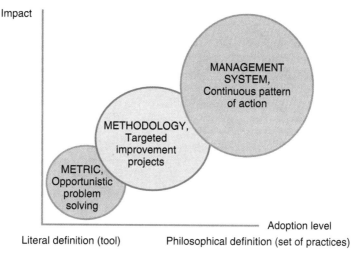

Figure 17.1 Use and Impact of Lean Six Sigma

kaizen events, the knowledge and skills of multiple employees are required to complete larger projects that will produce greater benefits for the organization. As more and more employees are involved and learn the value of Lean Six Sigma and its ability to improve processes and outcomes, it can be applied to ever-larger operations until it encompasses all employees and transforms the organization. The goal of Lean Six Sigma is to encourage and empower all employees to seek ways to enhance performance.

The A3 Report

Lean Six Sigma not only should improve processes and outcomes but should also improve the improvement process. The A3 report (**Figure 17.2**) provides a template that encapsulates the Lean Six Sigma process and goals. The A3 report documents the theme, background, current condition with flowchart, problems (identified with storm bursts in the flowchart), measures, root cause analysis findings, performance targets, the implementation plan including planned action, responsible parties, deadlines, costs, and follow-up activities including who, when, and how for a project. A database of A3s should be complied and studied to determine what actions are most successful and the employees who produce the results.

Insights Provided by Lean Six Sigma

Lean Six Sigma requires a revolution in how people approach work; while many of us believe we are effectively and efficiently performing our jobs, we seldom test our assumptions. Does our work satisfy others, whether final customers or downstream employees, and can we improve processes and products to increase the satisfaction of others? Likewise, is there a better way of doing our work that will take less time and resources and reduce costs? The Lean Six Sigma perspective and its tools lie outside the education and experience of most employees. Managers are taught how systems operate and healthcare providers how to treat patients, but neither are trained nor compensated to seek better approaches. Lean Six Sigma begins by recognizing what customers want and documenting how they are currently served to determine if things can be done better.

A performance improvement cycle should begin with what patients want (**Figure 17.3**). Our understanding of what we think patients want often varies substantially from what patients actually want. Wait times for emergency department care averaged 43.3 minutes in 2017.[3] Obviously, patients seeking emergency care expect faster

BACKGROUND:

- Contextual and background information.
- Impact on organization's goals.

CURRENT CONDITION:

- Value stream map, i.e., the diagram of how system works that should be understandable to all parties.
- Identification of major problems or opportunities
- Quantification of problem or opportunity, e.g., higher cost, lower revenue...

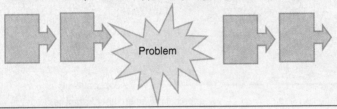

ROOT CAUSE ANALYSIS:
- List the main problem(s)
- Brainstorm potential major causes, e.g., manpower, materials, machinery, methods, mother nature (the 5 Ms)
- Brainstorm sub-causes under each major causes
- Select most likely sub-cause(s)

TARGET CONDITION:

- Value stream map of redesigned, restructured process.
- List of countermeasure(s) to address root cause(s).
- State expected improvement in the measure of interest (specifically and quantitatively)

IMPLEMENTATION PLAN:

- Actions required to realize the target condition, responsible party, and due date.
- Other factors relevant to the implementation, e.g., cost...

Action	Responsibility	Deadline
Action 1	Person 1	March 30
Action 2	Person 2	April 30
Action 3	Person 3	May 15
⋮	⋮	⋮
COST: no expenditures required		

FOLLOW-UP:

Plan	Actual
• Plan to measure the results. • When, how, and measured by whom.	• Results of implementation • Reviewer and date of follow-up

Figure 17.2 An A3 Report

treatment, as seen by the increasing numbers of patients leaving without being seen. Failure to provide timely care produces dissatisfied patients, reduces revenues, and creates a potential liability should a catastrophic medical outcome occur. The voice of the customer process affords an opportunity to return to basics. What do patients want, how do we know what they want, and how well are we satisfying them? Do we as healthcare providers place too much emphasis on technical

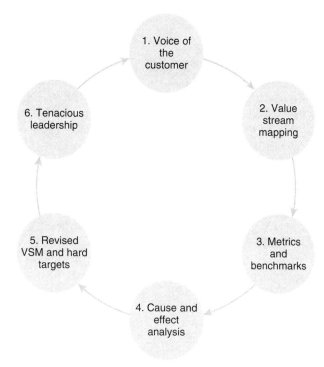

Figure 17.3 Performance Improvement Cycle

quality and fail to satisfy patients' desire for dignity, respect, and caring?

One cannot overestimate the value of value stream mapping. All of us work within systems that we do not fully understand. Whether you work in a hospital with more than $100 million in revenue or a physician office with $800,000 in revenue, you and your coworkers understand only a small part of what it takes to treat patients and keep the business operating. Our understanding of how systems work, like our understanding of what patients want, is often substantially different from actual system operation. Do ED physicians and managers know how long their patients wait?

Value stream mapping provides an opportunity to reexamine the systems we work in and our beliefs of how they work. Often we discover things occurring that we did not know, such as the total time needed to complete a process versus our part of the process and the outputs produced. Second, we learn that few people agree on how

systems work. The output of value stream mapping should be a better understanding of what is and is not done, and the identification of value-adding and non-value-adding steps. In addition, the mapping process should reduce differences in how people think the system works and assist in reaching consensus on where and what improvements should be made.

After establishing what patients want and how processes operate, the next step translates patient desires and expectations into quantifiable metrics. These measures must then be used to report performance. How much output is produced, what is the rate of defect, how long does it take to produce an output, what is the cost per unit, and how satisfied are patients? What services or products do patients want, what attributes should these products and services have, how quickly is treatment wanted, and what price are patients, third-party payers, and society willing to pay? We must answer these questions to determine where performance exceeds, meets, and falls short of patient expectations. Every healthcare organization provides services that can be improved to reduce cost and increase patient satisfaction, and furthermore, as patient expectations evolve, the things that presently satisfy may not continue to satisfy in the future—the need to identify and implement improvement never ends.

The value of quantifying data cannot be overestimated; "steady as she goes" is a comfortable direction when deficiencies and opportunities are not recognized. Without measurement, we cannot determine when improvement is desirable, so we default to continuing present practices. Quantifying past performance will answer whether performance has changed; have costs steadily increased, or are defects rates or delivery times increasing? Even when performance fully satisfies patients at one point of time, without continuous monitoring and benchmarking, we cannot know if current costs, defects, or performance times are too high. Has performance deteriorated and/or patients' expectations increased? We cannot even assume when performance is improving that we will retain patients if their expectations and/or the performance of competitors increases faster. Knowing the voice of the customer and benchmarking are essential to establishing targets and improving performance.

The limited results of past performance improvement initiatives can be attributed to their failure to incorporate changes into standard operating practices. Improvements are frequently recommended without considering how they interact with preceding and succeeding steps. A primary problem is detail avoidance. Improvements are presented without definitive expectations of how they interface with existing process and how much improvement should be expected. Lean Six Sigma's emphasis on cause-and-effect analysis and testing potential improvements prior to implementation increases the probability that changes will produce the desired results. A change at one point in a system may not produce any improvement if proceeding and succeeding work does not change (e.g., speeding up reporting of lab results to the ED may not reduce total time or cost in the ED if other processes do not change). Lean Six Sigma will overcome these problems if practitioners revise the value stream map (versus an e-mail, rewritten procedure, etc.); establish hard, measurable targets; measure performance; and follow up when performance does not meet targets.

The final point should not be underestimated. Tenacious managers are needed who will hold themselves and their employees accountable when targets are not reached. Managers must continually reinforce commitment to targets and work with employees to remove obstacles to success. Managers must be more than supervisors; they must be partners in achieving goals and encourage, if not drive, continuous improvement in their departments. Sustained improvement is not the result of one-time, poorly planned interventions. Lean Six Sigma provides a proven pathway to pursue improvement.

WRAP-UP

Summary

Lean Six Sigma provides a perspective to view and methodology to improve production processes. Lean Six Sigma focuses on reducing waste that arises from overproduction, unneeded processes, motion and transport, defects, excess inventory, idleness, and underutilized human resources. Understanding the sources of unnecessary cost is the first step to reducing cost.

Lean Six Sigma begins the process of improving efficiency by focusing on value. Workers should devote the majority of their efforts to producing the goods and services that customers want.

Once value-adding outputs are identified and non-value-adding outputs are reduced or eliminated, workers should examine how outputs are produced, activities should be performed in the most efficient manner, and the transition from one activity to another should be as smooth as possible. Value stream mapping and flow provide the means to understand what activities are performed and their interaction. Pull and perfection focus on when and how well activities are performed. Pull emphasizes that goods and services should be delivered when needed to ensure they are in fact wanted or needed and patients obtain them with minimal delay. Perfection stives for no errors but more importantly should encourage employees to continuously track defect rates and means to improve outcomes and patient satisfaction.

Improvement is difficult to achieve without a methodology to structure and monitor activities and results. The Define, Measure, Analyze, Improve, and Control (DMAIC) methodology provides a 21-step framework, but improvement does not require adhering to every step and gaining the support of every employee. Point kaizen highlights that every employee can improve their work by simply observing and restructuring their work or workspace. Kaizen events signal the emergence into broader and more impactful improvement that encompasses multiple workers, departments, and/or organizations. The broader scope demands a more structured process. Following the 21 steps will increase your chance of success by ensuring improvement team members understand the broad goal, the specific performance gaps to be closed, the potential of identified improvements to close these gaps, and how improvements will be implemented and maintained. Once the methodology is internalized, a kaizen system will arise in which improvement is a standard part of employee work.

Key Terms

Define, Measure, Analyze, Improve, and Control (DMAIC)
Eight Wastes
Flow

Jidoka
Kaizen
Kanban
Lean Six Sigma
Perfection

Pull
Value
Value Stream Mapping

Discussion Questions

1. Explain the objectives and method of Lean Six Sigma.
2. Describe the eight wastes.
3. Explain the five principles of Lean Six Sigma.
4. Describe each element in the Define, Measure, Analyze, Improve, and Control (DMAIC) methodology.
5. Explain the difference between point kaizen, kaizen events, and kaizen systems.

Notes

1. T. K. Ross, *Applying Lean Six Sigma in Health Care* (Burlington, MA: Jones and Bartlett Learning, 2021).
2. C. Protzman, G. Mayzell, and J. Kepchar, *Leveraging Lean in Healthcare* (Boca Raton, FL: CRC Press, 2011).
3. CDC, National Hospital Ambulatory Medical Care Survey 2017, https://cdc.gov, accessed June 30, 2021.

CHAPTER 18

The Time Value of Money

PROGRESS NOTES

After completing this chapter, you should be able to:

1. Explain why monies paid or received in the future must be decreased or increased to assess their likely value.
2. Calculate present values for single and multiple payments to be received in the future.
3. Calculate payback periods, net present values, and internal rate of returns.
4. Calculate the future values for investments made today (and in subsequent years) to be withdrawn in the future.

Overview: The Changing Value of Money

When is $1.00 not $1.00? The answer is when you are evaluating what money purchased in the past or will purchase in the future. For example, the average price of a Big Mac in 2020 was $4.95; the price when it was introduced in 1967 was 45¢.[1] In 2020, you needed 11 times more money to purchase a Big Mac than was needed in 1967, or you could say the dollar in 2020 was worth about 9¢ relative to $1.00 in 1967. **Inflation** (i.e., a general increase in the prices of goods and services) ensures that you and organizations will need more money in the future to purchase the same amount of goods and services as $1, $100, or $1 million will purchase today.

Managers have to evaluate whether planned investments in programs, equipment, and buildings that produce revenue over multiple years will generate more revenue than their cost. For example, spending $1 million today on a program that produces $100,000 per year for the next 10 years is not financially advantageous. The value of the $100,000 received in the tenth year of the program will only purchase $82,035 in goods and services as inflation erodes the purchasing power of money assuming 2% annual inflation. At any positive inflation rate, $1,000,000 today is more valuable than ten $100,000 payments received over the next 10 years. Managers must know how to compare the value of revenues and costs received in different years to ensure that prudent financial decisions are made.

Similarly, money invested today will grow based on the interest rate earned and the number of years invested. When you have future plans, you need to know whether you will have sufficient money to start and complete the expected actions. Healthcare managers also should know whether they will have the funds needed to maintain, improve, and expand operations and thus should know how much money the organization may have in the bank or investments in the future and how much it may have to borrow.

Present Value Analysis

The concept of **present value** analysis is based on the **time value of money** (i.e., the value of a dollar today is more than the value of a dollar in the future). The further in the future the receipt of your dollar occurs, the less it will purchase as inflation increases the prices of goods and services. Think of a dollar bill dwindling in size more and more as its receipt stretches further and further into the future. Present value discounts the value of future payments to recognize the declining purchasing power of money. The formula to determine the value of money received in the future is

$$PV = FV \div (1 + r)^n$$

where

PV = present value (i.e., the value today of money to be received in the future)
FV = **future value** (i.e., the amount of money received in the future)
r = the discount rate
n = the number of years in the future

Assume you will receive $100, future value, one year from today, n, and the discount rate is 5%. The present value of that payment is $95.24, $100 ÷ (1.05).[1] If the $100 is not received until the end of the fifth year, the payment may only purchase $78.35, $100 ÷ (1.05),[5] in goods and services.

Using this formula, it is possible to calculate the value of $1.00 to be received at the end of any year. Excel provides a convenient alternative to manual calculation via its present value formula:

=PV(rate, nper, pmt, [fv], [type])

where

Rate: discount rate (r)
Nper: number of years (n)

Pmt: a series of equal payments (**annuity**)
[fv]: a one-time payment (FV)
"[type]: 0 or blank if ordinary annuity (money received at the end of the year), 1 if annuity due (money received at the beginning of the year)" i.e., parathesis added after first year.

Entering =PV(0.05,1,,-1) = 0.9524 and =PV(0.05, 5,,-1) = 0.7835 calculates the present value of $1.00 at 5% over one and five years. Entering =PV(0.05,1,, -100) calculates the value of $100 received one year in the future at a 5% discount rate, $95.24. **Table 18.1** shows the present value for $100 received over five years at four different discount rates.

Table 18.1 shows that the value of money decreases the further out it is received in the future and the higher the discount rate. At a discount rate of 10%, $100 will purchase $90.91 of goods and services after one year; after five years, only $62.09 could be purchased. Likewise, $100 purchases $98.04 of goods and services with a discount rate of 2% after one year; only $83.33 can be purchased when the discount rate is 20%. **Figure 18.1** provides a visual representation of the declining value of money.

Annuities

An annuity is a series of equal payments received over time. Instead of receiving a single payment

Table 18.1 Present Value of $100

Payment [fv]	($100)		
	Discount Rate (rate)		
Year (nper)	2%	5%	10%	20%
0	$100.00	$100.00	$100.00	$100.00
1	$98.04	$95.24	$90.91	$83.33
2	$96.12	$90.70	$82.64	$69.44
3	$94.23	$86.38	$75.13	$57.87
4	$92.38	$82.27	$68.30	$48.23
5	$90.57	$78.35	$62.09	$40.19

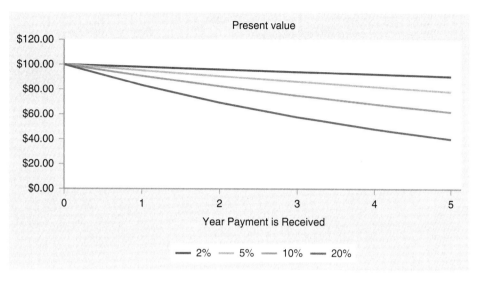

Figure 18.1 Present Value of $100

at one point of time, people and businesses often receive a series of payments. Assume you receive a gift of $100 to be paid at the end of each year for five years. The time value of money demonstrates that the value of the payment declines each year. **Table 18.2** shows what five payments of $100, $500 in total, will be worth given the discount rate.

By comparing Tables 18.1 and 18.2, you can see that the present value of these payments is the sum of the individual payments. For example, the value of the year 1 and 2 payments at 5% is $185.94 or the sum of the year 1 payment, $95.24, plus the year 2 payment, $90.70. Calculating the present value of an annuity using =PV function requires the user to enter the payment in the third argument, Excel will calculate the value of Nper or n payments instead of a single payment. Entering =PV(0.05,5,-100) = $432.95 and =PV(0.1,5,-100) = $379.08 calculates the present value of $100 over 5 years at 5% and 10%. **Figure 18.2** graphically shows the higher value of these payments, but you should recognize that the value declines as the discount rate increases.

Managers must assess when payments are received to ensure that the flow of payments over time exceeds the cost of investment given money that declines as either the discount rate or time of payment increases.

Table 18.2 Present Value of Five-Year Annuity of $100

Year	Nominal Payments	Discount Rate		
		2%	5%	10%
0	$0.00	$0.00	$0.00	$0.00
1	$100.00	$98.04	$95.24	$90.91
2	$200.00	$194.16	$185.94	$173.55
3	$300.00	$288.39	$272.32	$248.69
4	$400.00	$380.77	$354.60	$316.99
5	$500.00	$471.35	$432.95	$379.08

Evaluating Investments That Produce Future Revenue

Unlike the discussion of present value where future payments were simply received, obtaining future revenues generally involves an investment (i.e., individuals and organizations expend funds today to obtain future payments). Financial prudence requires that future payments exceed the cost of investment. This section examines three methods for assessing the return on an investment.

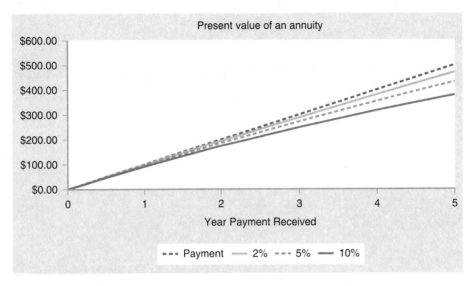

Figure 18.2 Present Value of Five-Year Annuity of $100

Payback Period

The **payback period** is the length of time required for the cash coming in from an investment to equal the amount of cash originally spent on the investment. In other words, if we invest $1,000 under a particular set of assumptions, how many years would it take to get our $1,000 back? The payback period concept is used extensively in evaluating whether to invest in equipment and/or facilities. For example, if the Curie Imaging Center invests $300,000 in a digital X-ray machine, how many years will it take to recoup their investment?

The assumptions are key to the computation of the payback period. In the case of equipment and facilities, the critical assumptions are output (or sales), revenue (output × price), and expenses, all of which are difficult to accurately predict. Therefore, it is prudent to run more than one payback period computation based on different circumstances (i.e., best-case, most likely, and worst-case scenarios).

The computation itself is simple, although it has multiple steps. The trick is to break it into segments. For example, the owner of the Curie Imaging Center has asked the practice manager to calculate the expected payback period for this

piece of equipment. The practice manager has made five assumptions: first, $300,000 purchase price; second, five-year useful life; third, $240,000 in annual revenue; fourth, $150,000 in annual direct operating costs associated with earning the revenue; and, finally, $60,000 in annual depreciation expense, $300,000 ÷ 5 years. Now that the assumptions are in place, the payback period computation can be made in three steps:

Step 1: Find the machine's expected net income after taxes.

Revenue (assumption 3)	$240,000
Less: Direct operating costs (assumption 4)	$150,000
Depreciation (assumption 5)	60,000
Total expense	$210,000
Net income before taxes	$30,000
Less: income taxes of 35% (>$209,425*)	$10,500
Net income after taxes	$19,500

Step 2: Find the net annual cash inflow after taxes the machine is expected to generate (in other words, convert the net income to a cash basis).

Net income after taxes	$19,500

Add: Depreciation (a noncash expenditure**) 60,000

Net annual net cash flow after taxes $79,500

Step 3: Compute the payback period.

Investment $300,000

Divide by: Net annual net cash flow after taxes $79,500

Payback period: 3.8 years

* Assumes Curie's net income is taxed at the owner's federal tax rate and the owner earns more than $210,000 per year. Also assumes clinic is located in a state with no personal income tax.

** Depreciation is a noncash expense. Cash was spent at the time of acquisition. Depreciation reduces taxable income but does not leave the practice.

The machine is expected to pay back its investment under these assumptions in 3.8 years. The practice owner must then determine if this is fast enough to warrant investment. Two other methods are now reviewed that begin with owners or managers establishing the acceptable rate of return on investment (i.e., the minimum acceptable discount rate).

Net Present Value

Net present value (NPV) determines if the discounted cash flows from a project will be equal to or greater than the investment made to undertake the project. In the payback period example, the equipment was expected to produce $79,500 of cash flow over five years, a total of $397,500. The equipment, however, is not worth $397,500, as the future cash flows must be discounted to determine their value today. We will assume the discount rate is 5%. **Table 18.3** shows the net cash flow by year, the present value factor (PVF $= 1 \div (1 + r)^n$), and the present value of the cash flow (PVCF = net cash flow × PVF). Summing the discount cash flows (PVCF) and subtracting the investment from the total discounted cash flow produce the NPV, $44,143.

Table 18.3 Expected Cash Flow and NPV from $300,000 Investment

Year	Net Cash Flow	PVF	PVCF
1	$79,500	0.9524	$75,714
2	$79,500	0.9070	$72,109
3	$79,500	0.8638	$68,675
4	$79,500	0.8227	$65,405
5	$79,500	0.7835	$62,290
	Total PVCF		$344,193
	Investment		-$300,000
	NPV		$44,193

The investment should be undertaken as long as the sum of the discounted cash flows is equal to or exceeds the cost of the investment. The $44,143 NPV indicates that this investment is expected to earn more than the 5% discount rate. If NPV were $0, it would earn exactly 5%, and if NPV is less than $0, it earns less than 5%. The next evaluation method, **internal rate of return**, calculates the rate of return on an investment.

Internal Rate of Return

The internal rate of return (IRR) calculates the interest rate that discounts future net inflows from the proposed investment down to the amount invested. The IRR recognizes the time pattern in which the earnings occur (i.e., the further in the future the cash is received, the less it is worth).

Manual calculation of the IRR is cumbersome, but fortunately Excel provides an easy-to-use formula, =IRR(values, [guess]). The manager must simply enter the range of cash flows including the negative outlay for the investment as values. [Guess] allows the manager to enter what they think may be the interest rate, but entering a guess is not required. The IRR for the machine is

=IRR(-300000,79500,79500,79500,79500,79500)
= 10.1783% or 10.2%

Table 18.4 shows how the IRR is calculated. The percentage 10.2% is used to discount each year's cash flow, and the total discounted cash flow (NPV) from year 1 through year 5 is almost equivalent to the year 0 investment of $300,000. The difference of –$166 is due to using 10.2% as the discount rate rather than the actual IRR of 10.1783%.

As 5% was established as the minimum required rate of return and the investment earns more than twice as much as the required minimum, it should be pursued. If the IRR had resulted in a rate less than 5%, the investment should not be undertaken.

Evaluating the use of resources in healthcare organizations is an important task. There are never enough resources to fulfill all the requests for funds, so it is important to use an objective process to evaluate which investments will be made by the organization. Understanding how the value of money decreases over time is the first step to ensuring that investments will increase the value of an organization. The second step is establishing a strong and consistent method for evaluating investments.

It is important to choose a method that is understood by the managers who will be using it. Understanding both the inputs required for the calculation and the information the output supplies is essential for sound financial decision-making. In summary, evaluations should be objective, the process should not be too cumbersome, and the responsible managers should understand how the computation was achieved.

Future Value Analysis

Managers must not only evaluate whether an investment is financially desirable, they must also know if they will have sufficient funds to complete an investment. While debt is regularly used for major, high-dollar investments, lenders typically are reluctant to finance 100% of an investment. Lenders want to know that borrowers have a stake in the success of an investment and will work hard to pay back a loan, so managers need to save a part of the annual profit or raise money by selling ownership interests or through donations to supply a portion of the expected outlay. If you own a home and have a mortgage, you may know that if you made less than a 20% down payment, your lender required private mortgage insurance (PMI) to ensure that the mortgage would be paid in the event of a default. When a borrower puts down a 20% down payment, the value of the property must decline by more than 20% before the lender's investment is at risk.

Future value calculates the interest earned on savings and thus can be used to calculate how much money you or an organization will have based on the interest rate and length of time invested. The power of investment comes from the compounding of interest. In future years, an investor receives interest not only on their original savings but also on the previous interest earned. The formula to calculate future value is

$$FV = PV \times (1+r)^n$$

An investment of $1,000 earning 10% annually would grow to $1,100 after year 1, $1,000 \times 1.1^1$ and $1,210 after two years, $1,000 \times 1.1^2$. Excel's future value formula can also be used to calculate future values:

Table 18.4 Calculating the IRR

Discount Rate	10.2%		
Year	Net Cash Flow	PVF	PVCF
1	$79,500	0.9074	$72,142
2	$79,500	0.8234	$65,464
3	$79,500	0.7472	$59,405
4	$79,500	0.6781	$53,906
5	$79,500	0.6153	$48,917
	Total PVCF		$299,834
	Investment		-$300,000
	NPV		($166)

=FV(rate, nper, pmt, [pv], [type])

where

Rate = discount rate (r)
Nper = number of years (n)
Pmt = series of equal investments (annuity)
[pv] = one-time investment (PV)
[type] = 0: ordinary annuity and 1: annuity due

Entering =FV(0.1,1,,-1000) = 1,100 and =FV(0.1,2,,-1000) = 1,210. The investment, −1000, is entered into the third argument, Pmt, as it is a one-time investment. When $1,000 is invested annually, an annuity, the amount would be entered into the fourth argument, and the third argument would be blank. The first investment of $1,000 is treated as being made on December 31 of year 0, so no interest is earned; in year 1, the year 0 investment earns interest, and year 1 investment of $1,000 is treated as if it is made on December 31. In year 2, the investor will have $1,210, $100 for interest earned in year 1 (10% × $1,000) plus $110 in interest for year 2 (10% × $1,100) plus the $1,000 year 1 investment, =FV(0.1,2,,-1000) = 1,210).

Examining **Table 18.5** shows that at a discount rate of 10%, $100 is earned on the $1,000 investment in year 1, but in year 2, the investor receives $100 on the initial investment and an additional $10 on the $100 of interest earned in year 1. Table 18.5 shows that in year 5, the

5% discount rate earns $172.20, $1,276.28 − $1,104.08, more in interest than the 2% investment, and when funds are invested at 10%, they will earn $506.43, $1,610.51 − $1,104.08, more in interest, highlighting the potential from higher-yield investments. **Figure 18.3** shows the difference in the amount of money available to the investor based on the interest rate and length of time invested.

Assume you want to purchase a $400,000 home with a minimum down payment of $20,000 (i.e., 5%). If you save $500 per month and earn 10% for the next 36 months, you will accumulate a down payment of $20,891 or your $18,000 investment will accumulate $2,891 in interest. If you believe three years is too long to wait based on increasing home prices, doubling your savings to $1,000 per month for 18 months will provide a $19,333 down payment.

Another way to view future value is it demonstrates the growth in the value of an organization based on its return on assets (ROA). Organizations with an ROA of 0% will be worth the same amount in five years as they are today. Organizations earning 10% over five years will see their assets increase by more than 60% from their value today. A 60% increase in assets will allow organizations to increase the amount of services and/or the quality of services.

The power of compound interest is more apparent when looking further into the future and making additional investments over time. Assume

Table 18.5 Future Value of $1,000

Future Value [pv]	$1,000			
	Discount Rate (rate)			
Year (nper)	0%	2%	5%	10%
0	$1,000.00	$1,000.00	$1,000.00	$1,000.00
1	$1,000.00	$1,020.00	$1,050.00	$1,100.00
2	$1,000.00	$1,040.40	$1,102.50	$1,210.00
3	$1,000.00	$1,061.21	$1,157.63	$1,331.00
4	$1,000.00	$1,082.43	$1,215.51	$1,464.10
5	$1,000.00	$1,104.08	$1,276.28	$1,610.51

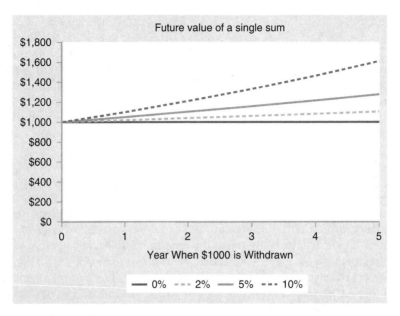

Figure 18.3 Future Value of $1,000

you save $1,000 a year at 10% over 40 years for retirement, an annuity. Your $40,000 investment, $1,000 × 40 years, will grow to $442,593, =FV(0.1,40,-1000). The power of compounding comes into play when money is invested for long periods of time at high discount rates. **Table 18.6** and **Figure 18.4** show what investing $1,000 per year over 40 years will grow to. At 10 years, the investment earning 10% is 146% more than the same investment at 2%, $15,937 ÷ $10,950. At 20 years, the difference grows to 236%, $57,275 ÷ $24,297, and at 40 years, the difference is 733%, $442,593. It bears repeating that each investment was funded by $40,000 in savings.

The increase in return from investing funds does not come without risk. Higher-return investments carry a higher risk of losing money. The stock market has earned close to 9.1% annually since 1987, but investors in the stock market recognize that the market can drop in value at any

Table 18.6 Future Value of an Annuity of $1,000

Year	Nominal Payments	Discount Rate		
		2%	**5%**	**10%**
0	$0	$0	$0	$0
10	$10,000	$10,950	$12,578	$15,937
20	$20,000	$24,297	$33,066	$57,275
30	$30,000	$40,568	$66,439	$164,494
40	$40,000	$60,402	$120,800	$442,593

time. The **risk/return trade-off** is a core principle of finance. Higher returns can only be achieved by accepting higher risk. In 2020, the stock market dropped 32% between February and March but recouped the loss by the fall and went on to record highs in 2021.

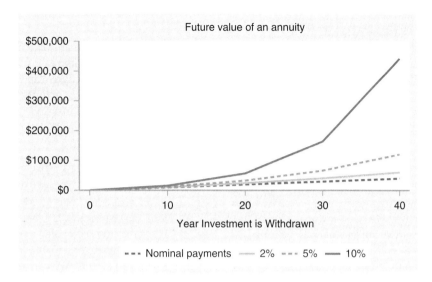

Figure 18.4 Future Value of an Annuity of $1,000

WRAP-UP

Summary

Investments in healthcare equipment and facilities require large cash outlays and produce cash over multiple years. The value of money declines over time due to inflation reducing the purchasing power of the dollar, so managers must incorporate the declining value of money into their analysis when evaluating potential investments. Present value analysis demonstrates that the value of future cash flows decreases the further in the future payment is received and the higher the discount rate.

Three evaluation methods are commonly used to equate the investment with future cash flows. The first, payback period, calculates the number of years needed to recoup the investment based on its annual cash inflow. Net present value

(NPV) discounts and sums future cash flows and subtracts the total from the initial investment. When NPV is equal to or greater than the cost of the investment, the investment should be undertaken. Internal rate of return (IRR) calculates the interest rate that equates future cash flows to the cost of the investment. An investment should be undertaken when IRR equals or exceeds the organization's discount rate.

Future value analysis calculates what savings will grow to based on the interest rate earned on the investment and the number of years it is invested. Future value analysis shows that growth is greater the higher the interest rate and the longer the period of investment.

Key Terms

Annuity	Internal Rate of Return	Present Value
Future Value	Net Present Value	Risk/Return Trade-Off
Inflation	Payback Period	Time Value of Money

Discussion Questions

1. Explain why the value of monies received in the future is lower than the value of the same money today.
2. Explain the differences among payback period, net present value, and internal rate of return. Which do think provides the best indicator of financial performance? Explain your reasoning.
3. Explain how the future value of investments changes with the interest rate and length of time invested.

Problems

1. Calculate the present value of the following single payments:
   a. $10,000 received five years in the future given a discount rate of 4%
   b. $10,000 received 10 years in the future given a discount rate of 4%
   c. $10,000 received five years in the future given a discount rate of 8%. How much different is the value compared to part (a)?
   d. $10,000 received 10 years in the future given a discount rate of 8%. How much different is the value compared to part (c)?
2. Calculate the present value of the following annuities:
   a. $10,000 received every year for five years given a discount rate of 4%
   b. $10,000 received every year for 10 years given a discount rate of 4%
   c. $10,000 received every year for five years given a discount rate of 8%. How much different is the value compared to part (a)?
   d. $10,000 received every year for 10 years given a discount rate of 8%. How much different is the value compared to part (c)?
3. Calculate the future value of the following one-time investments:
   a. $10,000 invested for five years given a discount rate of 4%. What is the total interest earned?
   b. $10,000 invested for 10 years given a discount rate of 4%. What is the total interest earned and how much different is the value compared to part (a)?

   c. $10,000 invested for five years in the future given a discount rate of 8%. What is the total interest earned, and how much different is the value compared to part (a)?
   d. $10,000 invested for 10 years given a discount rate of 8%. What is the total interest earned, and how much different is the value compared to part (c)?
4. Calculate the future value of the following annuities:
   a. $10,000 invested every year for five years given a discount rate of 4%. What is the total interest earned?
   b. $10,000 invested every year for 10 years given a discount rate of 4%. What is the total interest earned and how much different is the value compared to part (a)?
   c. $10,000 invested every year for five years given a discount rate of 8%. What is the total interest earned and how much different is the value compared to part (a)?
   d. $10,000 invested every year for 10 years given a discount rate of 8%. What is the total interest earned and how much different is the value compared to part (c)?
5. An investment requires a $1 million cash outlay in year 0 and produces $150,000 a year for eight years. Calculate the following:
   a. The net present value (NPV) using a discount rate of 5%
   b. The internal rate of return (IRR)

Note

1. M. DeMaria, "What a Big Mac Cost the Decade You Were Born", http://www.eatthis.com, accessed August 7, 2021.

CHAPTER 19

Constructing a Capital Budget

PROGRESS NOTES

After completing this chapter, you should be able to:

1. Explain why a capital budget is necessary.
2. Describe the major steps in creating a capital budget.
3. Calculate startup costs and expected cash flows from a capital expenditure for both nonprofits and for-profits.

Overview: Capital Budgets

Healthcare equipment and facilities cost millions of dollars and are used over many years, so before money is expended, managers should be confident that the investment will benefit the organization (i.e., the revenue generated by the investment will exceed its cost). Investments should be undertaken if NPV is equal to or greater than $0, IRR is equal to or greater than the discount rate, and/or the **payback period** is less than the desired number of years (see Chapter 18). The need for investment evaluation methods is more important when there are multiple potential capital expenditures and the organization has a limited amount of funds. Evaluation methods rank investments when decisions must be made

as to which projects will be pursued and which will be foregone.

Capital expenditures involve the acquisition of **capital assets** that are long-lasting, such as equipment, buildings, and land. **Capital budgets** are used to plan, monitor, and control long-term financial decisions. Operating budgets, on the other hand, generally deal with short-term revenues and expenses necessary to provide goods and services. For example, Codman Medical Center's operating budgets are created to cover the next year only (a 12-month period), while its[1] capital budgets may be created to cover a five-year or 10-year period.

The budget for capital expenditures is usually part of an overall, comprehensive financial plan. Responsibility for the comprehensive financial plan always rests with chief executive officers of the organization and is beyond the scope of this chapter.

Creating the Capital Budget

The capital budget, which may sometimes be identified by another name, such as *capital spending plan*, usually consists of two parts. The first part of the budget represents spending for capital assets that have already been acquired and are in place. This spending protects an existing asset; you are essentially spending money to protect that which you already have. The second part of the budget represents spending for new capital assets. In this case, you will be expending funds to acquire new assets such as equipment, buildings, and land.

The "existing asset" part of the budget focuses on whether existing equipment and buildings should be kept in their present condition including repair and maintenance, renovated, or replaced. Renovating equipment or buildings implies a large expenditure that would be capitalized. Capitalization means the expenditure is placed on the balance sheet as an additional capital cost that is recognized as an asset and depreciated over time versus repair and maintenance expenses that are included in the operating budget.

The "new capital asset" part of the budget forces more planning questions. The reasons for new asset spending may involve the following:

- Expansion of capacity in a department or program
- Creation of a new facility, department, or program
- New equipment to improve productivity
- New equipment or space to comply with federal or state requirements

Budget Construction Tools

How the capital budget is constructed may be predetermined by the requirements of the organization. Your facility or practice may have a template that must be used. This takes the decision out of your hands, but you should still understand the basic capital budgeting framework. When a format is not mandated, you will have to decide the structure and tools that will be most effective to build your capital budget.

One important tool is net cash flow reporting. The concept of **cash flow analysis**, usually an important part of the capital budget, is described later. But how will the cash flow be reported? Four methods are discussed in this section.

Cash Flow Concept

Cash flow analysis reports how a project's cash is expected to be received or paid over the life of an asset. Most analyses focus on the cash expenditure for the equipment, the outflow of funds, and the revenue earned from the investment, the inflow. In some cases, the analysis may focus only on cash expenditures.

For example, if a new piece of equipment will replace an old one and the replaced equipment will be sold for cash, the cash received from the sale will represent a cash receipt partially offsetting the cost of the new equipment. Cash flow must be reported as cumulative. **Cumulative cash flow** means the accumulated effect of cash inflows and outflows must be added and/or subtracted to show the overall net cash effect over the life of the asset.

Cash Flow Reporting Methods

Cash flow is typically reported using one of three methods:

- Payback method
- Net present value
- Internal rate of return

Chapter 18 explained and illustrated each of the three methods.

Payback Period

The payback period is based on cash flow, the difference between cash inflow and outflow. Payback period reports the number of years needed before the expected cash inflow recovers the initial cash invested (i.e., the outflow). The payback method is advantageous because it is easy to understand and highlights risks. However, it does not take either profitability or the time value of money into account.

Net Present Value

Net present value (NPV) is a discounted cash flow method. It is based on cash flows in that it takes all the cash (incoming and outgoing) into account over the life of the asset and incorporates the time value of money. NPV reports the total discounted amount of money expected to be gained (or lost) from an investment.

Internal Rate of Return

Internal rate of return (IRR) is also a discounted cash flow method that takes all incoming and outgoing cash into account over the life of the equipment (or the project) and incorporates the time value of money. IRR reports the interest rate that equalizes the cash inflows to the investment (i.e., it is the compound interest rate earned on an investment).

The use of IRR, NPV, and payback period is the vocabulary of capital budgeting and an important part of the language of finance. It is important to understand the differences between the three methods. Review Chapter 18 on the time value of money for more detail.

Budget Inputs

Capital budget inputs may have to be taken into consideration if the operating budget requires additional capital equipment or space renovations. **Figure 19.1** illustrates these potential inputs.

Startup Costs

If the proposal for capital expenditures incorporates operational expenses, the concept of startup costs must also be taken into consideration. In these cases, management believes the cost of starting up a new service line or a new program should be included as part of the original investment. Although such operational costs do not fall into a strict definition of capital budgeting, the requirement is common enough to warrant discussion.

Funding Requests
The Process of Requesting Capital Expenditure Funds

Institutions do not have an unlimited supply of funds, so different departments or divisions often have to compete for capital expenditure funding. A hospital's radiology department director may want new equipment, but so does the surgery department director, and so on. The various requests for

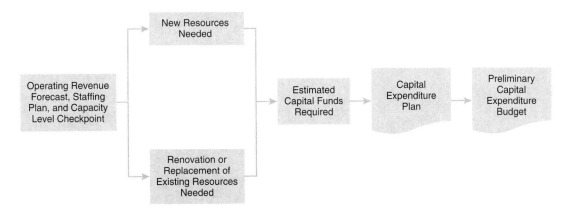

Figure 19.1 Capital Expenditures Budget Inputs

funding are often collected and reviewed to make decisions about where and to whom available capital expenditure funds will go. While senior management makes the overall decisions about future use of funds, departmental funding requests represent the first step in the overall process.

The process for requesting capital expenditure funding varies according to the organization. We would expect a large hospital or health system to have a more structured process than a two-physician practice. The corporate culture of the organization also plays a part. Some organizations are extremely formal, requiring managers to adhere to established policies and procedures, while others are more flexible in their management principles. In some facilities, politics and power play a part in the process of making and reviewing funding requests.

Types of Capital Expenditure Proposals

The type of proposal affects its size and scope. Proposal types commonly include the following types of requests:

- Acquiring new equipment
- Upgrading existing equipment
- Replacing existing equipment with new equipment
- Funding new programs
- Funding expansion of existing programs
- Acquiring capital assets for future use

Certain of these types may be paired as either/or choices in capital expenditure proposals versus multiple investments (e.g., upgrade or replace existing equipment or upgrade existing equipment or fund new programs). All six types of proposals are discussed in this section.

Acquiring New Equipment

The reason why new equipment is needed must be clearly stated. The acquisition cost must be a reasonable figure that contains all appropriate specifications. The number of years of useful life

that can be reasonably expected from the equipment is also an important assumption.

Upgrading Existing Equipment

The reason why an upgrade is necessary must be clearly stated. What is the impact? What will the outcomes be from the upgrade? The upgrade costs must be a reasonable figure that also contains all appropriate specifications. Will the upgrade extend the useful life of the equipment? If so, by how long?

Replacing Existing Equipment with New Equipment

The rationale for replacing existing equipment with new equipment must be clearly stated. Often a comparison may be made between upgrading and replacement in order to make a more compelling argument. The usual arguments in these comparisons revolve around improvements in technology in the new equipment that are more advanced than available upgrades to the old equipment. A favorite argument in favor of the new equipment is increased productivity and/or outcomes.

Funding New Programs

A proposal for new program capital expenditures must take startup costs into account. This type of proposal will generally be more extensive than a straightforward equipment replacement proposal because it involves a new venture without a previous history or proven outcomes.

Funding Expansion of Existing Programs

A proposal for expansion of an existing program is generally easier to prepare than a proposal for a new program. You will have statistics available from the existing program with which to make your arguments. In addition, any startup costs should be negligible for the existing program. The most difficult selling point may be comparison with other departments' funding requests.

Acquiring Capital Assets for Future Use

This type of proposal may be the most difficult to accomplish. Capital expenditures for future long-term use are often postponed by decision-makers in cash-strapped organizations who must first fulfill immediate demands for funding. Consider, for example, a metropolitan hospital that is hemmed in on all sides by privately owned property. The hospital will clearly need expansion space in the future. An adjacent privately owned property comes on the market at a price less than its appraised value. Even though expansion is not scheduled until several years in the future, it would be wise to consider this acquisition of a capital asset for future use.

Building a Capital Expenditure Proposal for a New Program

Various assumptions are made to determine whether an investment will generate a sufficient financial return (as seen in Chapter 18). We will return to the Curie Imaging Clinic to evaluate the request for a new imaging machine in greater detail. **Table 19.1** provides a seven-step capital budgeting process.

Curie's goal is to add a new service and generate a sufficient return on investment. First, we will begin by breaking down total revenue. Annual revenue remains $240,000 but now is the product of price and quantity, $100 per test × 2,400 tests. The office manager believes output price may increase 2% per year while output will grow by 2%. Optimistically, the manager believes 3% output growth may occur if the area continues to see high population and economic growth, and in the worst case, she expects growth to be no less than the rate of population growth in the United States (i.e., 1%). Based on most likely assumptions, revenue should grow to $281,198 in year 5 (**Table 19.2**).

Second, we will divide the $150,000 in direct operating costs into salary and supply expenses. Salary will be assumed to be a fixed cost while supplies will increase (and decrease) with output. As the investment will generate revenue and require resources over five years, we will include a growth rate for output and inflation rates for the

Table 19.1 Capital Budgeting Steps

1. Identify the desired goal and alternatives (see type of capital expenditure proposal).
2. Estimate output, output prices, and revenues, including when cash will be received.
3. Identify the type and quantity of resources needed, input prices, and when expenses will be paid.
4. Determine the discount rate and calculate the PV of future cash flows.
5. Select an evaluation measure (payback period, NPV, IRR) and calculate financial return.
6. Conduct sensitivity analysis.
7. Make recommendations (purchase/do not purchase).

Table 19.2 Investment Assumptions

Assumptions	Most Likely	Best Case	Worst Case
Quantity	2,400	2,640	2,160
Price	$100.00	$110	$90
Salaries	$120,000	$110,000	$130,000
Supplies	$12.50	$11.00	$14.00
Depreciation	$60,000	$60,000	$60,000
Discount rate	5.0%	5.0%	5.0%
Growth rate, output	2.0%	3.0%	1.0%
Inflation rate, output prices	2.0%	4.0%	0.0%
Inflation rate, expenses (not deprecation)	3.0%	1.0%	5.0%
Tax rate	35.0%	35.0%	35.0%

output price and expenses. Depreciation based on historical cost will be a constant $60,000 per year. Best-case, most likely, and worst-case outcomes for each assumption are shown in Table 19.2 (also see Chapter 18).

Salary expense is expected to be $120,000 per year and increase by 3% annually. Supply expense is expected to be $12.50 per test and increase by 3% per year. Year 1 supply expense should be $30,000, $12.50 × (1 + 0.03)$^{(year-1)}$ ×2,400 tests. The second factor, (1 + 0.03)$^{(year-1)}$, recognizes no inflation in the first year. In year 2, the supply expense should increase to $15.97 per test, $12.50 × (1 + 0.03)$^{(2-1)}$ or $31,212. As stated earlier, depreciation is $60,000 per year, $300,000 ÷ 5 years, and does not change.

Table 19.3 shows that net income before taxes, revenue − expenses, starts at $30,000 in year 1 and grows to $50,987 in year 5. If the organization is subject to tax, 35% of net income is subtracted to obtain net income after tax. Depreciation is then added back to net income after tax to obtain net cash flow. The outflow of funds for the investment, −$300,000 is recognized in year 0. Depreciation simply spreads this cost over the asset's useful life, and if depreciation is not added back, it would be double counted as an expenditure when the asset was acquired and again through annual depreciation.

The present value factor (PVF) is shown on the next line (i.e., what $1.00 would purchase in the future based on the assumed discount rate). The present value of cash flow (PVCF) is the product of net cash flow and the present value factor, net cash flow × PVF. Summing PVCF produces the net present value (NPV). Given NPV is $71,596, $371,596 discounted cash inflow − $300,000 cash outflow, the machine should be purchased. Table 19.2 provides the Excel formulas for NPV and IRR, =NPV(rate, range) − investment is used because the net cash flow is not constant. If the project had generated equal cash flows every year =PV(rate, nper, pmt, [fv], type) could have been used.

Table 19.4 shows the results of sensitivity analysis. In this case, the office manager believes the greatest risk lies with the initial output estimate. She believes in the best case initial output could be 2,640, 10% above most likely, and in the worst case, 2,160, 10% below. If 2,640 tests are produced, the practice could earn $135,418 over five years, an 89.1% increase over the most likely return. On the other hand, if the worst-case output is realized, NPV would fall to $7,773 or decline by 89.1% compared to most likely. Financial performance under worst-case initial output supports purchasing the equipment as NPV is greater than $0 and IRR, 5.9%, exceeds the discount rate.

Capital budgeting analysis is designed to make managers critically assess an investment *prior* to purchase. As seen in Table 19.3, explicitly defining key variables and working through the math determines if a project will earn an adequate return when assumptions are met. Capital budgeting analysis is both an art and a science as obviously, the best predictions of the future are subject to uncontrollable forces. After decisions are made to pursue a project, results should be regularly reviewed to assess performance. When performance is lower than expected, the manager should determine whether it is due to uncontrollable factors, controllable factors that can and should be improved, or poor assumptions. The goal of post-expenditure review is to improve management and future capital analyses.

Evaluating Capital Expenditure Proposals

Management planning must involve the allocation of available financial resources for projects that promise to reap returns in the future. This applies to both for-profit and not-for-profit organizations.

Hard Choices: Rationing Available Capital

Most businesses, including those providing healthcare services and products, have a limited

Table 19.3 Capital Budget Worksheet[2]

	Year 0	Year 1	Year 2	Year 3	Year 4	Year 5	Total
Investment	-$300,000						-$300,000
Price	$0	$100	$102	$104	$106	$108	
Quantity	0	2,400	2,448	2,497	2,547	2,598	
Revenue	$0	$240,000	$249,696	$259,784	$270,279	$281,198	$1,300,957
Expenses							
Salaries	$0	$120,000	$123,600	$127,308	$131,127	$135,061	$637,096
Supplies	0	30,000	31,212	32,473	33,785	35,150	$162,620
Depreciation	0	60,000	$60,000	$60,000	$60,000	$60,000	$300,000
Total Expense	$0	$210,000	$214,812	$219,781	$224,912	$230,211	$1,099,716
Net Income		$30,000	$34,884	$40,003	$45,367	$50,987	$201,241
Tax		$10,500	$12,209	$14,001	$15,878	$17,846	$70,434
Net Income After Tax		$19,500	$22,675	$26,002	$29,488	$33,142	$130,807
Plus: Depreciation		$60,000	$60,000	$60,000	$60,000	$60,000	$300,000
Net Cash Flow (CF)	-$300,000	$79,500	$82,675	$86,002	$89,488	$93,142	$130,807
Present Value Factor (PVF)	1.0000	0.9524	0.9070	0.8638	0.8227	0.7835	
Present Value of Cash Flow (PVCF)	-$300,000	$75,714	$74,988	$74,292	$73,622	$72,979	$71,596
Evaluation measure		**Excel formulas**					
NPV	$71,596	=NPV(B11,C37:G37)+B37		or	=NPV(0.05,795000...93142)-300000		
IRR	13.0%	=IRR(B37:G37)			=IRR(-300000...93142)		

Data from Ross, T. K. (2018). *A comprehensive guide to budgeting for health care managers.* Jones and Bartlett Learning; and Ross, T. K. (2021). *Practical budgeting for health care, a concise guide.* Jones and Bartlett Learning.

Table 19.4 Sensitivity Analysis

Best-case quantity (Q = 2,640)	ROI	% Change from Most Likely
NPV	$135,418	89.1%
IRR	19.7%	51.0%
Worst-case quantity (Q = 2,160)		
NPV	$7,773	−89.1%
IRR	5.9%	−54.6%

amount of capital available for purposes of capital expenditure, so available capital funds must be rationed. Different organizations approach the rationing process in different ways. However, most organizations will consider the following factors:

- Necessity for the request (community need, regulatory mandates, safety, etc.)
- Cost of capital to the organization
- Financial return that could be realized on alternative investments

These three factors will probably be considered in a descending sequence of decision-making. The overriding question is necessity. Necessity for the request pertains to the criticality of the need. What are the basic reasons for contemplating the capital expenditure? Are these reasons necessary? If so, how necessary?

While necessity is an overarching consideration, the cost of capital to the organization for the proposed capital expenditure is a key determinant of whether projects are funded (i.e., those

with expected returns above the cost of capital are funded, those below are not). The answer to "what is the cost of capital" is provided in the form of a computation. The discount rate depends on how a project is financed: debt, equity, or a combination. The cost of capital could be the cost of debt financing (typically the lowest rate), ROA, or ROE (the highest rate).

The third element in management's decision-making sequence is what return could be realized on alternative investments of the available capital. This concept is known as **opportunity cost** (i.e., the alternative foregone from choosing one action over another). Assume a rationing situation where unlimited funds are not available. Thus, when a choice is made to expend funds on capital project A, an opportunity is lost to expend those same funds on project B or C. The choice of A thus eliminates the opportunity to benefit from B or C, an either/or decision. Even though all three projects exceed the cost of capital, opportunity cost throws the choice to the project with the highest return.

Table 19.5 provides a list of five projects that Codman Medical Center could invest in. The total cost for all five projects is $11,250,000, but Codman only has $7,500,000 to invest, so choices must be made. The CFO also has established 5% as the discount rate. Project A offers the highest *dollar* profit, but it should not be the first project pursued.

Table 19.6 calculates return on investment (ROI), profit ÷ investment outlay, ranks the projects from highest to lowest ROI, and calculates the total capital outlay (i.e., the running budget). Project E should be pursued first

Table 19.5 Potential Projects (Investments)

Project	Investment Outlay	Revenue	Cost	Profit
A	$3,000,000	$5,400,000	$5,100,000	$300,000
B	$2,400,000	$4,000,000	$3,800,000	$200,000
C	$1,350,000	$2,400,000	$2,300,000	$100,000
D	$2,500,000	$3,100,000	$3,000,000	$100,000
E	$2,000,000	$3,850,000	$3,600,000	$250,000

Table 19.6 Investments Ranked by ROI

Project	Investment Outlay	Revenue	Cost	Profit	ROI	Running Budget
E	$2,000,000	$3,850,000	$3,600,000	$250,000	12.5%	$2,000,000
A	$3,000,000	$5,400,000	$5,100,000	$300,000	10.0%	$5,000,000
B	$2,400,000	$4,000,000	$3,800,000	$200,000	8.3%	$7,400,000
C	$1,350,000	$2,400,000	$2,300,000	$100,000	7.4%	$8,750,000
D	$2,500,000	$3,100,000	$3,000,000	$100,000	4.0%	$11,250,000

as it returns 12.5% for every dollar invested, followed by A and B. Pursuing E, A, and B exhausts the capital budget, $7,400,000, so no further projects can be pursued in the current year. Projects C and D may be carried over to the next year's capital budget, but they will again be ranked with other projects and only pursued when funds are available and their return is higher than the new projects.

Figure 19.2 provides a column chart of the investment options and adds the organization's cost of capital, 5%, to illustrate another point. If funds were unlimited, managers should pursue projects E, A, B, and C, but even with unlimited funds, they should avoid D as its

return is less than the organization's cost of capital, 4.0% < 5.0%.

Decision-makers must apply judgment in making investment decisions to ensure the financial well-being of their organization. This is a finance text, so the primary concern is return on investment, but managers must also recognize issues of community need, regulatory mandates, and so on when making investments.

The Review and Evaluation Process

The degree of attention paid to evaluation and the level of management responsible for making the decisions may be dictated by the overall availability of capital funding and the amount of funds requested. Evaluation of capital budget proposals may be objective or subjective. An impartial review process is most desirable.

An objective method usually involves scoring and/or ranking the competing proposals. In scoring, the approach generally focuses on a single proposal and evaluates it on a fixed set of criteria. In ranking, the proposal is compared with other proposals and ranked in accordance with a looser set of criteria.

The objective review and evaluation may first involve scoring to eliminate the very low-scoring proposals. The remaining higher-scoring proposals may then be ranked in accordance with still another set of criteria. The criteria may, in turn, contain quantitative items such as outcomes and/or productivity and qualitative items such as whether the proposal is in accordance with the

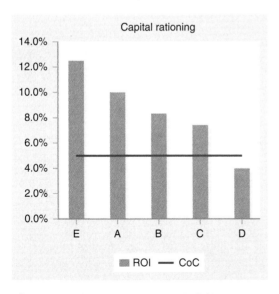

Figure 19.2 Ranking Investments by ROI

Table 19.7 Balancing Community Need and Financial Performance

Criteria	Widespread	Rare	Absent
Community need (availability of service)	1	2	3
	Below	**Equal**	**Above**
Return on investment	1	2	3
Organization with strong finances, 50% community need and 50% finance			
Project A: absent service and low ROI	2.00 =(0.5×3)+(0.5×1)	**Fund**	
Project B: widely available and average ROI	1.50 =(0.5×1)+(0.5×2)		
Organization with weak finances, 25% community need and 75% finance			
Project A: absent service and low ROI	1.50 =(0.25×1)+(0.75×2)		
Project B: widely available and average ROI	1.75 =(0.25×3)+(0.75×1)	**Fund**	

organization's core mission. **Table 19.7** shows two criteria, ranks two projects, and demonstrates the change in ranking based on the weight assigned to each criteria.

A financially strong hospital has the luxury of weighting community need equal to ROI and thus funds project A. A financially strapped organization must prioritize more profitable projects higher and thus weights ROI at 75%, shifting the choice to project B. Finally, some authorities believe the source of financing the project (whether it is internal or external, for example) should not be relevant to the investment decision. Real-world management, however, has a different view. How the project will be financed may be their first question in the review and evaluation process.

WRAP-UP

Summary

Equipment and facilities are large expenditures of organizational funds that require a structured review process to ensure they will recoup their cost. Capital budgeting analysis is a seven-step process beginning with defining the goal of the expenditure, estimating expected revenues and expenses, and ending with a purchase/do not purchase decision. Financial performance is based on assumptions, and managers should test these assumptions with sensitivity analysis to determine the robustness of the purchase decision.

While capital expenditure analysis estimates the return on a project, the returns on multiple projects must also be compared. Most organizations will have more requests for capital funds than available funds. Capital rationing ranks potential projects on return on investment. While this text emphasizes financial return, in the real world managers must also consider nonfinancial issues such as community need, synergy with existing programs, and other factors before making their final choice on investments.

Key Terms

Capital Budget

Capital Asset

Cash Flow Analysis

Cumulative Cash Flow

Internal Rate of Return

Net Present Value

Opportunity Cost

Payback Period

Discussion Questions

1. Explain why a capital budget is necessary.
2. Describe the different types of capital expenditures and how they affect the capital expenditure analysis.
3. Describe the differences between payback period, net present value, and internal rate of return.

4. Explain the three factors that affect capital budget decisions.
5. Explain the effect of limited funds (i.e., capital rationing) on the capital budgeting process.

Problems

1. A hospital is planning to build a nonprofit urgent care center next to its emergency department (ED) to siphon off nonemergent cases. The ED frequently operates beyond its designed capacity, creating patient and employee dissatisfaction. It is expected that the ED will not lose any patients if the center is built due to patients leaving before treatment is rendered and a growing demand for ED services. The center is expected to require a $4 million outlay in year 0. No depreciation expense is needed since the center is nonprofit and reaps no tax benefit.

The following table provides the best-case, most likely, and worst-case estimates for patient quantity, reimbursement, supply and other expenses per encounter, and growth rates for patient quantity, reimbursement, and expenses beginning in year 1. The ED and finance departments have estimated that the center will need five physicians earning an average of $240,000 in salaries and benefits, twelve nurses at $84,000 each, and nine other staff at $48,000 each. Create a five-year capital budget analysis and calculate the net present value (NPV)

Assumptions	Most Likely	Best Case	Most Likely	Worst Case	
Quantity	62,600	68,900	62,600	56,400	
Price	$100.00	$110	$100	$90	
Supplies	$30.00	$11.00	$12.50	$14.00	per unit (v)
Other	$10	$9	$10	$11	per unit (v)
Discount rate	6.0%	5.0%	5.0%	5.0%	constant
Growth rate, output	1.0%	3.0%	2.0%	1.0%	
Inflation rate, output prices	2.0%	4.0%	2.0%	0.0%	
Inflation rate, expenses (not depr)	3.0%	1.0%	3.0%	5.0%	
Tax rate	35.0%	35.0%	35.0%	35.0%	constant

and internal rate of return (IRR). In addition, calculate the NPVs and IRRs at best- and worst-case volume with all other variables at their most likely estimates.

2. A hospital is planning to build a for-profit MRI facility to expand its imaging services to compete with other local providers. The center is expected to require a $2 million outlay in year 0 to purchase the MRI and renovate the office space. The $2 million investment should be depreciated over five years.

The following table provides the best-case, most likely, and worst-case estimates for patient quantity, reimbursement, supply and other expenses per encounter, and growth rates for patient quantity, reimbursement, and expenses beginning in year 1. Physician salaries are $180 per image for reading and interpretation of images. The technician and other salaries are annual salaries and benefits. Create a five-year capital budget analysis and calculate the net present value (NPV) and internal rate of return (IRR). In addition, calculate the NPVs and IRRs at best- and worst-case volume with all other variables at their most likely estimates.

Assumptions	Most Likely	Best Case	Most Likely	Worst Case
Quantity	1,800	2,100	1,800	1,600
Price	$650	$700	$650	$550
Physician salaries	$180	$160	$180	$200
Tech salaries	$95,000	$90,000	$95,000	$100,000
Support salaries	$48,000	$44,000	$48,000	$52,000
Supplies	$70	$60	$70	$80
Other	$10	$9	$10	$12
Discount rate	6.0%	6.0%	6.0%	6.0%
Growth rate, output	1.0%	1.5%	1.0%	0.0%
Inflation rate, output prices	2.0%	3.0%	2.0%	0.0%
Inflation rate, expenses (not depr)	3.0%	1.0%	3.0%	5.0%
Tax rate	35.0%	35.0%	35.0%	35.0%

Notes

1. S. A. Finkler, "Flexible Budget Variance Analysis Extended to Patient Acuity and DRGs," *Health Care Management Review*, 10, no. 4 (1985): 21–34.
2. T. K. Ross, *A Comprehensive Guide to Budgeting for Health Care Managers* (Burlington, MA: Jones and Bartlett Learning, 2018); T. K. Ross, *Practical Budgeting for Health Care, A Concise Guide* (Burlington, MA: Jones and Bartlett Learning, 2021).

Evaluating Capital Investments

CHAPTER 20

Investing, Borrowing, and Statistics

PROGRESS NOTES

After completing this chapter, you should be able to:

1. Define cash equivalents.
2. Explain what the FDIC does and does not insure.
3. Describe the difference between stocks and bonds.
4. Describe the role of measures of central tendency and the differences among mean, median, and mode.
5. Describe the role of measures of dispersion and the differences among range, variance, and standard deviation.

Overview: Investing, Borrowing, and Statistics

Most organizations and individuals use debt to acquire assets, but many do not understand the fundamentals or costs of borrowing funds. At the same time, organizations and individuals may hold unneeded funds in low-yield instruments. For example, an individual may be holding $2,000 in their checking account paying them 0.01% in interest while carrying a credit card balance of $6,000 and paying 18% (or more) interest. The annual interest earned on the checking account is $0.20 while $1,080 in interest is paid to the credit card company. Obviously, individuals want to keep some funds in their checking

account for unanticipated expenses, but shifting $1,000 to the credit card balance will save the card holder $179.90 in interest per year. If the monthly interest savings of $14.99 are added to their minimum monthly payment, the card holder will save additional interest charges and pay off their debt sooner.

Organizations face the same choices: where to obtain financing at the lowest rate and where to invest unneeded funds to obtain the highest returns. The language of investment is an integral part of the finance world. Being knowledgeable about the meaning that lies behind investment terms gives you greater control over your finance transactions. This chapter explores investment terminology and related meanings for cash equivalents, long-term investments in bonds, investments in stocks, and company ownership (public or private) in the context of investing, along with investment indicators.

Investments are recorded as either current assets or long-term assets on the balance sheet of the organization. Current assets involve cash and cash equivalents, along with short-term securities, securities with a maturity of one year or less (see Chapter 4). Long-term investments, on the other hand, involve securities that mature in more than one year and are reported as long-term items on the balance sheet.

Cash Equivalents

Cash equivalents are liquid assets; that is, they can be liquidated and turned into cash on short notice when needed. Healthcare organizations need to keep money on hand to pay bills, but it is not usually optimal to hold those monies in a non-interest-bearing checking account. Instead, the chief financial officer (CFO) will probably decide to temporarily place the monies in some type of liquid asset (a cash equivalent) to earn interest.

Actual cash includes not just currency (the dollar bills in your wallet) but also monies held in bank checking accounts and savings accounts, plus coins, checks, and money orders. Cash equivalents with their interest rates as of October 3, 2021, include the following:

- Certificates of deposit (CDs) from banks, one year: 0.50 to 0.75%[1]
- Government securities, one year treasury bonds: 0.09%[2]
- Money market funds, one year: 0.30% to 0.55%[3]

All of these short-term investments should be very liquid and low risk. A prudent CFO should, of course, seek low-risk investments. Certificates of deposit can be purchased for various short periods of time: 30, 60, 90 days, and so on. The certificates earn interest and can be withdrawn (cashed) at end of the period without paying a penalty.

Government securities that rank as cash equivalents include Treasury bills and Treasury notes. Treasury bills are typically issued with maturities of 3, 6, or 12 months. There is a minimum dollar amount to purchase. A Treasury bill pays the full amount invested if redeemed at maturity. If the bill is redeemed prior to maturity, however, the amount received may be either higher or lower than your cost depending upon the current market. Treasury notes are typically issued with longer maturities—years instead of months. The shortest maturity period for a Treasury note is one year. A one-year note would be classified as short term and could be recorded as a current asset.

Money market funds are investments in conservative instruments such as commercial bank CDs and Treasury bills. A money market fund should invest in an assortment of conservative instruments. Portfolio managers, who are expected to manage responsibly, thus select only low-risk investments. Money market funds are somewhat of a hybrid, as these funds typically allow check-writing privileges. Thus, the investor is able to withdraw funds by writing what is actually a draft against the fund, although most everyone thinks of this draft as a check.

Governmental Guarantor: The FDIC

In the United States, the **Federal Deposit Insurance Corporation (FDIC)** "preserves and promotes public confidence in the U.S. financial system by insuring deposits in banks and thrift institutions ... by identifying and monitoring and addressing risks to the deposit insurance funds; and by limiting the effect on the economy and the financial system when a bank or thrift institution fails."[4] The FDIC insures deposits in banks and thrift institutions for $250,000 per depositor. Savings, checking, and other deposit accounts are combined to reach the deposit insurance limit. "Deposits held in different categories of ownership—such as single or joint accounts—may be separately insured. Also, the FDIC generally provides separate coverage for retirement accounts, such as individual retirement accounts (IRAs) and Keoghs."[5] It is important to note that not all

FDIC-Insured

- Checking Accounts (including money market deposit accounts)
- Savings Accounts (including passbook accounts)
- Certificates of Deposit

Not FDIC-Insured

- Investments in mutual funds (stock, bond, or money market mutual funds), whether purchased from a bank, brokerage, or dealer
- Annuities (underwritten by insurance companies, but sold at some banks)
- Stocks, bonds, Treasury securities or other investment products, whether purchased through a bank or a broker/dealer

Reproduced from the Federal Deposit Insurance Corporation. (2011). *The FDIC: Insured or not insured?: A guide to what is and is not protected.* https://www.fdic.gov/consumers/consumer/information/fdiciorn.html

institutions—and thus not all funds—are insured by the FDIC (see **Exhibit 20.1**).

Bonds

A bond is a long-term debt instrument under which a borrower agrees to make payments of interest and principal on particular dates to the holder of the debt (the bond). Bonds typically mature in 20 to 30 years, although there are exceptions. Interest rates are higher due to the longer duration, with 10-year treasury bonds paying 1.48%[6] and corporate bonds 2.35%[7] as of October 3, 2021. In general, interest is paid throughout the term, or life, of the bonds, and the principal is paid at maturity, but there are exceptions to this rule of thumb. There are three types of bonds.

Municipal bonds are long-term obligations that are typically used to finance capital projects. Municipal bonds are issued by states or political subdivisions. The political subdivision might be, for example, a county, a bridge authority, or the authority for a toll road project. General obligation bonds are backed, or secured, by the "full

faith and credit" of the municipality that issues them. This means the bonds are backed by the full taxing authority of the municipality that issues them. Revenue bonds, as their name implies, are backed, or secured, by revenues of their particular project (e.g., tolls collected on a bridge). Eligible not-for-profit healthcare organizations can sometimes issue revenue bonds through a local healthcare financing authority.

Mortgage bonds, as their name implies, are backed, or secured, by certain real property. When first mortgage bonds are issued, this means the first mortgage bondholders have first claim to the real property that has been pledged to secure the mortgage. If second mortgage bonds are also issued, this means the second mortgage bondholders will not have a claim against the real property until the claims of the first mortgage bondholders have been paid.

Debentures are bonds that are unsecured. Instead of being backed by real property, debentures are backed by revenues that the issuing organization can earn. Unlike bondholders, holders of debentures are unsecured. Subordinated debentures are even further unsecured, in that these debentures cannot be paid until any and all debt obligations that are senior to the subordinated debentures have been paid.

Stocks

Stocks represent equity, or net worth, in a company. Generally speaking, a bondholder is a creditor because bonds are liabilities to the issuing company. On the other hand, an individual or organization that buys stock in that company is an investor, not a creditor. Investors can purchase either common or **preferred stock**. Knueven reports that the S&P 500 has earned 13.6% annually between 2010 and 2020; returns of this magnitude do not come without risk, as the S&P fell 4.4% during 2018.[8] A purchaser of **common stock** buys an ownership interest in the company, shares proportionately in the net income (or loss) of the company, and votes for the board of directors and major issues. Any income earned may be distributed to shareholders or retained by the company. For example, HCA earned $10.93 per share in 2020 but paid a dividend of $1.92.

Preferred stock, as its name implies, has preference over common stock in certain issues such as payment of dividends (i.e., preferred stock dividends are paid before the common stock dividends). Preferred stock is a hybrid in that it generally has a fixed-rate dividend payment, like a bond's interest payment, and investors expect to receive a portion of net income of the company up to the amount of the fixed-rate dividend payment. Unlike common stock holders, preferred stock holders have no claim above the fixed-rate dividend payment. Convertible preferred stock is a type of preferred stock that can be exchanged for common shares. The exchange is usually at a particular time and price, and the exchange ratio of preferred to common is also stipulated.

Stock warrants allow the owner of the warrant to purchase additional shares of stock in the company, generally at a particular price and prior to an expiration date. Warrants do not pay dividends. They are often part of the compensation package awarded to executives.

Privately Held Versus Public Companies

Whether a stock is listed on a stock exchange is a function of ownership and size of the organization. These distinctions are described here.

Privately Held Companies

A small company with common stock that is not traded is known as a privately held company. Its stock is termed closely held stock.

Public Companies

Companies with publicly owned common stock are known as public companies. The stocks of many larger public companies may be listed on one of several stock exchanges. Stock exchanges exist to trade the stock of publicly held companies. At the time of this writing, besides multiple regional exchanges such as the Chicago Stock Exchange, there is the American Stock Exchange, known as AMEX, along with the New York Stock Exchange, known as the NYSE.

Smaller public companies, however, may not be listed on a stock exchange. The stock of these companies is considered to be unlisted; instead, their stock is traded "over the counter," or OTC. The National Association of Securities Dealers (NASD) oversees this market. The OTC stock market uses a computerized trading network called NASDAQ, which stands for the "NASD Automated Quotation system."

Published stock tables typically reflect the composite regular trading on the stock exchanges as of closing. A stock table will generally contain four columns: the first column is an abbreviation of the public company's name, the second column is the company's symbol (an alpha symbol), the third column is the stock's price as of closing for that day, and the fourth column is the net change of the stock price when compared to close of the previous day. Using healthcare organizations as examples, Johnson & Johnson's symbol is "JNJ," while Humana, Inc.'s symbol is "HUM."

The Securities and Exchange Commission

The overseer of the stock market in the United States is the **Securities and Exchange Commission (SEC)**. The mission of the SEC is to "protect investors, maintain fair, orderly, and efficient markets, and facilitate capital formation."[9] The SEC oversees "the key participants in the securities world, including securities exchanges, securities brokers and dealers, investment advisors, and mutual funds. Here, the SEC is concerned primarily with promoting the disclosure of important market-related information, maintaining fair dealing, and protecting against fraud."[10]

Statistics

It is important to understand that our usage of statistical terms in the world of healthcare finance is a specialized view. For example, on HospitalCompare differences in quality outcomes, such as mortality rates, are only identified when the difference is statistically significant. Hospitals can have large differences in outcomes but still be grouped in the same category. In other words, we need enough information to understand the general process and what the terms mean in general usage. As such, the following definitions are not technical but instead are intentionally generalized.

The Field of Mathematics Versus the Discipline of Statistics

The field of mathematics is broad and varied. The National Council of Teachers of Mathematics (NCTM) has developed a set of mathematical standards for teaching and learning mathematics. These standards are important because they help the user understand the breadth and depth of mathematics.

The NCTM has set two categories of standards: thinking math and content math. Thinking math standards cover problem solving, communication, reasoning, and connections. Content math standards cover statistics and probability, fractions and decimals, estimation, number sense, geometry and spatial sense, measurement, and patterns and relationships.[11]

- Statistics is the branch of mathematics that deals with collecting, summarizing, and analyzing numerical data, along with estimating probability and interpreting analytical results.
- Arithmetic, on the other hand, is the branch of mathematics that covers the basic functions of multiplication, division, addition, subtraction, and so on.

In other words, statistics often provides sophisticated analytical results, while arithmetic provides the results of basic calculations.

Commonly Used Statistical Terms

The two most important concepts in statistics are central tendency and dispersion. Central tendency reports the "average" outcome for a group, and dispersion reports how far individual observations lie from the average. Understanding these two concepts allows you to determine if an organization's performance is common or exceptional, exceptional meaning substantially better or worse than "average" performance.

Mean, Median, and Mode

Mean, **median**, and **mode** are measures of central tendency. To begin our description of the mean, median, and mode, review **Table 20.1**, where the operating margins for 10 community hospitals are recorded. The numbers are arranged, or ranked, in order. In this case, the operating margins are arranged from the lowest to the highest, but they could also be reported from highest to the lowest.

Table 20.1 Illustration of Mean, Median, and Mode

Hospital	Margin
1	−5.0%
2	−1.0%
3	1.0%
4	3.0%
5	4.0%
6	4.0%
7	5.0%
8	6.0%
9	8.0%
10	13.0%
Mean	3.8%
Median	4.0%
Mode	4.0%
Range	18.0%
Variance	0.2%
Standard deviation	4.9%

Mean: The mean is the average of numbers, or values. To obtain the average, all the values are added together to obtain the total and the total is divided by the number of items to obtain the mean, $38\% \div 10 = 3.8\%$. This method is known as the arithmetic mean and is the most commonly used.

Median: The median occupies a position in a ranked series of values (numbers) in which the same number of values appear above and below the median. In this case, the median is 4.0%, as there are four hospitals with operating margins less than and greater than 4.0%. In a situation where there is no one middle number (as is possible when there are an even number of values), the median instead is the average of the two middle numbers within the ranked series of values.

Mode: The mode is the number, or value, that appears the most times (is the most frequent) within a series of numbers or values. The mode is 4.0%, two occurrences versus only one occurrence of the other eight numbers. In this case, the mean, median, and mode are the same, indicating few extreme observations.

Range, Variance, and Standard Deviation

Range, **variance**, and **standard deviation** are measures of dispersion that assess how much difference there is between observations. When assessing operating margin or cost per discharge, dispersion answers the questions "Do different hospitals have similar or dissimilar performance? Is the cost per discharge difference between the highest and lowest cost institutions $200 (unimportant) or $2,000 (extremely important)?" Managers should identify the reasons for large differences and rectify the differences in their control that lead to lower financial performance. The first measure of dispersion is the range. Range is the maximum value in the data set minus the minimum, 18%, 13% to −5%. A large range indicates that there is a substantial difference in performance; in this case, 18% is large as it is four and a half times larger than the mean.

Variance is the sum of the square of the differences between each individual value in a data set and the mean divided by the number of observations−1, 0.2%. The variance is mainly used to calculate the standard deviation. Standard deviation is the square root of the variance. In a normally distributed population, 68% of all observations fall within one standard deviation and 95% within two standard deviations. The standard deviation for the 10 hospitals is 4.9%, so 68% of hospitals should have an operating margin between −1.1% (3.8% − 4.9%) and 8.7% (3.8% + 4.9%). Examining Table 20.1 shows that 70% of hospitals, seven of 10, fall in this range. The remaining three hospitals lie within two standard deviations, −6.0% through 13.8%. Only 2.5% of hospitals should fall more than two standard deviations from the mean, in this example no hospitals fall outside two standard deviations to meet the strict criterion of statistical significance. The performance of hospital 1 is unacceptable. Hospital 1's negative margin of 5.0% will create future problems, so managers should assess the performance of "average" hospitals, if not hospital 10, the best-performing hospital, to determine how they can improve performance. Likewise, the managers of hospital 10 should assess their own performance to determine if they can sustain their exceptional performance.

Illustrating the Difference

The mean operating margin is 3.8%, the median is 4.0%, four hospitals have operating margins above and below 4.0%, and the mode is 4.0% (two hospitals reported 4.0% operating margins). The similarity of the mean, median, and mode indicate that the group is normally distributed; 3.8% is a valid indicator of the average operating margin, and the distribution is not skewed.

The measures of central tendency and dispersion can be used to predict what is likely to happen and the amount of confidence you should have in the prediction (i.e., how likely will it occur?). For example, managers may want to identify potential quality issues based on the length of stay (LOS) for patients with a particular condition (DRG). Cases to investigate could be identified as those patients with an LOS more than two standard deviations above or below the average for all patients. Since occurrences beyond two standard deviations should be 5% or less, a high rate of these cases may indicate treatment problems.

Other Statistical Analysis Terms

Algorithm: A problem-solving, step-by-step process or a set of formulas used in calculations, particularly in computer programs.

Domain: A subgroup of a whole group that is of particular interest for research or for measurement purposes. For example, the domain of safety is one subgroup of an entire patient care grouping.

Measure: A unit of analysis, such as a measurement standard.

Measurement: The process of assigning numbers to something, such as to variables. In other words, measurement is how we get the numbers we analyze using statistical methods.

Standardized measure or scale: A statistical method that can compare data measured on different scales or instruments.

For example, the method of comparison could be a score or a percentage.

Statistically significant: In general terms, a result or relationship is found to be reliable, and thus statistically significant, if it is either bigger or smaller than if the equivalent result could be attributed to chance alone. Typically, a value is deemed statistically significant if the probability that it would arise from chance is 5% or less.

Variable: A finding or quantity that can vary or is apt to vary. Examples of variables include just about anything that is capable of being measured. Note that a constant is the opposite of a variable because it does not vary.

Terms About Distributions

These descriptions pertain to distribution terms, such as those used to explain scoring methodology.

Frequency distribution: A count of how many times (how frequently) a value appears in a group of values (**Figure 20.1**).

Decile: A distribution into 10 classes, each of which contains one-tenth of the whole; any one of the 10 classes is a decile.

Quartile: A distribution into four classes, each of which contains one-quarter of the whole; any one of the four classes is a quartile.

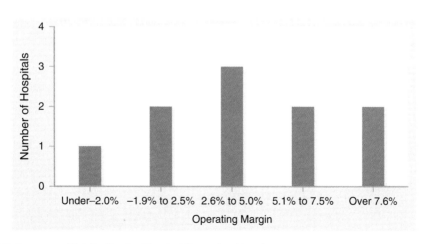

Figure 20.1 Frequency Distribution for Hospital Operating Margins

Terms About Data

These descriptions pertain to data. Note that the word *data* is plural.

Data: The factual information being analyzed. This information is typically used to measure and/or calculate, although it may also be used for reasoning and/or discussion.

Database (also data base): A particular set of computerized data organized in a manner designed for efficient retrieval.

Data entry: The process of recording data, generally by electronic means.

Data mining: A process used by organizations to turn raw data into useful information.

Data processing: Generally speaking, taking raw data and converting them into a form that can be readily used by computer software (processing). The processing can take place in magnetic, optical, or mechanical form.

Data set: A group of data (a set) gathered together for a like purpose.

Data standardization: The process that converts data into a standard, such as the creation of standard scores.

Big data: Large data sets that are analyzed for patterns or trends.

Terms About Time Measurements

These descriptions pertain to terms about time measurements.

Period: A unit of time.

Baseline period: A unit of time (period) used as a basis for comparison.

Base year: A 12-month unit of time (year) used as a basis for comparison.

Performance period: A unit of time during which performance is measured.

WRAP-UP

Summary

Whether an organization is borrowing or investing funds, it is faced with a wide variety of options. The return from investing funds depends on the length of time invested so cash equivalents typically pay less than long-term investments. The return also depends upon whether the organization invests in lower-risk and return bonds or higher-risk and return stocks. Understanding the differences between financial instruments is the first step toward value-maximizing borrowing and investing decisions.

Statistics describes the performance of systems. Measures of central tendency describe the average outcome in a system. While the mean, median, and mode provide information on performance, measures of dispersion are needed to understand how likely the average will occur. Managers should understand range, variance, and standard deviation to differentiate commonly occurring outcomes from low-frequency events to institute action to prevent undesirable low-frequency events and maintain beneficial ones that are within their control.

Key Terms

Common Stock	Median	Range
Debentures	Mode	Securities and Exchange
Decile	Money Market Funds	Commission (SEC)
Federal Deposit Insurance	Municipal Bonds	Standard Deviation
Corporation (FDIC)	Quartile	Stock Warrants
Mean	Preferred Stock	Variance

Discussion Questions

1. Do you know if your own monies on deposit are FDIC insured? If you do not know, how would you go about finding out?
2. Do you know of a healthcare company whose stock is publicly held? If you do not know, how would you go about finding out?
3. Do you know if any healthcare company that you have worked for (now or previously) has issued revenue bonds that were purchased by investors? If you do not know, how would you go about finding out?
4. Do you agree with the distinction between thinking math and content math? What type(s) of mathematics have you ever studied?

Problems

1. Given the following table, calculate the mean, median, mode, range, variance, and standard deviation for average length of stay (ALOS) across the 15 hospitals. Create a frequency distribution for profit. Is the distribution normal?

Hospital	ALOS
1	4.50
2	6.50
3	4.00
4	3.00
5	9.00
6	3.50
7	5.50
8	3.00
9	4.00
10	4.00
11	6.00
12	10.50
13	7.00
14	8.50
15	3.50

2. Given the following table, calculate the mean, median, mode, range, variance, and standard deviation for inpatient reimbursement and cost per discharge across the 15 hospitals. Profit per discharge ranges from $1,248 to –$957 per discharge. Is the difference in profit due to variation in reimbursement, cost, or both? Create a frequency distribution for profit. Is the distribution normal?

Hospital	I/P Reimb	I/P Cost	Profit
1	$5,239	$5,717	–$478
2	5,533	5,502	31
3	5,531	6,117	–586
4	5,678	5,508	170
5	5,531	5,310	221
6	5,778	5,557	221
7	5,607	5,589	18
8	5,986	5,927	59
9	6,102	5,447	655
10	6,408	5,758	650
11	6,221	5,952	269
12	6,965	5,717	1,248
13	5,958	5,941	17
14	6,456	7,413	–957
15	6,284	6,245	39

Notes

1. M. Goldberg, "Best 1-Year CD Rates, October 2021," https://bankrate.com, accessed October 3, 2021.

2. U.S. Department of the Treasury, "Daily Treasury Yield Curve Rates," https://www.treasury.gov, accessed October 3, 2021.

3. M. Goldberg, "10 Best Money Market Account Rates for October 2021," https://bankrate.com, accessed October 3, 2021.

4. Federal Deposit Insurance Corporation, "Who Is the FDIC?," http://www.fdic.gov/about/index.html.

5. Ibid.

6. U.S. Department of the Treasury, "Daily Treasury Yield Curve Rates," https://www.treasury.gov, accessed October 3, 2021.

7. St. Louis Federal Reserve Bank, "10-Year High Quality Market (HQM) Corporate Spot Rate," https://fred.stlouisfed.org, accessed October 3, 2021.

8. L. Knueven, "The Average Stock Market Return over the Last 10 Years," https://www.businessinsider.com, accessed October 3, 2021.

9. U.S. Securities and Exchange Commission, "The Investor's Advocate: How the SEC Protects Investors, Maintains Market Integrity, and Facilitates Capital Formation," http://www.sec.gov/about/whatwedo.shtml, last modified June 10, 2013.

10. Ibid.

11. "What Is Mathematics?", p. 1, http://www.2.ed.gov/pubs/EarlyMath/whatis.html, accessed July 12, 2016.

CHAPTER 21

Business Loans and Financing Costs

PROGRESS NOTES

After completing this chapter, you should be able to:

1. Explain capital structure and how it affects the cost of acquiring assets.
2. Describe four sources of capital.
3. Calculate loan payments and create and explain an amortization schedule.
4. Describe loan costs.

Overview: Loans and Financing Costs

Acquiring assets requires money, and businesses must raise it from owners and/or creditors. Business loans, as the term implies, represent debts incurred to acquire resources. Numerous borrowing instruments are available with varying interest rates that will substantially affect the cost of acquiring assets. The decisions to take on debt, the amount of debt to take on, and what borrowing instruments to use are common and necessary parts of financial planning.

Capital Structure

Capital represents the financial resources of the organization, and **capital structure** defines the proportion of debt and equity within an organization. The phrase *capital structure* refers to the debt–equity relationship. When a physician practice has $1,000,000 in assets and owes $500,000 in debt, it has $500,000 in equity and a 50-50 debt–equity relationship.

Different industries have different debt–equity relationships. Industries that have stable customer demand such as health care and utilities tend to rely on more debt than riskier industries, such as entertainment and information technology, that see wide swings in sales. In large healthcare organizations, the chief executive officers are usually responsible for guiding decisions about the proportion of debt the organization will use. Owners make these decisions in smaller organizations.

Sources of Capital

There are four common sources of funds:

- Borrowing from a lending institution
- Borrowing from investors

- Direct investment by owners or donors
- Retaining net income (i.e., the excess of revenues over expenses)

Borrowing from a lending institution (e.g., a bank) is generally classified by the length of the loan. **Short-term borrowing** is commonly expected to be repaid within a 12-month period. **Long-term borrowing** is regularly used to purchase land, buildings, and/or equipment. Long-term borrowing for these purposes is usually accomplished by obtaining a mortgage from the lending institution. The amount paid for borrowed funds varies based on the type of debt and length of loan. Short-term interest rates are typically lower than long-term rates.

Borrowing from investors assumes the organization is big enough and has the proper legal structure to do so. A common example of borrowing from investors is that of selling bonds. **Bonds** represent the company's promise to pay at a future date. When bonds are sold, the purchaser expects to receive a certain amount of annual interest and that the bonds will be redeemed on a certain date, several years in the future. Interest rates tend to increase with the duration of the bond (e.g., 30-year bonds pay a higher interest rate than 10-year bonds). Aaa bonds—the highest-quality, lowest-risk bonds, on August 29, 2021, paid 1.86% on 10-year bonds and 3.57% on 30-year bonds.[1]

Direct investment includes owners investing their own funds in an organization and acquiring the rights to any profit. While purchasing a right to the profits can only occur in for-profit organizations, nonprofit organizations can raise capital from private citizens through donations. Once established, a for-profit organization can sell additional interests in the organization, often by selling additional shares of common stock. Not-for-profit organizations cannot sell an interest, so they often use fundraising to increase equity.

Retaining net income (i.e., the excess of revenues over expenses) is another way to increase equity. For-profits can distribute their net income to their owners or retain it to expand the business. A not-for-profit organization is supposed to use its funds for public purposes and is prohibited from using its funds to benefit those with a close relationship to or control of the organization.

The Costs of Financing

Interest Expense

Payments on a business loan typically consist of two parts: principal and interest expense. The principal portion of the loan payment reduces the loan itself, while the rest of the payment is made up of interest on the remaining balance due on the loan.

The amount of principal and the amount of interest contained in each payment are illustrated in an **amortization schedule**. For example, assume equipment is purchased for $60,000, monthly payments will be made over a three-year period, and the annual interest rate is 6%. Excel provides the =PMT formula to calculate the loan payment based on the interest rate (rate), loan term (nper), and principal (pv):

=PMT(rate, nper, pv, [fv], [type])
=PMT(0.06/12,36,-60000) = $1,825.32

Note that the rate is entered as the monthly interest rate, 6% ÷ 12, and nper is the loan term in months, 3 years × 12 months, contrary to earlier work that used annual interest rates and years. The amortization schedule for this loan is illustrated in **Table 21.1**.

The interest expense for each monthly payment is computed on the principal balance remaining after the principal portion of the prior month's payment has been subtracted. The Balance column shows the declining balance of the principal. The difference between the payment and interest is the paydown on the principal (e.g., month 1's payment of $1,825.32 – $300.00 interest on $60,000 = $1,525.32 principal payment). The starting balance for month 2 is $58,474.68, $60,000 – $1,525.32. The interest payment declines and the principal payment increases as the principal is paid off. In month 36, the payment reduces the principal balance to zero; $9.08 is paid in interest, and $1,816.24 pays off the remaining balance. Not all amortization schedules are set up in the same configuration. If you use =PMT to calculate your mortgage payment, you will probably see it does not equal your payments as banks often add property taxes and insurance to the payment. =PMT calculates only the amount due for the loan.

Table 21.1 Loan Amortization Schedule

Month	Loan Payment	Interest	Principal Payment	Balance
1	$1,825.32	$300.00	$1,525.32	$58,474.68
2	1,825.32	292.37	1,532.94	56,941.74
3	1,825.32	284.71	1,540.61	55,401.13
4	1,825.32	277.01	1,548.31	53,852.82
5	1,825.32	269.26	1,556.05	52,296.77
6	1,825.32	261.48	1,563.83	50,732.94
7	1,825.32	253.66	1,571.65	49,161.29
8	1,825.32	245.81	1,579.51	47,581.78
9	1,825.32	237.91	1,587.41	45,994.37
10	1,825.32	229.97	1,595.34	44,399.03
11	1,825.32	222.00	1,603.32	42,795.70
12	1,825.32	213.98	1,611.34	41,184.37
13	1,825.32	205.92	1,619.39	39,564.97
14	1,825.32	197.82	1,627.49	37,937.48
15	1,825.32	189.69	1,635.63	36,301.85
16	1,825.32	181.51	1,643.81	34,658.04
17	1,825.32	173.29	1,652.03	33,006.02
18	1,825.32	165.03	1,660.29	31,345.73
19	1,825.32	156.73	1,668.59	29,677.14
20	1,825.32	148.39	1,676.93	28,000.21
21	1,825.32	140.00	1,685.32	26,314.90
22	1,825.32	131.57	1,693.74	24,621.16
23	1,825.32	123.11	1,702.21	22,918.95
24	1,825.32	114.59	1,710.72	21,208.23
25	1,825.32	106.04	1,719.28	19,488.95
26	1,825.32	97.44	1,727.87	17,761.08
27	1,825.32	88.81	1,736.51	16,024.57
28	1,825.32	80.12	1,745.19	14,279.37
29	1,825.32	71.40	1,753.92	12,525.46
30	1,825.32	62.63	1,762.69	10,762.77

(continues)

Table 21.1 Loan Amortization Schedule *(continued)*

Month	Loan Payment	Interest	Principal Payment	Balance
31	1,825.32	53.81	1,771.50	8,991.26
32	1,825.32	44.96	1,780.36	7,210.90
33	1,825.32	36.05	1,789.26	5,421.64
34	1,825.32	27.11	1,798.21	3,623.43
35	1,825.32	18.12	1,807.20	1,816.24
36	1,825.32	9.08	1,816.24	0.00
=PMT(0.005,36,–60000)			=PMT(rate,nper,pv,[fv])	

Loan Costs

The term **loan costs** covers expenses necessary to close the loan. Loan closing costs generally include some expenses that would be reported in the current year and other expenses that should be spread over several years.

Suppose Salk Family Practice bought a tract of land for expansion purposes. The practice made a 20% down payment and obtained mortgage financing from a local bank for the remainder of the purchase price. When the loan was closed, meaning the transaction was completed, the statement that lists closing costs included prorated real estate taxes and "points" on the loan. Points represent a percentage of the loan amount that is paid to the bank to cover the costs of processing the loan.

The prorated real estate taxes represent an expense to be reported in the current year by the practice. The points, however, would be spread over several years. How would this multiple-year reporting be handled? The total cost of the points would be placed on the balance sheet as a liability not yet recognized as expense. Each year a certain portion of the liability would be charged to current operations as an "amortized expense." Amortization expense is a noncash expense that is assigned to multiple reporting periods in the same way as depreciation expense.

Management Considerations About Real Estate Financing

Real estate financing typically occurs in the form of real estate mortgages. Management must take several important considerations into account when contemplating a real estate purchase that involves a mortgage. These considerations include the following:

- What would the return on investment (ROI) be for this purchase?
- What is the cost of money (i.e., the interest rate) for the mortgage?
- What would the return of capital (equity) be for this purchase?
- What is the liquidity prospect (i.e., the ability to sell this property)?
- What are the potential risk factors, if any, involved in the purchase and/or mortgage financing?
- Is there an income tax factor to be considered? If so, what is the impact?

Repayment of a mortgage is typically a long-term liability, and this fact is yet another element in management's decision-making process.

Management Decisions About Business Loans

Decisions concerning how to obtain capital and minimize financing costs are an important part of financial management decision-making. Chapter 19 on capital budgeting discussed how new capital often has to be rationed within an organization. Repaying long-term loan obligations will impact the facility's cash flow for years to come, and decisions to undertake a large debt load should not be made lightly. Most large, multimillion-dollar organizations have a formal approval process in place that begins with the chief financial officer and his or her staff and may require the board of trustees' approval depending on the amount of the expenditure. Management decisions about investment and debt are often interwoven with strategic planning due to the size of the expenditure and its long-term implications on the organization.

WRAP-UP

Summary

This chapter reviewed debt and equity sources for obtaining funds. The different debt instruments have different interest rates based on length of debt and the type of debt used, which thus changes the cost of acquiring assets. When debt is used to acquire assets, managers should understand the financial burden it will place on the organization. The chapter demonstrated how to calculate debt payments and create an amortization schedule to display how loan payments are divided into principal, reducing the outstanding loan, and interest payments.

Key Terms

Amortization Schedule
Bonds
Capital

Capital Structure
Loan Costs
Long-Term Borrowing

Short-Term
 Borrowing

Discussion Questions

1. Explain capital structure and how it affects the cost of acquiring assets.
2. Describe four sources of capital to purchase assets.
3. Describe the factors that determine the amount of a loan payments.
4. Explain how interest rates typically change with the length of a loan.

Problems

1. Redwood Hospital must replace its energy plant including the heating and air-conditioning systems and backup electrical systems due to a series of breakdowns. The replacement cost is $20,000,000, and the local bank will provide a 20-year loan at 4.0%. Calculate the annual loan payment and create the 20-year amortization schedule. What are the total payments over the life of the loan and the total interest paid?

2. Instead of the 20-year loan in Problem 21–1, Redwood Hospital can obtain a 10-year loan for $20,000,000 at 3.5%. Calculate the annual payment, the total payments over the life of the loan, and the total interest paid. How much will the hospital save in interest by taking the 10-year loan rather than the 20-year loan in Problem 21–1? What factor may prevent the hospital from using the 10-year loan?

3. Salk Family Practice needs to upgrade its appointment, medical record, and billing system at a cost of $100,000. The local bank will provide a three-year loan for 3%. Calculate the monthly debt payment and create a 36-month amortization schedule. What are the total loan payments and total interest expense?

4. The office manager for Salk Family Practice wants to explore a longer-term loan to upgrade its appointment, medical record, and billing system. The local bank will provide a five-year, $100,000 loan for 3.5%. Calculate the monthly debt payment and create a 60-month amortization schedule. What are the total loan payments and total interest expense? How much more will the practice pay in interest expenses compared to the three-year loan in Problem 21–3? Why should the practice owner consider the longer loan given the higher interest expense?

Note

1. Fidelity Investments, "Fixed Income Bonds & CDs," https://www.fidelity.com, accessed August 29, 2021.

CHAPTER 22

Purchasing Versus Leasing

PROGRESS NOTES

After completing this chapter, you should be able to:

1. Explain the two types of leases.
2. Calculate the cost of purchasing (owning) and leasing equipment for a for-profit organization.
3. Calculate the cost of purchasing (owning) and leasing equipment for a nonprofit organization.
4. Explain the factors that affect the desirability of purchasing and leasing.

Overview: Purchasing Versus Leasing

Healthcare providers require hundreds of thousands or millions of dollars of equipment and buildings to provide treatment. How these assets are obtained affect their operating cost. Managers can choose to purchase assets using organizational funds or debt. Debt may be required when organizational funds are limited, but managers should be able to assess the difference in expense from both methods and select the lowest cost option when circumstances allow.

For brevity, the discussion will focus on equipment. Purchasing equipment means taking title to, or assuming ownership of, the item; the asset is then recorded on the organization's balance sheet. The purchase could take place by paying cash from the organization's cash reserves, or the organization could finance all or part of the purchase. When financing occurs, the resulting liability is recorded on the balance sheet. The alternative to purchase is leasing, in which a third party retains ownership and the organization simply rents the asset for a period of time.

Leasing Equipment

When is a lease not a lease? When it is a lease-purchase, in which the lessee has an option to own the equipment at the end of the lease. On the other hand, the organization may enter into an **operating lease** to use equipment for a defined period of time and the equipment remains the property of the lessor.

The **lease-purchase** is a formal agreement that may be called a lease but is really a contract to purchase. A contract-to-purchase is also called a **financial lease**. The important difference is the equipment must be recorded on the books of the organization as a purchase, a process called "capitalizing" the lease. Generally speaking, a lease must be capitalized and placed on the balance sheet as an asset, with a corresponding liability, if the lease contract meets any one of the following criteria:

1. The lessee can buy the asset at the end of the lease term for a bargain price.
2. The lease transfers ownership to the lessee before the lease expires.
3. The lease lasts for 75% or more of the asset's estimated useful life.
4. The present value of the lease payments is 90% or more of the asset's value.

The other type of lease is an operating lease, in which the cost is considered an operating expense. Operating leases do not have to be capitalized and placed on the balance sheet because they do not meet the criteria described previously.

An operating lease is treated as an expense of current operations. This is in contrast to the financial lease just described that is treated as an asset and a liability. Payments on operating leases are an operating expense within the time period the payment is made.

Buy-or-Lease Management Decisions

When analyzing **buy-or-lease decisions**, it is usually assumed that the money to purchase the equipment will be borrowed. In some cases, however, this is not true. The organization may use cash from its own funds to make the purchase. This decision would, of course, change certain assumptions in the comparative analysis.

Another differential in comparative analysis concerns service agreements. Sometimes the service contracts or service agreements to maintain and/or repair the equipment are part of the lease agreement. This feature and its expense would need to be deleted from the total agreement before the comparison between leasing and purchasing can occur because the service agreement would be an expense regardless of whether the equipment would be leased or purchased.

The question for our example is whether a clinic should purchase or lease equipment. We examine two clinics: Morton Clinic, a for-profit corporation, and Lister Clinic, a not-for-profit corporation. Both clinics need to upgrade their electronic medical record system, and the cost is $50,000 if purchased and $11,000 per year for five years if leased. The system is not expected to generate any additional revenue or reduce expenses, so the only choice to be made is how to finance the acquisition. Even if revenues or expenses changed, it would be irrelevant to the financing decision as long as the change was the same for each option. The analysis will look at the difference between the present values of the cash flows based on purchasing or leasing using a 6% discount rate. The lease or purchase analysis differs from capital budgeting as the expenditure *will* be made unlike capital budgeting's focus on determining whether an investment *should* be made.

Analyzing the Purchase or Lease Decision for a For-Profit Organization

When the equipment is purchased, we must make assumptions about depreciation. For the initial year of acquisition (year 0), we assume the half-year method of depreciation, whereby the amount will be one-half of $10,000 ($50,000 ÷ 5 year life), or $5,000. Straight-line depreciation in the amount of $10,000 will be recorded for years 1 through 4. We further assume the equipment can be sold for its salvage value, $5,000, 10% of its purchase price, on the first day of year 5.

The difference between the for-profit Morton and the not-for-profit Lister Clinic is the for-profit pays income tax so any expense reduces its net income and taxes. We assume the federal and state income taxes are 35%, so the depreciation expense results in a tax savings amounting to 35% of the total expense in each year. The depreciation expense and its equivalent tax savings are shown by year in **Table 22.1**. Similarly, the $11,000 leasing expense in the for-profit organization will reduce taxes by 35% or $3,850 (i.e., the net cash outflow is $7,150, $11,000 − $3,850).

Table 22.1 Cost of Owning, Morton Clinic

	Year 0	Year 1	Year 2	Year 3	Year 4	Year 5	Total
Purchase price	−$50,000						−$50,000
Depreciation expense	$5,000	$10,000	$10,000	$10,000	$10,000	$0	$45,000
Depreciation expense tax savings	$1,750	$3,500	$3,500	$3,500	$3,500	$0	$15,750
Salvage value	—	—	—	—	—	$5,000	$5,000
Net cash flow	−$48,250	$3,500	$3,500	$3,500	$3,500	$5,000	−$29,250
Present value factor (6%)	1.0000	0.9434	0.8900	0.8396	0.7921	0.7473	
Present value of cash flow	−$48,250	$3,302	$3,115	$2,939	$2,772	$3,736	−$32,386

The $45,000 of depreciation expense reduces total taxes by $15,750 and increases cash flow by $3,500 per year in years 1 through 4. The present value of the cash flow, the last line, shows the cost of purchasing the system is $32,386 over five years.

Comparing the Present Value of Purchasing and Leasing

When equipment is leased rather than purchased, the year 0 outlay is reduced from $48,250 to $7,150, 65% of $11,000. Subsequent years'

cash flows are also $7,150 as the lease expense reduces taxable income and increases cash flow. **Table 22.2** shows the present value of the cash flow based on $11,000 per year lease payments paid on the first of year.

Table 23–2 shows that the lease payments after tax savings total −$35,750, $7,150 per year, and the present value of the cash flow is −$31,926. Leasing costs $460 less than purchasing due to the $50,000 cash outlay required for purchasing in year 0 (i.e., it is less expensive to pay $11,000 a year than commit $50,000 in year 0). The net advantage to leasing is $460, and the difference is

Table 22.2 Cost of Leasing and Comparison with Owning, Morton Clinic

	Year 0	Year 1	Year 2	Year 3	Year 4	Year 5	Total
Lease (rental) payments	−$11,000	−$11,000	−$11,000	−$11,000	−$11,000	—	−$55,000
Lease expense tax savings	$3,850	$3,850	$3,850	$3,850	$3,850	—	$19,250
Net cash flow	−$7,150	−$7,150	−$7,150	−$7,150	−$7,150	—	−$35,750
Present value factor (6%)	1.0000	0.9434	0.8900	0.8396	0.7921	—	
Present value of cash flow	−$7,150	−$6,745	−$6,363	−$6,003	−$5,663	—	−$31,926
Present value cost of owning							−$32,386
Present value cost of leasing							−$31,926
Difference							−$460

so small that it might be disregarded and the two methods of financing considered as equivalent. Of course, the importance of evaluating the cost of purchasing and leasing increases and decreases with the amount of money to be invested. The next section demonstrates the importance of evaluating financing alternatives to a nonprofit.

Analyzing the Purchase or Lease Decision for a Nonprofit Organization

The Lister Clinic is a nonprofit that does not pay income taxes, but its manager should still attempt to minimize financing costs so more money can be devoted to patient care. **Table 22.3** differs from Table 22.1 in that depreciation expense and

tax savings are irrelevant to nonprofits. The desirability of owning and leasing is determined solely by the investment or lease payments (cash outflows) and salvage value. The $50,000 purchase (cash outflow) in year 0 is partially offset by the $5,000 salvage value payment (cash inflow) in year 5. The present value of a $5,000 payment after five years at 6% is $3,736. Thus, the cost of purchasing is $46,264.

Table 22.4 shows that the cost of leasing is determined by the present value of the lease payments. The lease payment of $11,000 per year is due on the first of the year, so the first payment is entered into year 0 and no discounting is recognized. Discounting the annual lease payments at 6% reduces the cost from $55,000 to $49,116 and shows leasing is $2,852 more expensive than

Table 22.3 Cost of Purchasing—Lister Clinic

	Year 0	Year 1	Year 2	Year 3	Year 4	Year 5	Total
Purchase price	-$50,000						-$50,000
Depreciation expense tax savings	$0	$0	$0	$0	$0	$0	$0
Salvage value	$0	$0	$0	$0	$0	$5,000	$0
Net cash flow	-$50,000	$0	$0	$0	$0	$5,000	-$45,000
Present value factor (6%)	1.0000	0.9434	0.8900	0.8396	0.7921	0.7473	
Present value of cash flow	-$50,000	$0	$0	$0	$0	$3,736	-$46,264

Table 22.4 Cost of Leasing and Comparison with Owning, Lister Clinic

	Year 0	Year 1	Year 2	Year 3	Year 4	Year 5	Total
Equipment lease (rental) payments	-$11,000	-$11,000	-$11,000	-$11,000	-$11,000	—	-$55,000
Lease expense tax savings	n/a	n/a	n/a	n/a	n/a	—	$0
Net cash flow	-$11,000	-$11,000	-$11,000	-$11,000	-$11,000	—	-$55,000
Present value factor (6%)	1.0000	0.9434	0.8900	0.8396	0.7921		
Present value cash flow (PVCF)	-$11,000	-$10,377	-$9,790	-$9,236	-$8,713	—	-$49,116
Present value cost of owning							-$46,264
Present value cost of leasing							-$49,116
Difference							$2,852

purchasing. Lister's manager should purchase the EMR to reduce expenses.

The purchase or lease decision should consider the amount of the expenditure and the organization with a goal of minimizing financing costs. The importance of analysis increases with the size of the investment, and the ultimate decision should consider cash holdings (those with limited funds may have no option but to lease), differences in purchase price and lease expense, the useful life of the asset, the discount rate, and tax status. A change in one variable can change the decision, as demonstrated by the tax status of the Morton and Lister Clinics.

Accounting Principles Regarding Leases

One of the advantages of operating leases was the ability to reduce reported liabilities (i.e., the organization could acquire equipment and commit to rental payments over multiple years but avoid reporting a long-term liability). Beginning December 15, 2019, organizations must include the leases as liabilities and equipment as assets on their balance sheets.[1] This change may encourage purchases over leasing as it is generally believed that healthcare providers can borrow at a lower cost than leasing.

The change in accounting standards has encouraged the growth in other options. **Managed services agreements** (MSAs) offer healthcare providers an alternative that preserves the ability to expense equipment, avoids recognizing a liability, and increases flexibility. MSAs often bundle hardware, software, maintenance, ability to upgrade or downgrade equipment, and change contract duration.[2] These agreements are structured as service agreements rather than loans whereby the provider does not have to worry about maintenance, can change the equipment in use based on demand, and can terminate the contract. The added features of MSAs increase the expense relative to traditional purchase and lease agreements but may fit providers' abilities and current and future needs. Managers should consider all options—purchase, lease, and MSAs—to ensure that the best option is used to meet the organization's resources and needs.

WRAP-UP

Summary

Managers should examine operating and financial leases when assets are needed to ensure that operating costs are minimized. The major factors in the lease-versus-purchase decision are the amount of the investment, the amount of the expenditure, and the operating and financial lease terms. Managers in for-profit organizations should also consider taxes in their decision.

Key Terms

Buy-or-Lease Decisions
Financial Lease
Lease-Purchase
Managed Services Agreements
Operating Lease

Discussion Questions

1. Explain the two types of leases.
2. Describe how taxes affect the purchase or lease decision in a for-profit organization.
3. Explain why a nonprofit organization should evaluate purchase and lease options.
4. Explain the factors that affect the desirability of purchasing and leasing.

Problems

1. The Morton Clinic needs to replace its radiology equipment. The vendor will sell the needed equipment for $100,000 or lease it for five years for $24,000 per year. Morton is a for-profit organization that pays 30% tax. The equipment will be placed into service on the first day of the first year, be depreciated $20,000 per year, and have zero salvage value at the end of year 5. Calculate the cost of purchasing and leasing using a 4% present value. Should Morton purchase or lease?

2. The Morton Clinic has received a revised leasing offer from their equipment vendor (which wants to grow its leasing business) that lowered the annual lease payment to $23,000. If the purchase price remains $100,000 and all other factors are the same as Problem 22–1, recalculate the cost of purchasing and leasing. Does the lower lease payment change the purchase or lease decision?

3. The Lister Clinic also needs to replace its radiology equipment and received the same offer from its vendor to purchase the needed equipment for $100,000 or lease it for five years for $24,000 per year. Lister is a nonprofit organization, so no consideration of tax savings needs to be considered in the purchase or lease decision. The salvage value will be zero at the end of year 5. Calculate the cost of purchasing and leasing using a 4% present value. Should Lister purchase or lease?

4. After informing its sales representative that it would purchase its radiological equipment, the Lister Clinic received a revised lease option from its sales representative that lowered the annual lease payment to $23,000. If the purchase price remains $100,000 and all other factors are the same as Problem 22–3, recalculate the cost of purchasing and leasing. Does the lower lease payment change the purchase or lease decision?

Notes

1. T. Bannow, "Rent or Own? Change to Accounting Standard Could Encourage More Buying," https://www.modernhealthcare.com, accessed February 8, 2021.

2. J. R. Ross, "Buy, Lease or Make Another Arrangement?," https://www.radiologybusiness.com, accessed February 8, 2021.

Data Analytics, Planning, and Payment Systems

CHAPTER 23

Understanding the Impact of Data Analytics and Big Data

PROGRESS NOTES

After completing this chapter, you should be able to:

1. Define data analytics and describe healthcare analytics.
2. Define big data and data mining.
3. Explain the differences among retrospective, predictive, and prospective analytics.
4. Describe the improvements analytics has made in healthcare.

Overview: Data Analytics

Advancements in information technology offer managers the ability to understand what patients want, monitor their condition, and reach out to them with needed or desirable services. Similarly, information technology offers the ability to better understand how patient care is delivered and the results of treatment. Medical care can move away from the historical focus on single patients toward a population health orientation where providers can identify best practices and ensure appropriate services are delivered when needed. Improved coordination of care and better outcomes will arise as healthcare workers develop their data analytic skills.

Data Analytics

Data analytics is the process of examining **big data** to uncover hidden patterns, unknown correlations, and other useful information that can be used to make better decisions.[1] **Data analytics** applied to the healthcare industry is referred to as **healthcare analytics**. In addition to helping reveal and understand historical patterns of service use and outcomes, healthcare analytics enables new approaches to strategic forecasting, environmental analyses, competitor assessments, needs assessments, patient-centered care, and improving market knowledge about population health.

Big data refers to large data sets that an organization analyzes for patterns or trends.[2] In other words, big data enhances data analytics by applying more sophisticated analysis techniques, by using new tools, and by sharing expanded data sets that go beyond traditional claims data and are obtained from multiple sources.[3]

Big data typically refers to volumes of data so large that traditional health information technologies and systems can no longer manage or process the information. Another characteristic of big data is the speed at which data is created and must be processed as well as the array of different data sources and formats. The basic unit of data measure is the byte. A word is typically 2 bytes, and larger measures are generally expressed in ascending order, beginning with the byte. Thus, 1,024 bytes equal one kilobyte (KB), 1,024 kilobytes equal one gigabyte (GB), 1,024 gigabytes equals one terabyte (TB), and 1,024 terabytes equal one petabyte (PB). For reference, a gigabyte may hold approximately 536,770,912 words. The volume measures actually continue upward, as 1,024 petabytes equal one exabyte and so on through zettabytes and even yottabytes. **Exhibit 23.1** illustrates these data measure units.

We need to know data volume amounts to ensure adequate data storage. While gigabytes used to be adequate, terabytes are fast becoming the standard for data storage. Such storage needs will only continue to grow. Consider, for example, Kaiser Permanente: This health network, with over 9 million members, is believed to have between 26.5 and 44 petabytes of data from electronic health records (EHRs) including annotations, images, and figures.[4] To put such volume into perspective, using a byte converter app, we find that one

terabyte equals 1,099,511,627,776 bytes.[5] Can you imagine how many bytes are in just one petabyte?

Managers should focus on the relevance of the data rather than the volume of data collected. Using the data to help reduce costs and improve patient care should be of paramount importance.

Big Data in the Healthcare Industry

Healthcare industry data are of many types and are derived from many sources. A sampling of these sources includes the following:

- Physicians' written notes and prescriptions
- Medical imaging
- Laboratory data
- Pharmacy data
- Insurance and other administrative data
- Patient data in electronic patient records
- Machine-generated and/or sensor data, such as from monitoring vital signs
- Social media posts (Twitter feeds, blogs, and status updates on Facebook)
- Website pages
- Information that is non-patient specific (emergency care data, news feeds, and medical journal articles)[6]

This totality of data related to patient health care and well-being makes up big data in the healthcare industry. Its appropriate use should lead to better-informed decisions.

Retrospective and Prospective Data Analytics

Retrospective analytics identifies trends and problems. It looks at what has already happened (past actions) and draws empirical conclusions. Thus, retrospective analytics, sometimes called descriptive analytics, deals with historical information. The retrospective analytics approach can readily identify variations and provide the foundation for standardizing care. It can be extremely

Exhibit 23.1 Data Volume Measures

1,024 bytes	=	1 kilobyte (KB)
1,024 kilobytes	=	1 megabyte (MB)
1,024 megabytes	=	1 gigabyte (GB)
1,024 gigabytes	=	1 terabyte (TB)
1,024 terabytes	=	1 petabyte (PB)
1,024 petabytes	=	1 exabyte (EB)

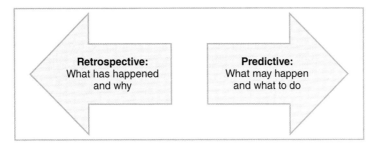

Figure 23.1 Two Basic Approaches to Data Analytics

effective in dealing with healthcare tasks such as inventory control, staffing, and billing.[7]

Predictive analytics attempts to extract value from data to determine future action. It cannot not tell you what will happen in the future but analyzes the probability of what is likely to happen in the future. We can think of the predictive approach as looking forward while the retrospective approach looks back. **Figure 23.1** illustrates these approaches.

Working with many sets of data provides different views of the organization's operations that are not possible when examining one set of data at a time. Analyzing data sets or using data analytics helps find relationships that exist in the data. Finding relationships such as new correlations and business trends, in turn, may lead to opportunities to improve care, reduce costs, and improve health outcomes.

Prospective Analytics: A Subset of Predictive Analytics

Prospective analytics is a decision-making tool that can deliver value by providing evidence-based solutions. The following example highlights the differences among retrospective, predictive, and prospective analytics.

Every year on Amateur Rodeo Night, an emergency department (ED) would get many more patients—mostly orthopedic patients—than an average day. Retrospective analytics allowed the hospital to see how many patients were treated on Rodeo Night compared to the previous 20 or 30 Saturday nights. In other words, retrospective analytics was used to quantify the likely increase in ED patients.

Predictive analytics told the hospital what the likelihood was that it would need an increase in certain services that would be relevant to these emergency room injuries—for example, X-rays, casting, operating rooms, and so on. In other words, predictive analytics is used to anticipate demand.

When prospective analytics is performed, the hospital sees how to adjust resources for the overload. For example, if the X-ray suites were all full, the analytics could suggest which cases should have portable X-rays brought to the bedside instead of using the suites. In other words, prospective analytics could provide possible solutions to the problems identified by retrospective analytics and anticipated by predictive analytics.

Data Analytics Serves Many Purposes

Using Predictive Analytics to Answer a Patient Population Question

From a demographic perspective, predictive analytics can help answer a primary question: Who are the most likely candidates for health services? For example, one hospital learned that its self-pay population was split equally among men and women, with their ages falling mostly between 18 and 26 years old, which led to bad debt problems as well as patients who were less compliant with their care than other age groups. The hospital addressed the issue starting with incentives to reduce bad debt and putting a program in place in which the patients agreed to be compliant with their care if the provider helped them pay the cost of their prescriptions.[7-8]

Using Predictive Analytics in the Human Resources Department

An emerging domain for the application of big data is human resources. The practice of "people analytics" is already transforming how employers hire, fire, and promote.[9] The application of predictive analytics to people's careers is illustrated by the following example. In 2010, Xerox switched to an online evaluation for job applicants that incorporated personality testing, cognitive-skill assessment, and multiple-choice questions about how applicants would handle specific scenarios that they might encounter on the job. An algorithm (a process or set of rules used in calculations) behind the evaluation analyzed the responses, along with factual information gleaned from the candidates' applications—as used in conjunction with in-person interviews.

Using a Combination of Retrospective and Prospective Data Analytics

The use of analytics has allowed hospitals to correlate the patient risk of readmission with the actual readmission rate, the total cost of readmissions, and the clinical drivers of readmissions. Analytics can also provide a financial model that calculates the overall impact of readmission rate reductions on reimbursement, cost, and value-based purchasing payments.[10]

Using an Analytics Approach to Combat Prescription Drug Fraud

Express Scripts, a national pharmacy benefit management organization, has created the Express Scripts Fraud, Waste, & Abuse Team. The team uses "...industry-leading, proprietary data analytics to uncover patterns of potential fraud or abuse, and scans for behavioral red flags to identify when someone is involved in wrongdoing."[11] The proprietary data analytics are combined with Express Scripts' Health Decision Science platform (behavioral sciences, clinical specialization, and actionable data) to identify 290 potential indicators of pharmacy fraud.[12]

One case uncovered by the team involved a couple of whom in just eight months the wife obtained over 2,800 tablets from eight physicians and five pharmacies and the husband obtained almost 4,000 tablets from nine physicians and 12 pharmacies. The tablets included oxycodone, Endocet, and hydrocodone.[13] The team reported that "...upon contacting several of the physicians we found that in several instances, the couple had signed agreements that prohibited obtaining narcotics from other doctors. However, none of the physicians was aware of the couple's visits to the others."[14]

Data Mining

The big data "revolution" encompasses yet another semantic variant: data mining. **Data mining** is a process used by organizations to turn raw data into useful information. Managers and analysts use software, such as Excel, to look for patterns in large batches of data to learn more about their patients, develop effective marketing strategies, increase utilization, and decrease costs. Data mining depends on effective data collection and working with many sets of data in what is often called a data warehouse.

Sloan Kettering Use of Data Mining for Clinical Research

A noteworthy application of data mining to clinical medicine is occurring at Memorial-Sloan Kettering (MSK) Cancer Center in New York City. MSK scientists leverage the massive amount of data produced by tumor sequencing to learn more about the biology of cancer.[15] They use that information to make the genetic discoveries that lead to more precise, timely, and cost-effective treatments for people with cancer.

Boston Children's Hospital Use of Data Mining for Patient Safety Research

Boston Children's Hospital teamed with the nonprofit, federally funded MITRE Corporation research center to tackle patient safety issues.[16] In harnessing big data to boost patient safety, they pulled data together from multiple sources—electronic health records, safety event reports, physiologic monitors, and so on—to gain insights into what may have caused patient harm.

Developing a Treatment Protocol Through Data Mining

Using a combination of clinical experience and big data analytics research, the University of Michigan Health System developed a protocol for the administration of blood transfusions. The effort led to a 31% reduction in transfusions and monthly savings of $200,000.[17]

Associating Clinical Data with Cost Data

Kaiser Permanente generated a key data set by associating clinical data with cost data. The result of this important analysis led to the discovery of adverse drug effects from Vioxx, an anti-inflammatory drug, which led to its withdrawal from the market.[18]

Impacts of Healthcare Analytics

Corporate Acquisition

Noteworthy regarding the growth in the data analytics and cloud computing business is IBM's recent acquisition of Truven Health Analytics for $2.6 billion. The magnitude of the purchase is reflected in the enhanced capabilities of the company's Watson Health Unit, which is a digital repository of health-related information for approximately 300 million patients. Truven's contribution is to add patient-related payment information to a database that already includes data from patients' electronic medical records and medical imaging software.[19] The ultimate goal is to have Watson's artificial intelligence software assist physicians and administrators in improving care and curbing costs.

The Big Data Revolution

Big data creates opportunities and challenges. It's revolutionary insofar that it gives healthcare professionals the ability to use the data to solve problems more quickly and in new ways to gain greater business insight. It is a disruptive change for healthcare organizations in that it requires new business models.[20]

New tools and statistical techniques are used to extract meaningful information from what was unstructured data. An algorithm, or set of rules or processes, governs the greatly enhanced speed with which problems are solved. The potential benefits in the realm of public health and medicine are being defined in real time.

Collaborative Efforts

By necessity, the generation and utilization of big data in health care involves collaboration between organizations. Optum Labs, a collaborative research and innovation center, has been instrumental in integrating data, generating new knowledge, and translating knowledge into practice. This has necessitated a shift in current patient care practices. Optum's efforts have focused on enabling physicians to utilize big data to improve the care of patients with comorbidities or chronic illnesses.[21] A challenge for Optum amid its collaborative efforts is to ensure an appropriate level of privacy regarding patient information.

Thus, analytics provide the data to reshape healthcare environments in the transition from fee-for-service to value-based reimbursement and in so doing can help by strategically targeting patients who need preventive care. The upshot is more effective patient-volume forecasting. Other impacts that result from enhanced data analytics and related data sharing include better coordination of patient care, better use of available resources, better claims and benefit management, and improved prevention of fraud and abuse.

Challenges for Healthcare Analytics

The human resources challenge in the use of big data is well illustrated by AT&T's Vision 2020 Plan. The essence of the challenge is to retrain its 280,000 employees to enable them to learn coding skills and make quick business decisions based upon huge volumes of data that are all sorted through software managed in the cloud.[22] In an effort to keep up with competitors such as Google and Amazon, AT&T executives are urging staff to spend five to 10 hours a week in online learning relative to cloud computing. The company is willing to fund a good part of that training. The new systems facilitate collecting more data, quickly analyzing information about what people and things are doing, and taking action on the knowledge gained.

An ongoing challenge in the use of data analytics is to weigh progress versus privacy: Balancing the promise of big data with consumer privacy and security is an essential consideration. Along with rising digital expectations of practitioners and patients, healthcare IT executives know they face strict requirements related to patient privacy and data protection, leaving them to ponder how to transform their infrastructures and keep data secure.

WRAP-UP

Summary

Data analytics is the process of examining large data sets to uncover patterns, correlations, and other information to improve decisions. Healthcare analytics is the use of data analytics to improve treatment and outcomes and reduce costs. Better decisions and outcomes are the result of using big data that integrates data from multiple sources and more sophisticated data mining techniques.

Managers should be familiar with and use retrospective, predictive, and prospective analytics to advance their work. Retrospective analytics examines historical data to determine what has happened in the past, find out why it happened, and improve future outcomes. Predictive analytics examines what is likely to occur, and in tandem with prospective analytics providers can develop action plans to handle the possible outcomes (i.e., how to adjust staffing, inventory levels, etc.).

Healthcare analytics is in its infancy and has already led to improvements in cancer treatment by greater understanding of the biology of cancer, reduced patient harm, lower treatment costs by improved treatment protocols, and identified adverse effects of pharmaceuticals. Healthcare analytics promises to drive faster identification of disease and superior treatment processes based on the outcomes the treatments achieve to ensure all patients receive the best evidenced based medicine.

Key Terms

Big Data	Healthcare Analytics	Prospective Analytics
Data Analytics	Predictive Analytics	Retrospective Analytics
Data Mining		

Discussion Questions

1. Define data analytics and describe healthcare analytics.
2. Define big data and data mining.

3. Explain the differences among retrospective, predictive, and prospective analytics.
4. Describe the improvements analytics has made in health care.

Notes

1. SAS, "Big Data Analytics," http://www.sas.com/en_us/insights/analytics/big-data-analytics.html, accessed November 15, 2015.
2. Z. Budryk, "5 Health IT Terms Every Hospital CEO Must Know," http://www.fiercehealthcare.com/healthcare/5-health-it-terms-every-hospital-ceo-must-know, accessed September 17, 2016.
3. D. Hillblom, A. Schueth, S. M. Robertson, L. Topor, and G. Low, "The Impact of Information Technology on Managed Care Pharmacy: Today and Tomorrow," *Journal of Managed Care & Specialty Pharmacy, 20* (2014): 1076.
4. Institute for Health Technology Transformation (IHTT), "Transforming Health Care Through Big Data: Strategies for Leveraging Big Data in the Health Care Industry," http://c4fd63cb482ce6861463-bc6183f1c18e748a49b87a25911a0555.r93.cf2.rackcdn.com/iHT2_BigData_2013.pdf.
5. What's a Byte?, http://www.whatsabyte.com/P1/byteconverter_App.htm, accessed February 17, 2016.
6. W. Raghupathi and V. Raghupathi, "Big Data Analytics in Healthcare: Promise and Potential," *Health Information Science and Systems, 2* (2014): 3, http://www.hissjournal.com/content/2/1/3.
7. A. Bickmore, "Prospective Analytics: The Next Thing in Healthcare Analytics," http://www.healthcatalyst.com/using-prospective-analytics-to-improve-outcomes, accessed February 17, 2016.
8. *Healthcare Finance News,* June 6, 2015.
9. D. Peck, "They're Watching You at Work: What Happens When Big Data Meets Human Resources?," *The Atlantic,* December 2013.
10. http://www.mentorhealth.com/control/category/~category_id=W_HOSPITAL/~status=live, accessed December 16, 2016.
11. Express Scripts, "INFOGRAPHIC: Prescription Drug Fraud and Abuse," http://lab.express-scripts.com/insights/drug-safety-and-abuse/infographic-prescription-drug-fraud-and-abuse, accessed February 16, 2016.
12. Ibid.
13. Express Scripts, "Rx Addiction: One Family's 7,000 Pills," http://lab.express-scrpts.com/insights/drug-safety-and-abuse/rx-addiction-one-faily's-7000-pills/, accessed February 16, 2016.
14. Ibid.
15. E. Kiesler, "Tumor Sequencing Test Brings Personalized Treatment Options to More Patients," Memorial Sloan Kettering Cancer Center News, https://www.mskcc.org/blog/new-tumor-sequencing-test-will-bring-personalized-options-more-patients, accessed February 2015.
16. M. Stempniak, "Big Data Applied to Patient Safety in Children's Hospitals," Hospitals and Health Networks, http://www.hhnmag.com/articles/3335-big-data-applied-to-patient-safety-in-children-s-hospitals, accessed July 14, 2015.
17. W. Raghupathi, and V. Raghupathi, "Big Data Analytics in Healthcare: Promise and Potential," https://link.springer.com, accessed October 3, 2021.
18. Institute for Health Technology Transformation, "Transforming Health Care Through Big Data: Strategies for Leveraging Big Data in the Health Care Industry," http://c4fd63cb482ce6861463-bc6183f1c18e748a49b87a25911a0555.r93.cf2.rackcdn.com/iHT2_BigData_2013.pdf.
19. S. Lohr, "IBM Buys Truven for $ 2.6 Billion, Adding to Trove of Patient Data," http://www.nytimes.com/2016/02/19/technology/ibm-buys-truven-adding-to-growing-trove-of-patient-data-at-watson-health.html, accessed February 18, 2016.
20. J. Shaw, "Why 'Big Data' Is a Big Deal," March–April 2014, http://harvardmagazine.com/2014/03/why-big-data-is-a-big-deal.
21. N. D. Shah and J. Pathak, "Why Health Care May Finally Be Ready for Big Data," *Harvard Business Review,* https://hbr.org/2014/12/why-health-care-may-finally-be-ready-for-big-data, accessed December 3, 2014.
22. Q. Hardy, "AT&T's New Line: Adapt, or Else," http://www.nytimes.com/2016/02/14/technology/gearing-up-for-the-cloud-att-tells-its-workers-adapt-or-else.html?_r=0, accessed December 16, 2016.

CHAPTER 24

Strategic Planning and the Healthcare Financial Manager

PROGRESS NOTES

After completing this chapter, you should be able to:

1. Describe the six major components of strategic planning.
2. Understand the purpose and relationship between mission, vision, and value statements.
3. Describe the strategic planning cycle and its process flow.
4. Identify the four components of SWOT analysis.

Overview: Strategic Planning

Strategic planning is designed to set an organization on a sustainable path by establishing its mission and goals and identifying the actions needed to fulfill the goals. This chapter covers the six major components of planning and their process flows, along with examples of mission, value, and **vision statements**, and discusses strategic planning tools, including **situational analysis** and **financial projections**.

Strategic planning is vital for any organization. There are multiple approaches to accomplish such planning, and there is often confusion about the terminology used in these different approaches. In the next section, we describe the typical components of strategic planning and the confusion about differences in approach and terminology.

The Six Major Components of a Strategic Plan

The ultimate result of strategic planning is an actual plan, presented in report form. The major components of a strategic plan include the following:

- Mission statement
- Vision
- Organizational values

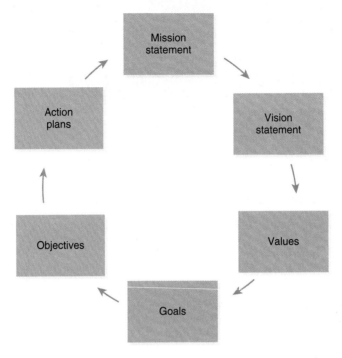

Figure 24.1 The Six Major Components of Strategic Planning
Courtesy of J.J. Baker and R.W. Baker, Dallas, Texas.

- Goals
- Objectives
- Action plans, performance plans, and initiatives

These components are illustrated in **Figure 24.1** and are further described as follows.

Mission Statement

The **mission statement** explains the purpose of the organization (i.e., its reason for existing). It identifies target customers, services, and geographic areas as well as aspirations and image. Generally speaking, the mission statement covers a period of three to five years.

Vision

The **vision statement** explains "what we want to be" or perhaps "what we aspire to be." It is a look further into the future, perhaps 10 years from now. A vision statement should be clear (understandable and hopefully inspiring), coherent (follows mission), and consistent (reflected in decision-making). Not all organizations publicize a vision statement.

Organizational Values

Values express the philosophy of the organization, often addressing ethics, quality, and teamwork. There seem to be two approaches to expressing values: Either they are summarized into just a few meaningful phrases, or they are quite lengthy and "wordy."

Goals

A **goal** includes "…a statement of aim or purpose included in a strategic plan."[1] Goals support the mission statement. While strategic goals are necessarily broad in nature, nevertheless each goal should tie directly into an element of the mission statement. Every goal should be considered an outcome that can be accomplished in the future, and the total number of goals should be limited to focus employees' attention and ensure goals are met.

Objectives

A **strategic objective** further defines intended outcomes in order to achieve a goal. Each objective must support—and thus tie directly into—a particular strategic goal. Objectives should challenge employees, establish the measure by which success will be measured, set the time period for completion, and be realizable. There are typically several objectives associated with each goal.

Action Plans

An **action plan** is a detailed plan of operations that shows how one part of a particular objective will be accomplished. It supports a subcomponent of the overall objective. It is a short-term plan that provides details (actions) about how a specific area of a particular objective will be carried out. Action plans are often called by other names, such as operational plans, performance plans, or initiatives.

Approaches to Strategic Planning

How strategic planning is approached may be affected by the organization type and/or the program or project type.

Governmental Versus Nongovernmental

Governmental entities are guided by regulatory restrictions. Among these restrictions are federal regulations that mandate strategic planning. These regulations apply to federal governmental organizations and specify the format, contents, and timing of the required strategic plans. On the other hand, nongovernmental entities are not covered by these mandated requirements.

For-Profit Versus Not-for-Profit

A for-profit company is in business to make a profit and is answerable to its owners. Its owners may be shareholders (for corporations), partners (for partnerships), or possibly sole proprietors. A not-for-profit organization, on the other hand, is expected to have a mission that is broadly charitable in nature. It is typically answerable to the stakeholders, patients, employees, their community, and others who are impacted by its mission, goals, and actions.

Specific Programs or Projects

The type of program, project, or initiative may also define the basic approach to strategic planning. Funding sources and/or regulations may require an explicit planning process. For example, in some states, construction of healthcare facilities is controlled by a regulatory Certificate of Need process. In these states, strategic planning for a new facility would be a specific project. Whether the project will be approved is uncertain, so the project would be specially treated within the strategic plan.

Mission, Vision, and Value Statements

This section introduces various types of mission, vision, and **value statements**. The structure and the length of these statements vary. Their terminology and their emphasis can also vary. The first examples recognize a special status or focus, others a financial emphasis, and the third shows how messages are relayed.

Recognizing a Special Status or Focus

Recognizing Nonprofit Status: Sutter Health

Sutter Health is a network of doctors and hospitals located in Northern California. Sutter's mission statement specifically points out its not-for-profit commitment.

Mission

"We enhance the well-being of people in the communities we serve through a not-for-profit commitment to compassion and excellence in healthcare services."

Vision

"Sutter Health leads the transformation of health care to achieve the highest levels of quality, access and affordability."

Values[2]

Figure 24.2 reports Sutter's values and emphasizes the centrality of honesty and integrity.

Recognizing For-Profit Status: Tenet Healthcare Corporation

Tenet Healthcare Corporation is a publicly held corporation that is listed on the New York Stock Exchange (NYSE: THC). As a for-profit corporation operating a healthcare delivery system, Tenet specifically mentions providing a return to its shareholders.

Mission

"Our Mission is to provide quality, compassionate care in the communities we serve. Creating ethos of good health, wellness and responsibility is central to our mission and an everyday commitment to our neighbors and families."

Values

"Our Values define who we are, what we stand for and what we CARE about: Compassion and respect, Acting with integrity, Results and Embracing inclusiveness."[3]

Recognizing the Vision and Intent of Their Founders: Mayo Clinic

The Mayo Clinic, a large nonprofit organization with a long history, provides medical care, research,

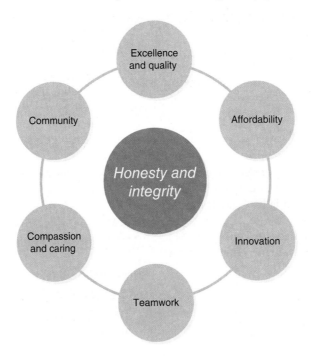

Figure 24.2 Sutter Health Values

and education at locations including the Midwest, Arizona, and Florida. The Mayo Clinic is research oriented and is known for treating difficult cases.

Mission

"To inspire hope and contribute to health and well-being by providing the best care to every patient through integrated clinical practice, education, and research."

Primary Value

"The needs of the patient come first."

Values

"These values, which guide Mayo Clinic's mission to this day, are an expression of the vision and intent of our founders, the original Mayo physicians and the Sisters of Saint Francis."[5]

Financial Emphasis within the Statements

A Medical Practice Network Emphasizes Financial Structure: Texas Oncology

Texas Oncology specializes in oncology patients through a network of physicians that covers the state of Texas. This organization places its vision first and mission second, as follows. Note also that evidence-based, or scientific, care is contained within the mission statement.

Mission

"To provide excellent, evidence-based care for each patient we serve, while advancing cancer care for tomorrow."

Vision

"To be the first choice for cancer care."

Values

Texas Oncology has three Core Values, consisting of Patient Care, Culture, and Business. The Business Core Value is of particular interest to us. At the

time of this writing, it reads as follows: "Business— Our practice values professional management that:

- Promotes convenient access at rural and urban sites.
- Provides leadership in efficient care delivery and improves all aspects of cancer care.
- Provides a financial structure to expand services to our patients.
- Is competitive in all aspects of our business."[5]

These values recognize that an organization must have the financial structure and resources to endure and to succeed.

Relaying the Message

The results of strategic planning as expressed in the mission statement, vision, and values are of little use unless people know about them and what they say. This section focuses upon relaying a message.

Explaining the Terms: Good Samaritan Society

The Good Samaritan Society is the largest not-for-profit provider of senior care and services in the United States.

There is an important paragraph that appears before Good Samaritan's strategic statements. That paragraph explains the purpose of each term contained with the statements, as follows:

- "Our Mission states why the Society exists.
- Our Vision defines the desired outcome of our work.
- Our Strategic Direction defines where we want to be as an organization.
- And our Hallmark Values and related Core Principles identify the values that we strive to integrate into all aspects of our work."[6]

Mission Expressed as a Motto

Mottos are an effective way to communicate the organization's mission. However, composing such a short piece is much more difficult than it seems at first.

Good Samaritan Society

The Good Samaritan Society has also created a pithy concise motto consisting of only six words: "Grounded in Mission Centered in Values."[7]

Providence Healthcare Network

Providence Healthcare Network is a member of Ascension Health, the largest Catholic and largest nonprofit health system, and uses a three-phrase motto:

- "A mission of compassion.
- Compassion is perfected by excellence.
- Because excellence goes beyond the will to help others by providing the determination and tools to succeed where the heart takes you."[8]

The Message Available as Website Downloads

Duke Medicine

The umbrella term *Duke Medicine* actually covers three components—the Duke University Health System, the Duke University School of Medicine, and the Duke University School of Nursing, all based in the Raleigh-Durham area of North Carolina. Duke Medicine has created both a mission and a vision that encompass all these components. Then each component also has its own strategic plan that feeds in turn into the combined plan.

At the time of this writing, an overview of these plans was available in booklet form. The booklet, titled "Thinking Big," could be downloaded from the Duke Medicine website as a PDF file.[9] Summaries of each strategic plan could also be downloaded. Thus, Duke provides transparency and useful summaries in a readily accessible electronic format.

The Strategic Planning Cycle and Its Process Flow

The basic elements of strategic planning can be visualized as a series of process flows. Thus, by visualizing the process involved, the planning function can be broken into its various manageable components.

Process Flow for Creating Goals, Objectives, Action Plans, and Performance Measures

Figure 24.3 illustrates these initial three components of the strategic plan.

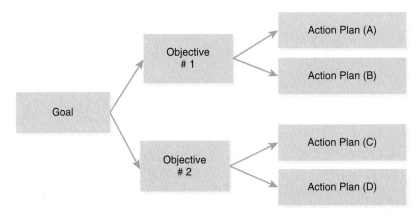

Figure 24.3 Process Flow for Creating Goals, Objectives, and Action Plans
Courtesy of J.J. Baker and R.W. Baker, Dallas, Texas.

Establishing Goals

You will recall that a goal is a statement of aim or purpose. In order to establish such a goal, it is important to define how it will accomplish a particular segment of the mission statement. Establishing the actual goal involves the following:

- Define the goal.
- Determine that there is a clear and distinct connection to the mission statement.
- Decide how long it will take to accomplish this goal; that is, will it take one year, two years, three years?
- Compose and condense final wording of the goal to properly express it in a concise manner.

Broad Goals Become Narrower Objectives

A strategic objective further defines a particular strategic goal. Thus, a single broad goal is segmented into several narrower and more defined objectives, as illustrated in Figure 24.2.

Narrower Objectives Become Detailed Action Plans

You will also recall that an action plan provides a detailed plan of operations that shows how to achieve one part of a particular objective. Thus, a single defined objective is segmented into a number of even more detailed action plans. This step shows how part of the objective will actually be accomplished. The action plan's relationship to objectives and to goals is also illustrated in Figure 24.3.

Detailed Action Plans Specify Performance Measures

Ultimately the action plans should specify how success will be measured. Performance measures detail what, how, and when performance will be measured and should specify expected outcomes. While Figure 24.2 only develops

the action plans and performance measures for objective 1 and 2, the reader should recognize that in the real world there will be more than two objectives with multiple action plans and performance measures.

The Planning Cycle Over Time

The ideal strategic planning cycle is a never-ending process. In other words, a completed plan is not set in stone, never to change. Instead, there should be a "refresh and renew" approach to such planning. Incidentally, planning cycle segments may be called by different names, but they are still in a cycle. Look past the names to see the "skeleton" of the overall process.

Goals, Objectives, and Action Plans Interact and Repeat

The interaction of goals, objectives, and action plans should take feedback into account. This feedback should be obtained as is appropriate from all levels of management within the organization. However, internal managers are not the only stakeholders involved with the strategic plan.

Planning Revisions and Updates Are Necessary

The capability for planning revisions and updates should ideally be built into the plan. Unanticipated events can occur—both internally and externally—that require major revisions if the plan is to be kept operational. Updates, on the other hand, are to be expected, and allowances should be made for them to meet goals.

Stakeholders Provide Input Within the Cycle

Stakeholders can be both internal and external. In order to maintain a manageable planning cycle, questions need to be answered. For example, how many external stakeholders need input into the plan? Who, specifically are they? How will they provide this input?

Likewise, how many internal stakeholders need to provide input and/or feedback to the plan? Who, specifically, are they? What departments or divisions do they represent within the organization? Is this representation a good balance? And how will they provide this input?

Programming and Budgets Support the Planning Cycle

Planning should be supported by budgets (i.e., funding must be provided to acquire the resources needed to reach goals). It is also logical that programming, specifying the type and number of services to be delivered, should be integral to establishing budgets. We can then ask, "What goal and what objective do this particular program and this budget support?"

Financial Aspects of the Plan

A plan must, above all, be feasible (i.e., the organization must have sufficient financial resources to support the planned actions). How will this financial support be provided? Will another division or project be cut in order for this to happen? Can the consequences be predicted? If so, what will they be?

Related Time Frames

Necessary time frames are appropriate for the particular portion of strategic planning. For example, the plan itself typically covers a period of four to five years. If there is a vision statement, it should be much further into the future, perhaps out to 10 years. Yet the managers' accountability should be at least annually and in fact may be quarterly.

Managers' Responsibilities

Planning

The manager may contribute to planning by gathering data or by analyzing the data to provide specific information that is desired and necessary for the plan. In other words, the manager is participating in the planning function by doing their part in the preliminary segment of the process.

Decision-Making

The manager may or may not be able to participate in the actual decision-making for the plan, depending upon their position within the organization. However, they may be assigned to work on a planning committee or a task force that contributes directly to the decision-makers in the organization.

Providing Accountability

Managers can contribute to the planning process by suggesting criteria for performance measures. The action plan will require performance measures to provide accountability, and managers are the best people to understand what measures are needed within their department or division.

A well-designed planning process will also include milestones. The milestones signify the completion of plan segments within a designated time frame for completion of the entire plan. The manager can and should be responsible for assisting in reaching certain milestones on a timely basis. This function (one hospital CEO called it "ramrodding") is another type of accountability responsibility.

Management Responsibilities within the Planning Cycle

This section concludes with a generalized view of planning responsibilities by three levels of management. **Figure 24.4** illustrates the three levels. Any planning cycle should reflect these levels, as does the previous example.

Senior-Level Responsibilities

Senior management represents those individuals at the top of the organization chart (i.e.,

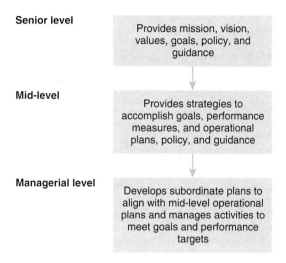

Senior level

Provides mission, vision, values, goals, policy, and guidance

Mid-level

Provides strategies to accomplish goals, performance measures, and operational plans, policy, and guidance

Managerial level

Develops subordinate plans to align with mid-level operational plans and manages activities to meet goals and performance targets

Figure 24.4 Primary Planning Responsibilities by Management Levels

chief executive officer, chief operating officer, chief financial officer). These individuals should provide overall direction for the organization's mission, vision, and strategic framework. They should be responsible for policy making and supervisory guidance issues.

Mid-Level Responsibilities

Mid-level individuals are accountable to those senior managers. They often hold director titles and are responsible for multiple departments while they operate in a supervisory mode to those below them in the organization chart. Mid-level management should typically provide the strategies to accomplish goals, performance measures, and operational plans.

Managerial-Level Responsibilities

Managers typically are responsible for a department and are accountable to all those above them on the organization chart. The managerial level should typically develop the subordinate plans that will align with mid-level operational plans. Other responsibilities include managing the activities that are designed to meet strategic goals, initiatives, and performance targets.

Tools for Strategic Planning: Situational Analysis and Financial Projections

A **situational analysis** reviews the organization's internal operations for strengths and weaknesses and explores the organization's external environment for opportunities and threats. A **situational analysis, or strengths-weaknesses-opportunities-threats (SWOT) analysis**, provides a framework to examine the major factors that may affect an organization's performance.

SWOT Analysis as a Strategic Tool

A **SWOT analysis**, properly performed, can be an excellent strategic tool. The four components of a SWOT analysis are the following:

- Strengths
- Weaknesses
- Opportunities
- Threats[10]

The SWOT matrix is illustrated in **Figure 24.5**. Here we see that the "Strengths" and "Weaknesses" sectors of the matrix are labeled "Internal," while

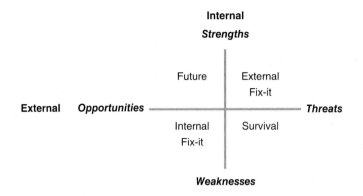

Figure 24.5 SWOT Matrix

the "Opportunities" and "Threats" sectors are labeled "External."

The internal strengths and weaknesses of an organization are determined by assessing its services, management and culture, finances, and resources. The goal is to determine what an organization *can* do based on an assessment of the overall organization. As this is a finance text, we will explore net income and net worth. An organization with high net income and no debt would be extremely strong and thus able to undertake bold initiatives. On the other hand, an organization running losses with high debt load would be extremely limited in what it could undertake. Of course, the net strength of weakness of the organization and a strength in one area, services, may be offset by a weakness in another area (e.g., finance). Strategic choices are based on value judgments given most organizations are a combination of strengths and weaknesses that must be weighed to conclude how strong or weak an organization is.

The external assessment is based on a review of economic, demographic, political/regulatory, technology, and competitive issues at the national, industry, and local levels. The goal is to determine what the organization *should* do based on its operating environment. An opportunistic environment would be one with a favorable political, regulatory, and economic environment that provides more generous reimbursement and a growing patient population. On the other hand, even when national factors are favorable, a stagnant local economy with a shrinking population would be unfavorable.

Figure 24.5 shows the potential conclusions from a SWOT analysis. Quadrant 1, future, is for organizations that are predominantly strong operating in an opportunistic environment. These organizations can and should take bold action. Expansion through increasing services to existing markets, horizontal and vertical integration, product and market development, and diversification are key strategies. A strong organization operating in a threatening environment, quadrant 2, external fix-it, should take more conservative action due to the external challenges. Its action may seek to correct the external problems before pursuing strengths (i.e., move the organization from quadrant 2 to quadrant 1).

A weak organization operating in an opportunistic environment, quadrant 3, internal fix-it, must also take conservative action. In this case, the first step should be to correct internal problems before pursuing opportunities (i.e., move the organization from quadrant 3 to quadrant 1). The worst situation is a weak organization operating in a threatening environment, quadrant 4, survival. Organizations in this situation should take defensive actions including reducing the size of the organization through harvesting, retrenchment, divestiture, or liquidation to raise money and/or eliminate money-losing operations.

Sequential Steps in the SWOT Analysis Project

The following steps pertain to both the internal and external components of the analysis:

1. First, identify the fundamental factors that determine the strengths and weaknesses of an organization and the environmental factors that present opportunities or threats.
2. Gather necessary information on each factor.
3. Reach agreement, or consensus, on the final score for each factor.
4. Summarize the scores for each factor.
5. Summarize the overall score for the internal (strength or weakness) and external (opportunity or threat) components (i.e., where will the task force or committee place the organization on the SWOT matrix) (Figure 24.4).
6. Report the results.

Commencing the SWOT Analysis Project Process

In order to commence the SWOT analysis project's process, a number of decisions must be made. They include the following:

1. What type of task force or committee does the project need?
2. Who will be appointed to this task force?
3. What types of data/information should be gathered for this project?
4. Who will gather the information that is needed?
5. Will the scoring process be subjective, objective, or both? This may depend on the amount and type of available data.
6. Will the same task force members who are involved in recording the worksheet information also be involved in the scoring process, or will a separate group be appointed to carry out the scoring function?
7. Who prepares the final report?
8. Who receives the report?
9. Who is responsible for taking appropriate action after the analysis and its report are completed?

Financial Projections for Strategic Planning

The type of **financial projection** that we discuss in this section is produced internally. These projections are intended for internal planning purposes and are not intended for use outside the organization. Projections are views into the future. We "project" future events, projects, or operations using a set of presumed, or hypothetical, assumptions.

Projections are different than forecasts, although both are considered to be "prospective" (thus, "future") financial statements. Forecasts are based on assumptions that are expected to exist and that reflect actions that are expected to occur.[32] Projections, on the other hand, are often prepared to answer a "what if" question, such as "What if this service, program, or initiative is adopted?" In these "what if" situations, several projections may be prepared, each based on a different set of hypothetical assumptions and each reflecting the actions that might occur based on such assumptions.[11]

Building a Financial Projection

Building a financial projection is a seven-step process for internal planning purposes as illustrated in **Table 24.1** and usually developed by the finance department under the direction of senior management.

Determine the Time Horizon

What should the future start and end dates be for this projection? Is the time period to be covered long enough, or is it too long for reasonable assumptions to be made? Strategic plans commonly use a five-year horizon, but as seen in capital budgeting, equipment and facility planning may expand to 10 or 20 years in the future.

Table 24.1 Building a Financial Projection

1. Determine time horizon
2. Determine focus
3. Gather information
4. Make and document assumptions
5. Prepare projected financial statements
6. Review for reasonableness
7. Create alternative scenarios

Determine the Focus

Focus on what the plan (or planner) needs to know to go forward. Let that focus determine the direction your search for information will take. You should also recognize that focus can change based on information collected and/or new or reprioritized goals.

Gather Information

You will need enough information to make informed decisions about your projection. The range of subjects may vary, but the information should be as up-to-date as possible.

Make and Document Assumptions

A reasonable assumption is one that is likely to be achieved. An unreasonable assumption would be to double revenue by the fourth quarter of next year. Assumptions for output, revenue, and expenses growth rates should follow past history unless strong justifications can be provided to support large increases or decreases. Assumptions used for the projection are key to its success. Documenting the assumptions allows everyone to understand and possibly question the assumptions, thus adding to the validity of the final product.

Prepare the Projected Financial Statements

Projected income statements and balance sheets are then assembled using the documented assumptions to determine if the organization will have sufficient resources to complete the plan. Will future net income increase or decrease, and where will money come from to purchase any planned additions to equipment or facilities? Will additional debt be needed, and if so, where can it be obtained at the lowest cost?

Review for Reasonableness

For example, ask: "Is this assumption reasonable for an organization of my type and size?" This type of review may be subjective, but it is a logical part of the process. Appropriate members of the organization may also perform reviews to highlight weak spots within the assumptions.

Create Alternative Scenarios

It is often helpful to produce multiple versions of the projections (i.e., best-case, most likely, and worst-case scenarios). Key output, revenue, and expenses assumptions are changed in each scenario to answer the "what if" questions.

Financial Projections as Strategic Tools

Financial projections should be used to make informed decisions. When properly constructed, they can provide information that is laid out in a logical format, supported by assumptions that are properly explained for the knowledgeable reader.

WRAP-UP

Summary

Strategic planning begins with the mission statement and ends with a set of action plans to ensure an organization's vision, values, goals and objectives are fulfilled. An organization mission statement is its reason for being and should be integral to its vision, goals, and objectives as well as supported by its values.

The process flow of strategic planning should establish clear goals and provide linkages between the organization's broad goals and narrower objectives and between the objectives and the detailed action plans that show how one or more objectives will be achieved.

The action plans should clearly recognize the strengths and weaknesses of the organization (i.e., what it is capable of achieving) and the opportunities and threats posed by the environment in which it operates (i.e., what it should do). The SWOT matrix provides a format to weigh the four factors and develop strategies. After a strategy has been developed, financial projections should be developed to evaluate the strategy (i.e., does the organization have the resources to complete the planned actions, and if successful, will the organization be stronger?).

Key Terms

Action Plan
Financial Projection
Goal
Mission Statement

Situational Analysis
Strategic Objective
situational analysis, or
    strengths-weaknesses-

opportunities-threats
    (SWOT) analysis
Value Statement
Vision Statement

Discussion Questions

1. Describe the six major components of strategic planning.
2. Understand the purpose and relationship between mission, vision, and value statements.
3. Describe the strategic planning cycle and its process flow.
4. Identify the four components of a SWOT analysis.

Notes

1. Department of Veterans Affairs (VA), VA Directive 6052 Appendix A (April 23, 2009).
2. Sutter Health, http://www.sutterhealth.org/about/mission (accessed May 31, 2012).
3. Tenet Health, A Community Built on Care, http://www .tenethealth.com/about/pages/missionandvalues.aspx (accessed August 29, 2021).
4. Mayo Clinic, http://www.mayoclinic.org/about/mission values.html, accessed July 30, 2012.
5. Texas Oncology, http://www.texasoncology.com/about -txo/vision-mission-history.aspx, accessed December 3, 2012.
6. Good Samaritan Society, http://www.good-sam.com/index .php/about_us/, accessed July 30, 2012.
7. Ibid.
8. Providence Healthcare Network, http://www.providence .net/about/, accessed January 16, 2013.
9. Duke Health, http://www.dukemedicine.org/AboutUs, accessed July 30, 2012.
10. L. E. Swayne, W. J. Duncan and P. M. Ginter, *Strategic Management of Health Care Organizations*, 6th ed. (San Francisco, CA: Jossey-Bass, 2008).
11. American Institute of Certified Public Accountants (AICPA), "Financial Forecasts and Projections" AT Section 301 (c) (d), http://www.aicpa.org/Research/Standards/Audit Attest/DownloadableDocuments/AT-00301.pdf.

CHAPTER 25

Creating a Business Plan

PROGRESS NOTES

After completing this chapter, you should be able to:

1. Describe the steps in preparing a business plan.
2. Explain the purpose of the organization and personnel section of a business plan.
3. Describe the elements in a marketing plan.
4. Explain the purpose of the projected income statement, balance sheet, and cash flow statement in the business plan.

Overview: Business Plans

Assume you are asked to develop a plan to provide more services in your current market, provide new services to your existing patients, or begin operations in a new market. You will need to collect and analyze data on current utilization and the need for more services in the current and/or new markets to determine how many additional services could be produced, the additional revenues that will be earned, and the cost of additional labor, supplies, equipment, and facilities. A **business plan** is a document typically prepared to obtain funding and/or financing. A traditional business plan typically contains four major elements: an executive summary; a description of the company or department; a **marketing plan**; and financial projections. The overall business plan is built up as these individual segments are completed.

Elements of the Business Plan

A business plan typically contains four major elements:

- Executive summary
- Description of the organization, personnel, product, and required resources
- Marketing plan (target market, quantity, price, challenges)
- Financial projections (performance and funding)

The executive summary will be described last as it is generally the last element written because it draws on the information developed in the other three elements. The description of the organization, personnel, product, and required resources provides an overview of the plan to be developed in the marketing plan and financial projections. The product section should provide a clear and concise description of the service and/or good to be produced and sold as well the resources required deliver the products to customers. The marketing plan identifies the target market and projects expected sales, the prices to be received for products, actions to be taken to reach sales projections, and challenges. The financial projections show how the project is expected to operate over the life of the business plan. It is important to begin the business plan with an executive summary that outlines key points.

Preparing to Construct the Business Plan

The planning stage will shape a business plan's content. The initial decisions, such as those shown in **Exhibit 25.1**, will determine your approach to the plan. For example, if your organization requires a certain type of format and preexisting blank spreadsheets, many of the initial decisions have already been made for you. Otherwise, the checklist contained in Exhibit 25.1 will assist you in making initial decisions for the business plan's approach.

It is important to note that the level of sophistication for the overall plan should be based on the decision-makers who will be the primary audience (i.e., know and write to your audience). Another practical consideration involves creating a grid or matrix to assist in gathering all necessary information. The grid or matrix could also include which individuals are responsible for helping create or collect the required information. Finally, it

---

Exhibit 25.1 Initial Decisions for the Business Plan

- Outline necessary format
- Decide on length
- Decide on level of sophistication
- Determine what information is needed
- Determine who will provide each piece of information

Courtesy of J.J. Baker and R.W. Baker, Dallas, Texas.

---

is important to create a file at the beginning of the project in which all computations, backup information, dates, and sources are kept together in an organized fashion. This file will save time when revisions are required.

Organization, Personnel, Product, and Required Resources Section

The description of organization, personnel, product, and required resources should provide background on the organization, management team, and other key personnel. It should provide a picture of current operations including the history of the organization, what it produces, and its goals. The personnel section should describe who is employed, their skills and prior accomplishments, and the authority and decision-making structures. Who will be charged with the new budget? Who will be responsible for the controls and reporting for this proposal? It is important to provide a clear picture that informs decision-makers about how the proposed acquisition will be managed. Visual depictions of the chain of authority and supervisory responsibilities are helpful in this section.

The Product

The product section should define the product to be produced. What does it do for whom, and why do or why will customers purchase it (i.e., why do patients need the treatment)? When others produce similar products, attention should be given to explain how the proposed product will be different than competitors' products. For new products, the report should document the stage of development. Is it in a conceptual stage or ready to launch and the result of market tests? The product section should also describe how the proposed good, service, or equipment fits into the organization, including advancing the mission and relationship to existing goods and services. Will the new product complement existing goods and services, or will it substitute for or replace them, leading to a loss of sales?

Required Resources

The required resources section describes the labor, equipment, and facilities that will be needed to produce and deliver the proposed good or service. The product and required resources sections should describe what the heart of the business plan is about. If the business plan is for a new project or service line, then this description should be expanded to include the entire project or the overall service line. Basic information for the organization, personnel, product, and required resources section is shown in **Exhibit 25.2**.

The test of a good description is whether an individual who has never been involved in your planning can read the description and understand the objective and resource needs without asking additional questions.

The Marketing Plan

The marketing plan should describe the available market, the portion of the market the product should attract, and the portion of the market occupied by the competition. This segment should achieve a balance between describing those individuals who will be availing themselves of the product and a description of the competition. The four P's of marketing—product, price, physical distribution (or place), and promotion—will

Exhibit 25.3 Information in the Marketing Plan

- Product: patient wants and needs, product design and image (pricing and packaging)
- Price: patient mix and reimbursement
- Physical distribution: availability, times, and location
- Promotion: advertising plans
- Other: decision-makers, competition and its impact, and estimated sales and portion of the market to be captured

determine which customers will purchase the product (**Exhibit 25.3**).

The product should describe the medical condition it serves and how it will treat the condition. The product will determine the size of the market, who will want the product, and in many cases reimbursement. In many industries, managers can use price to appeal to a large group of customers or attract high-income customers willing to pay high prices. In health care, the patients and their payers will have a major impact on how much is received for services. Given that the majority of patients are covered by managed care, Medicare, and Medicaid, this part of the marketing plan may require determining the patient mix and the fixed payment these payers will reimburse. Likewise, physical distribution (where services will be provided) will have a major impact on the type of patient attracted. Will services be broadly available or at a single location? Will facilities be located in poor or wealthy areas? Finally, promotion defines how services will be brought to the attention of potential patients.

The marketing plan should also identify who will be responsible for the marketing, how competition is expected to respond, and the goal in terms of units sold and market share. Managers should strive for a realistic and objective appraisal of the situation. Of all areas of the business plan, the marketing segment is most likely to be overly optimistic in its assumptions. It is wise to be conservative about estimations of physician and patient acceptance and usage and realistic when assessing the competition and its likely impact.

Exhibit 25.2 Information for the Organization, Management, Product, and Required Resources Section

- History of the organization: date founded, current products, sales, and revenue, expense, and net income history
- Composition of the management team: number of managers, work and educational background, previous accomplishments
- Product, what it is and does, who will purchase (if relevant), differentiation from other available products
- Personnel, equipment, and facility requirements to implement plan

The Financial Plan

The financial segment lays out the expected revenues and expenses that illustrate how the project is expected to operate over period of time. Financial plans may range from a projected period of one year to as long as 10 years. One-year projections will seldom be able to determine whether a project will cover its costs, whereas a 10-year projection of sales and costs may be too long to meaningfully forecast. Your organization will usually have a standard length of time that is accepted for these projections. The standard forecasted periods for high-tech equipment often range from three to five years because advances in technology may render equipment obsolete in five years or less. Therefore, the forecast is set for a realistically short time period.

The financial projections for a business plan should contain a forecast of operations. The forecast may be simple, such as a cash flow statement, or it may be more extensive. A more extensive forecast would also require a balance sheet and an income statement. The required statements and schedules will depend on two factors: the cost and complexity of the project and the usual procedure for a business plan presentation that is expected in your organization.

The Projected Cash Flow Statement

The purpose of projecting a cash flow statement is to show how cash will be affected over the life of the business plan. Previous chapters have emphasized the difference between cash inflows and outflows and revenues and expenses. Assuming investments in equipment, facilities, accounts receivable, and/or inventories are needed in the first year of the business plan, cash outflows may exceed inflows while revenues exceed expenses. The cash flow statement should identify where money will come from to fund increases in assets (i.e., will the organization need to borrow funds to support the business plan?). In any case, the cash flow statement can be complex, with many detailed line items, or condensed. The condensed

type of statement is most often found in a business plan. Keep in mind, however, that a detailed worksheet—the source of the information on the condensed statement—should be filed in the supporting work papers for the project. Cash flow assumptions are illustrated in **Exhibit 25.4**.

The Projected Income Statement

The purpose of projecting an income statement is to show whether the business plan will increase or decrease an organization's net income (i.e., revenues and expenses for each year of the business plan and the total return expected over the life of the business plan). The basic assumptions for a healthcare project's income statement are illustrated in **Exhibit 25.5**.

The "revenue sources" refer to how many payers will pay for the service and/or drug and device and in what proportion, such as Medicare

Exhibit 25.4 Assumptions for Business Plan Cash Flow Statement Projections

- Capital asset purchase or lease information (equipment and facilities)
- Changes in short-term assets (accounts receivable and inventories)
- 1. Cash inflow
- 2. Cash outflow

Exhibit 25.5 Assumptions for Business Plan Income Statement Projections

- Sales (or output from marketing plan)
- Revenue source(s) (i.e., payer mix)
- Revenue amount, reimbursement by payer
- Total revenue
- Expenses:
  - Labor
  - Supplies
  - Equipment
  - Space occupancy
  - Overhead
- Total expense
- Net income

50%, Medicaid 5%, managed care 25%, and other 20% (e.g., commercial and self-pay). The "revenue amount" refers to how much each payer is expected to pay for the service or good. The total amount of revenue can then be determined by multiplying each payer's expected payment rate times the percentage of the total revenue expected from that payer.

The expense portion translates the required resources into expected dollar outlays. Labor expenses in Exhibit 25.5 are determined by staffing assumptions. The required staffing should be set out by the type of employee and the pay rate for each type of employee. The number of full-time equivalents (FTEs) for each type of employee will then be established, and the FTEs will be multiplied by the assumed pay rate to arrive at the expected labor cost.

"Supplies" refer to the necessary materials required to perform the procedure or service. The labor, supplies, and cost of drugs or devices are costs that can be directly attributed to the service that is the subject of the business plan. Likewise, "equipment" refers to the annual depreciation expense of any equipment that is directly attributed to the service that is the subject of the business plan.

"Space occupancy" refers to the overall cost of occupying the space required for the service or procedure. Space occupancy is a catchall phrase including depreciation expense (if the building is owned), rent expense (if the building is leased) of the square footage required for the service, utilities, maintenance, housekeeping, insurance, and security. The actual forecast might group these expense items into one line item, or the forecast might show each individual expense (depreciation, housekeeping, etc.) on a separate line. If the expenses are grouped, a footnote or a supplemental schedule should show the actual detail that makes up the total amount.

"Overhead" refers to the remaining expenses of operation that are necessary to produce the service but that are not directly attributable to that service. Examples of such overhead in a physician's office might include items such as insurance and licensing fees. This amount of indirect overhead may be expressed as a percentage; for example, 10% of labor, supplies, equipment, and space occupancy. Whether overhead is reported as a single amount or detailed in the forecast will probably depend on how large the amount is in relation to the other expenses or the usual format that your organization expects to see in a business plan that is presented to management.

The Projected Balance Sheet

The purpose of projecting a balance sheet is to show where an organization expects to be if the business plan is followed (i.e., the anticipated changes in assets, liabilities, and net worth). Where will money come from to fund increases in assets? The basic assumptions for a healthcare project's balance sheet are illustrated in **Exhibit 25.6**. The elements of a balance sheet (assets, liabilities, and equity) were described in Chapter 11. If a full projected set of financial statements is required for the business plan, the balance sheet entries will in large part be a function of the income statement projections discussed in the preceding section of this chapter. For example, accounts receivable would be primarily determined by the revenue assumptions, while accounts payable would be primarily determined by the expense assumptions. Likewise, acquisition of equipment or other capital assets will affect capital assets (property and equipment), while their funding assumptions will affect liability and/or net worth totals on the projected balance sheet.

Exhibit 25.6 **Assumptions for Business Plan Balance Sheet Projections**

- Cash
- Accounts receivable
- Inventories
- Property and equipment
- Total assets
- Accounts payable
- Accrued current liabilities
- Long-term liabilities
- Total liabilities
- Net worth (equity or fund balance)

The purpose of the financial plan is to flesh out the operating and marketing plans to determine if the project will benefit the organization. As stated earlier, business plans are often used to obtain financing for a project. Investors in a project, whether within or outside the organization, want to know if a project will cover its costs and generate a sufficient return.

The "Knowledgeable Reader" Approach to Your Business Plan

We believe a good business plan should answer the questions that occur to a knowledgeable reader. Thus, the information you include in the business plan should reflect the choices that you made in selecting the assumptions for your financial analysis. For instance, an example of considerations for forecasting an equipment acquisition is presented in **Exhibit 25.7**. The content of the final business plan should touch upon these points in describing your assumptions that underlie the financial analysis.

Exhibit 25.7 Considerations for Equipment Acquisition

- Single purpose or multipurpose equipment?
- Technology: new, middle-aged, old (obsolete versus untested)?
- Equipment compatibility?
- Purchase or lease?
- If purchase, new or used (refurbished)?
- If lease, number of years or lease on a pay-per-procedure deal?
- Location(s)?
- How much staff training is required?
- Certification required?
- Square footage required for equipment?
- Is the required square footage available?
- Medical supply cost?
- Cleaning methods and equipment?
- Repairs and maintenance expense?
- Total capital investment?

Courtesy of J.J. Baker and R.W. Baker, Dallas, Texas.

The Executive Summary

The executive summary should contain a well-written and concise summary of the entire plan. It should not be longer than two pages; many decision-makers consider one page desirable. Some people like to write the executive summary first to use as an outline to guide the rest of the content. More commonly the executive summary is written last when the writer knows all the detailed content from the other three sections. In either instance, the executive summary should tell the entire story in a compelling manner to gain the support of decision-makers for the plan.

Assembling the Business Plan

The business plan should be assembled into a suitable report format that is determined by many of your initial decisions, such as length and level of sophistication. A sample format appears in **Exhibit 25.8**. When an appendix is desired, it should contain detail to support certain contents in the main part of the business plan. In preparing the final report, certain other logistics are important. It is expected, for example, that the pages should be numbered. You might also want to add the date in the footer and perhaps a version number as well. Although the report may or may not be bound, it should have all pages firmly secured.

Exhibit 25.8 Sample Format for a Business Plan

- Title page
- Table of contents
- Executive summary
- Description of organization, management, product, and required resources
- Marketing plan
- Financial projections
- Appendices (optional)

Presenting the Business Plan

You may be asked to present your plan more than once. Sometimes you will have to prepare a short form and a long form of the plan, depending on the audience. Tips on presenting your business plan are given in **Exhibit 25.9**. It is especially important to practice your presentation in advance. When you leave time for questions and for discussion, you also want to be well prepared for anticipated questions. By constructing a well-thought-out business plan, you have substantially increased your chances for a successful outcome.

Exhibit 25.9 Tips on Presenting Your Business Plan

- Determine who will be attending ahead of time
- Determine how long you will have for the presentation
- Be sure you have a copy for each attendee
- Decide on whether to use audio/visual aids
  - LCD projector and PowerPoint slides?
  - Flip chart and markers?
  - Other methods?
- Practice your presentation in advance
- Leave time for questions and for discussion

Courtesy of J.J. Baker and R.W. Baker, Dallas, Texas.

Strategic Aspects of Your Business Plan

Your business plan must fit into your organization's strategic plan. To begin to do so, you might answer the following questions:

- How does my business plan fit into the overall strategic plan (the "master plan") for my organization?
- How does my business plan specifically fit into my department or division's segment of the organization's overall strategic plan/master plan?
- Does the proposed timing of my business plan coincide with the strategic plan's time frames?
- Does the proposed funding of my business plan fit into available funding resources mentioned in the strategic plan?
- What competition will my business plan face, strategically speaking, within my organization? Does my plan provide a good defense against this competition?
- Are there external competition and/or legislative aspects mentioned in my business plan that are also addressed within the strategic plan? If so, does my plan's treatment of these external aspects coordinate with that of the strategic plan? If not, have I explained why not?

The previous chapter explored strategic planning in some depth. Many aspects discussed in that chapter may also be applicable to your business plan.

WRAP-UP

Summary

A business plan describes how a desired project is expected to perform in order to gain approval and financial support for the project. A business plan often contains four major parts beginning with the executive summary, which outlines the major points to the project. The writers of the business plan should invest energy in writing the summary as many readers will not read the entire report.

The second part of the plan describes the organization and personnel to highlight the mission, history, and successes of the organization and the skills and successes of employees. After describing the organization and personnel, the project, including the good or service to be delivered to customers and why customers will be attracted to the product, is discussed. The next section describes the additional resources, labor, equipment, and facilities the organization will need to produce the good or service.

The marketing plan is the third part. The marketing plan discusses the characteristics of the product to be delivered, the expected price at which it will be sold, where customers can purchase the product, and how the product will be brought to the attention of potential purchasers (i.e., the 4 P's of product, price, physical distribution, and promotion). In addition, the marketing plan should identify who will be in charge of marketing, how competition is expected to respond, and sales targets.

The final part of the plan is the financial projections. The financial section calculates the expected revenue that will be generated given the sales target and prices and the cost of the additional resources needed to complete the project. Projected cash flow statements, income statements, and balance sheets are often prepared to assess the impact of the project on cash, profitability, and net worth.

Key Terms

Business Plan

Marketing Plan

Discussion Questions

1. Describe the steps in preparing a business plan.
2. Explain the purpose of the organization and personnel section of a business plan.
3. Describe the elements in a marketing plan.
4. Explain the purpose of the projected cash flow statement, income statement, and balance sheet.

CHAPTER 26

Healthcare Delivery Systems, Finance, and Reimbursement

PROGRESS NOTES

After completing this chapter, you should be able to:

1. Define healthcare delivery systems.
2. Define the area of healthcare finance.
3. Understand the strategic relationship between healthcare delivery systems and finance.
4. Understand the strategic relationship between finance and reimbursement.
5. Recognize the strategic relationship between third-party reimbursement and government expenditures.
6. Recognize a new focus on the relationship between finance and healthcare delivery.

Overview: Delivery Systems, Finance, and Reimbursement

We begin this chapter by defining three areas—**healthcare delivery systems, finance,** and **reimbursement**—to illustrate where finance and reimbursement fit into the overall system and then describe the various strategic relationships that are involved. By its very nature, the complexion and purpose of a healthcare delivery system cannot be considered separately from the range of values and issues surrounding finance and reimbursement, including the magnitude of government involvement. Healthcare finance is the linchpin of the healthcare delivery system in the United States as well as other countries. While there are some similarities to corporate finance (i.e., budgeting, variance analysis, capital budgeting, etc.), there are also major differences.

Healthcare Delivery Systems

A healthcare delivery system typically contains different levels of patient care and sites of service operating under a central administrative structure. A more formal definition is:

A delivery system that "provides or aims to provide a coordinated continuum of services to a defined population and are willing to be held clinically and fiscally accountable for the outcomes and the health status of the population served."[1]

A successful health system that functions properly needs the six following elements:

- Trained and motivated workers
- A well-managed infrastructure
- A reliable supply of medicines and technologies
- Adequate funding
- Evidence-based policies
- Strong, updated strategic plans[2]

Who Are the Stakeholders in Healthcare Delivery Systems?

Stakeholders, people with an interest in the operation of an organization, in healthcare delivery systems can be divided into internal and external groups. Internal stakeholders consist of those receiving care (patients), those delivering care (clinicians), and those supporting the care deliverers (administrators).

External stakeholders are varied and numerous. Their motivations may vary, but their interests still center upon the delivery of care within the internal system. **Figure 26.1** illustrates 12 different types of external stakeholders. They include the following:

- Insurance companies
- Government providers
- Government policy makers
- Government regulators (overseers)
- The pharmaceutical industry
- The medical device industry
- Other health industry suppliers
- Professional organizations
- Educators
- Investors
- Caregivers
- Consumers

Insurance providers include such organizations as Aetna, United Health, and more. Government providers include federal agencies such as Medicare, Medicaid, and TRICARE, along with state agencies. Government policy makers include Congress and supporting federal agencies such as the Office of Management and Budget (OMB), while individual states also determine relevant

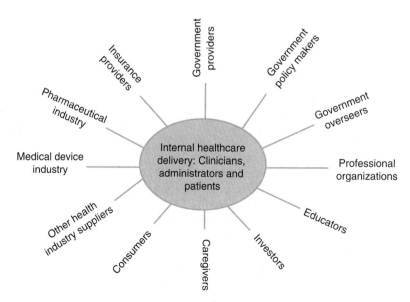

Figure 26.1 Stakeholders in Health Delivery Systems

health policy. Other government agencies regulate various elements of our public health including the Centers for Disease Control and Prevention (CDC), the National Institutes of Health (NIH), and others.

Health care is a largest employer in the United States and consumes 17.7% of the country's gross domestic product (see Chapter 1). Numerous professional organizations provide support for clinicians and administrators; examples include the American Hospital Association (AHA) and the American Medical Association (AMA), there are many more and they all play important supporting roles. Colleges and universities are stakeholders for their role in training future doctors, nurses, allied health personnel, and managers.

Investors, whether equity holders, donors, or creditors, play an important stakeholder role, as they provide funding. Caregivers, the families and friends of patients, have a personal interest in the health delivery system. Consumers in their roles of workers and taxpayers are stakeholders because they are impacted by rising healthcare costs. Finally, various organizations supply goods and services to healthcare providers such as pharmaceutical firms and medical supply and equipment industries as well as food service, housekeeping, and **information technology (IT)** companies.

Healthcare Finance

There are four major responsibilities typically associated with healthcare finance. They include:

- Planning
- Organizing and directing
- Controlling
- Decision-making[3]

Healthcare finance can be thought of as "a method of getting money in and out of the business." You now understand that the money coming in must at the very least equal if not exceed the money flowing out. Finance is primarily responsible for ensuring the continued operation of the organization (i.e., maximizing revenue and minimizing expenses).

What Are the Duties Associated with Finance?

The duties associated with healthcare finance revolve around the successful management of planning, organizing and directing, controlling, and decision-making. Specific duties for financial officers depend upon the organizational structure where they work.

For example, is the organization large and consolidated with a head office? If so, some or all of the decision-making and planning may be handled in the head office. Onsite financial officers' duties will then mostly center on operational matters such as organizing, directing, and controlling. Large organizations may have a treasurer in addition to a chief financial officer who focus on planning and decision-making. When the organization is smaller, a single person may have to direct all financial matters—planning and decision-making in addition to day-to-day operational matters.

The individual performing these duties may have one of several different job titles. A description of three such titles follows.

- *Chief financial officer*: Responsible for operations (administrative, financial, and risk management), including both financial and operational strategies; determining the metrics that are related to the strategies; and developing and monitoring internal control systems[4]
- *Controller*: Responsible for the organization's accounting functions; includes producing accurate financial reports that adhere to appropriate standards, maintaining the accounting system, and overseeing controls and budgets[5]
- *Treasurer*: Responsible for a higher level of the organization's financial activities, mainly centering upon financial liquidity, investments, and risk management[6]

Healthcare Reimbursement

The term *reimbursement* basically means the method of paying a healthcare provider for services or procedures provided. Payment is made upon receipt of a claim (bill) from the service provider. This claim typically contains codes for specific procedures and services that tie to relevant payment amounts. Payment of the claim may be made by a third-party payer or by the patient directly.[7]

What Are the Responsibilities Associated with Reimbursement?

There are three major responsibilities associated with reimbursement:

- Preparing a correct and complete claims
- Submitting claims to the correct payer(s) in a timely manner
- Collecting the proper payment that is due in a timely manner

In addition, the reimbursement personnel are responsible for carrying out any directives received from the finance department, including those of strategic planning.

What Are the Duties Associated with Reimbursement?

Reimbursement duties within the system may be split up into different positions. The following job titles may typically be responsible for these duties. Note that other job titles also exist that describe these same duties.

- *Data entry clerk*: Enters codes and insurance information
- *Medical coder*: Enters service and procedure codes onto a claim
- *Medical biller*: Verifies the patient's insurance coverage; prepares the bill (claim form); reviews unpaid claims and/or appeals those that are denied
- *Billing supervisor or coordinator*: Oversees scheduling, monitoring, and training of personnel
- *Medical claims specialist or examiner*: Reviews samples of claims for accuracy; documents information for legal actions; provides legal

support when required (this position functions outside the regular day-to-day operations and may work directly from the finance department)

Other reimbursement duties involve management of monies received or not received. Incoming payments of claims must be reconciled and matched to the organization's records of billings. Non-payments (past-due bills) require collection efforts. These payment duties are typically handled by different personnel.

It is also possible that the billing and collection duties may be performed by an outside contractor. In 2020, outsourced medical billing was a $10.2 billion industry.[8]

Medical information and billing information can now be generated in real time. For example, a doctor may have a data entry person in the exam room recording the physician's observations and services provided. This may be a nurse who has other duties or a "scribe" whose only job is data entry. The doctor dictates medical notes as they perform their examination, and the assistant enters the information into the computer. At the end of the visit, they refer to the **super bill** that contains procedure and diagnosis codes specific to a particular practice and/or specialty. A super bill allows information to be recorded quickly and efficiently. The physician calls off the codes to be billed for the examination plus any lab work ordered and so on. The data entry assistant enters this coding information into the computer. The billing codes are then transmitted electronically, either to the internal billing department or to the outside billing service. When transmitted externally, the outside billing service is then typically responsible for all billing and collection—for a fee, of course.

While the preceding description encapsulates the essence of healthcare reimbursement, two caveats are worth mentioning. When healthcare reimbursement involves a third party, consumers may be largely unconcerned with the costs of their care, knowing that their bills are paid by another party. Moreover, third-party transactions may also reduce provider concerns about the cost of care, as they may not need to confront a patient covered by insurance with the actual charges, no matter how high. One may hope that third-party concerns about the price and amount of services will be mitigated by the implementation of value-based purchasing.

The Strategic Relationship Between the Healthcare Delivery System and Finance

This relationship can be described as a circular cause and effect. That is, finance department actions affect the delivery system, and the delivery system in turn affects the finance department. We illustrate this cause and effect with an example. In this example, particular elements of the overall delivery system affect the strategic positioning of the finance department.

Value-based programs are an important current trend in payment for U.S. healthcare services. Briefly, the programs rely upon digitally recorded performance measures, including quality measures, to assess the value of services provided. High-value care is rewarded with a bonus payment, and low-value services receive lower payment.

It follows, then, that accurate and timely recording of such quality measures will ultimately affect total payments, which will affect the finance department's financial strategic planning. The finance department has no control over how (or when) these measures are recorded; they happen elsewhere within the system. This strategic relationship is illustrated step-by-step in **Figure 26.2**. Note that the information generated in this example is used internally and externally. Steps are as follows:

Step 1: A medical service is performed by a clinician assigned to a medical department somewhere within the system.

Step 2: The data generated from this service is recorded within an **electronic health record (EHR)** including the service itself plus specific quality information (measures).

Step 3.1: The data is reported in two parts. First, the medical service portion is transmitted to patient accounting, which then bills the third-party payer.

Step 3.2: In the second part of this step, the quality measures portion of the data is transmitted to the third-party payer, which accumulates it for future analysis.

Step 4: At a future point in time, the third-party payer analyzes the accumulated quality measure data.

Step 5: The outcome of this analysis becomes actionable by the payer, as shown by the data analytics.

Step 6: The resulting action may be a pay-for-performance bonus or penalty.

Step 7: Higher or lower payments then impact the finance department's revenues, budgets, and forecasts.

Step 8: The resulting financial impact affects strategic positioning by the finance department.

The resulting financial impact also impacts the financial position of the overall system. Thus, the strategic relationship of the entire system and finance department is cause and effect. Accurate reporting of good quality measures by an entirely separate department trickles down to affect the dollars received or not received, which affects the finance department and entire system.

Strategic Analysis Relationships Within the System

The previous example illustrated a relationship that resulted in payment from a payer outside the health delivery system. However, the same data can and should be analyzed for internal strategic uses. **Figure 26.3** illustrates this type of analysis as follows:

1. The medical service data is generated and recorded via EHRs using software installed by the organization.

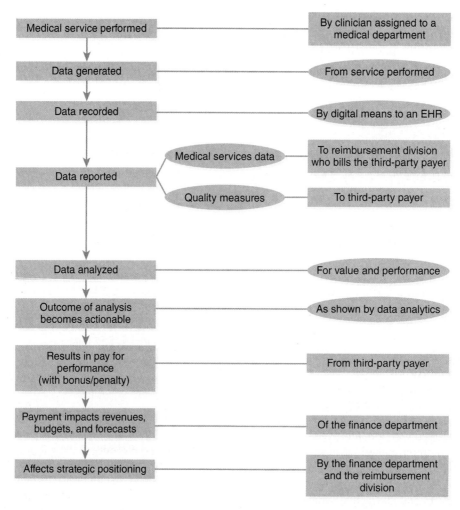

Figure 26.2 The Strategic Relationship of Value-Based Programs, Quality Measures, Finance, and Reimbursement

2. The accumulated data is analyzed for value-based purposes. This analysis may be performed internally by the IT department or by an outside contractor.
3. The outcome of such analysis, as shown by data analytics, becomes actionable. This is an internal analysis, generated for internal use.
4. The strategic action plan is then revised. Revisions are undertaken by the personnel who are responsible for strategic planning within the system.
5. Strategic positioning results from plan revisions.

Such analysis highlights strategic relationships between and among the various departments within the system. While the positioning in this example may be most likely to affect the finance and patient accounting departments (i.e., reimbursement), as shown, that might not always be the case. The result of the internal strategic analysis may reveal faults in the process and workflow at the clinical level. Strategic relationships should then be activated to remedy the faults, wherever they may lie.

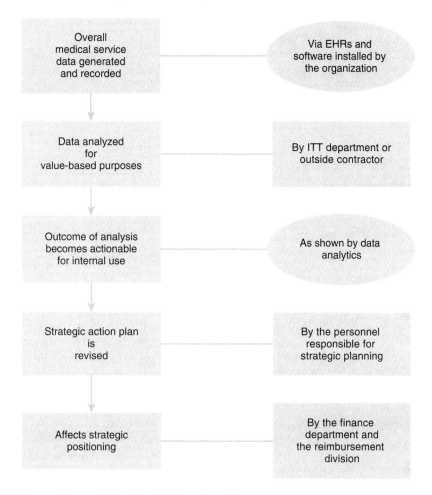

Figure 26.3 Internal Strategic Analysis for Value-Based Programs

The Strategic Relationship Between Finance and Reimbursement

At first glance, the strategic relationship between finance and reimbursement seems like a one-way street. That is, finance personnel provide the lead in strategy and reimbursement personnel must follow.

However, what happens if the patient account department fails in its responsibilities? Answer: Cash flow for the organization is reduced, and in some cases, the reduction in cash flow can be significant. When cash flow is reduced, finance must react to the reimbursement situation instead of providing the lead. Finance personnel will have to find funding to make up the cash shortfall. Strategic planning must be revised while remedial action is taken.

Inasmuch as the chief financial officer (or vice president of finance in a larger organization) is responsible for all finance activities within the organization, it is incumbent upon that person to raise the necessary funds and to ensure that those funds are effectively used. Specific applications may include the acquisition of capital, cash and debt management, and lease financing among strategic alternatives.

It is worth noting that some things are beyond the organization's control. A case in point is the Centers for Medicare and Medicaid Services' (CMS) Readmission Reduction Program. CMS data shows that 2,545 hospitals may face penalties for excessive readmissions in fiscal 2021 with 41 facing the maximum 3% reduction.[9]

Third-Party Reimbursement and Government Expenditures

Reliance on third-party reimbursement sets healthcare finance apart from other industries. Reimbursement plays the dominant role in the configuration of finance in the healthcare industry. Without third-party reimbursement, inclusive of private insurance carriers, healthcare finance and the delivery system that it supports would take on a very different complexion, one that would not be sustainable.

Reimbursement Methods Have Evolved

Historically, different methods of reimbursement have had attendant risks and incentives associated with them. They have gone through an evolution of sorts, beginning with the retrospective cost-based or cost-plus method, moving on to charge-based methods (using negotiated rates that sometimes reflect discounts), and evolving into the prospective payment system that pays a predetermined, fixed amount.[10] Retrospective reimbursement pays *after* the service is provided, while the prospective payment system pays *before* the service is provided. These three types of reimbursement mechanisms are indicative of a fee-for-service framework.

Two additional types of reimbursement that are relevant to the interplay between health delivery systems and finance are **capitation** and **pay-for-performance (P4P)**. Under capitation, the provider is typically paid a fixed per-member-per-month payment for each covered participant.

This payment covers all medical services that have been contracted for the period.[11] In P4P, providers receive payment incentives when they meet specific performance measures that show they are delivering high-quality, efficient care. Thus, pay-for-performance is also referred to as value-based purchasing in that it "...connects reimbursement to the quality of patient care rather than just the quantity of services received."[12]

Government Support in Healthcare Spending

The magnitude of government support, of which third-party reimbursement is a central feature, is illustrated by the following data. Healthcare spending in the United States grew 4.6% in 2019, reaching $3.795 trillion or $11,582 per person. As a share of the nation's **gross domestic product (GDP)**, health spending accounted for 17.7%, up from 17.3% in 2010.[13] **Figure 26.4** provides a visual representation of the distribution of the $3.795 trillion across payers.

Currently, Medicare's major role in the health delivery system is illustrated by its accounting for 21.1% of total health spending in 2019 while Medicaid accounted for 16.2%. By comparison, in fiscal year 2014, Medicare and Medicaid

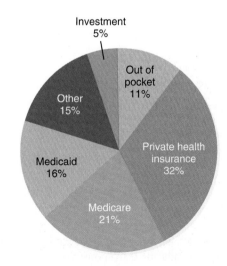

Figure 26.4 National Healthcare Expenditure by Payer, 2019

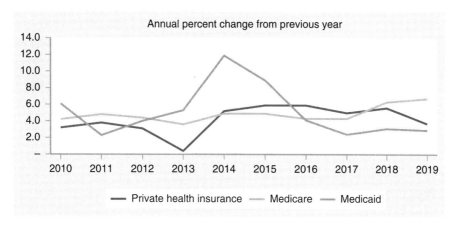

Figure 26.5 Annual Percent Change from Previous Years by Major Payers

accounted for 20.5% and 16.6%. Private health insurance covered 31.5% of all expenditures, up from 30.8% in 2014.[14] **Figure 26.5** illustrates the annual percent change in expenditures for the three major payers from 2010 through 2019. CMS predicts annual healthcare costs will be $6.0 trillion by 2027 and consume 19.4% of GDP.[15]

From 2010 through 2019, private health insurance increased 4.2% per year versus 4.8% for Medicare and 5.1% for Medicaid. The rate of increase in annual healthcare expenditures has slowed compared to 2000 through 2009 when these payers saw annual increases of 6.8%, 9.1%, and 7.6%.

A New Focus on the Relationship Between Finance and Healthcare Delivery

Medicare and Medicaid turned 50 in 2015 and had more of an impact on American health care and well-being than any other programs. That said, it should be noted that the Affordable Care Act (ACA), signed into law in March 2010, created insurance plans for those not covered by Medicaid, expanded Medicaid coverage, and sought to tie payment closer to outcomes. The ACA is the largest change in healthcare financing and accessibility to health care since 1965.

CMS unveiled its Accountable Care Organization (ACO) program in 2012. The ACO model stresses primary care coordination, primarily for the chronically ill, and beneficiary engagement opportunities, as well as advancing the managed care concept by rewarding providers for measurably improving care quality and efficiency rather than simply for saving money.[16] The groups of providers who are integral to ACOs come together voluntarily. Recent revisions are designed to test whether stronger incentives can improve outcomes and cut costs for Medicare beneficiaries. As of July 2015, there were over 750 ACOs.[17]

The New Finance–Delivery Link Is a Challenge

As such, this new focus on the finance–delivery link reflects the ongoing challenge for healthcare leaders to integrate clinical and business data. It's the shift to value-based care that is making this integration an imperative. An important part of this shift entails at-risk payments, such as those that characterize the aforementioned ACOs, both upside risk (sharing in savings) and downside risk (reimbursement penalties).[18] The presence of risk causes providers, such as physician organizations, to increase their dependence on analytics modules. Providers need to know the cost of care when they're going to be at risk.

Reimbursement and Physicians: An Ongoing Strategic Challenge

Healthcare finance and reimbursement is anathema to many physicians. Aspects of Medicare illustrate the complexity that many physicians contend with. An ongoing feature of the program has been the **sustainable growth rate (SGR),** which was used by CMS to control growth in Medicare physician service expenditures. Generally, this was a method to ensure that the yearly increase in expense per Medicare beneficiary did not exceed the growth in the GDP.[19]

On March 1 of each year, the physician fee schedule was updated accordingly. This was euphemistically known as a "doc fix." Physician groups, including the AMA and the American Osteopathic Association (AOA), lobbied for a permanent reform to the SGR so that physician payment rates would not be subject to annual cuts—a permanent doc fix.

The SGR Has Been Replaced

A 1.5% or less annual update in payment rates has been common over the past 10 years.[20] Predictably, these low increases in Medicare payments have consequences: Fewer physicians take on new Medicare patients, and others have withdrawn entirely from the program. On April 14, 2015, Congress ended the doc fix by passing the Medicare Access and Children's Health Insurance Program (CHIP) Reauthorization Act (MACRA). This act put an end to the SGR physician payment formula. Providers would have seen Medicare reimbursement rates drop by 21% starting on April 15, 2015, had this legislation not been enacted. The act establishes an automatic 0.5% raise annually in provider reimbursement rates from 2015 through 2019.[21]

The New Performance-for-Payment Reimbursement Method Presents Different Physician Challenges

From 2019 on, payments to providers are adjusted based on performance under a two-part Quality Payment Program (QPP). The QPP thus includes certain payment adjustments under the Merit-Based Incentive Payment System (MIPS). The program also provides certain payment adjustments for "Advanced" Alternative Payment Model (APM) entities. What QPP underscores, potentially further vexing physicians, is CMS's objective to tie the majority of reimbursement to quality outcomes and increased beneficiary access to quality care.

The program may also present practice management challenges to providers and their business partners. For example, starting in 2019, MIPS mandated negative payment adjustments for providers who fall below certain performance thresholds. By 2022, some providers may see payments cut by up to 9%. For more detail about QPP, see Chapter 28, "New Payment Methods: MIPS and APMs."

Physician Leadership Is Needed

Concurrent with the change to value-based payment and the resulting value-focused organization should be a shift in leadership roles that involves more physicians as leaders. Physicians have unique insight into the needs of the patient population. Their knowledge of optimal patient outcomes and how to achieve them is critical to effectively adopting to the new reimbursement climate based on value. Building an effective "physician enterprise" wherein new management structures are physician directed and led requires that the resulting organization be both flexible and transparent enough to achieve both cost reduction and better outcomes.[22]

In conclusion, CMS's attempt to remake the nation's healthcare finance system based upon value-based payments is a "sea change." Strategic relationships are very much affected by this sea change. Recognizing the importance of such change and how it impacts various areas of the organization is an important step in revising the strategic plan.

WRAP-UP

Summary

This chapter highlighted the strategic relationship between the healthcare delivery system, finance, and reimbursement. Under retrospective, fee-for-service reimbursement, healthcare providers did not have to consider the impact of their actions on the money flowing into an organization. The advent of pay-for-performance and value-based purchasing requires all members of an organization to understand how their actions can increase or decrease the amount of money received for services and therefore the viability of the organization.

Key Terms

Capitation

Electronic Health Record (EHR)

Finance

Gross Domestic Product (GDP)

Healthcare Delivery System

Information Technology (IT)

Pay-for-Performance (P4P)

Reimbursement

Super Bill

Stakeholder

Sustainable Growth Rate (SGR)

Discussion Questions

1. If you work in a healthcare organization, describe how your finance operation is organized, if not, describe the finance operation of your employer or the university where you are enrolled.
2. Discuss the essence of the relationship between the healthcare delivery system and third-party reimbursement.
3. Do you think that the transition from fee-for-service payment to value-based payment is feasible?
4. If you work in a healthcare organization, what percentage of your revenue is derived from third-party reimbursement, if not, research and report the current percentage of third-party revenues for one type of providers.

Notes

1. F. Lega, "Organizational Design for Health Integrated Delivery Systems: Theory and Practice," *Health Policy, 81* (2007): 258–279.
2. World Health Organization (WHO), "Health Systems Service Delivery," http://www.who.int/healthsystems/topics/delivery/en/, accessed December 15, 2016.
3. Note that these areas of responsibility are more fully discussed under "The Elements of Management" in Chapter 1.
4. Accounting Tools, "Chief Financial Officer (CFO) Job Description," http://www.accountingtools.com/job-description-cfo, accessed March 1, 2016.
5. Ibid.
6. Ibid.
7. The term *reimbursement* implies that a claim is being paid, or reimbursed, for services already rendered. We now have prospective reimbursement whereby payment may be made for services that will be rendered in the future. Nevertheless, *reimbursement* is still being used as a descriptive term even though the payment method may be prospective.
8. Grandview Research, "Medical Billing Outsourcing Market Size, Share and Trends by Component, by Service, by End Use, by Region, and Segment Forecasts 2021–2028," https://www.grandviewresearch.com, accessed October 4, 2021.
9. R. Daly, "Medicare Readmission Reduction Program Penalizes Hospitals Inaccurately, Study Finds," https://www.hfma.org, accessed July 16, 2021.
10. Health Care Financing & Organization (HCFO) & Robert Wood Johnson Foundation (RWJF), "Learning from Medicare: Prospective Payment," May 2011; CMS, "Hospital Value-Based Purchasing," http://www.cms.gov/Medicare/Quality-Initiatives-Patient-Assessment-Instruments

/hospital-value-based-purchasing/, accessed June 28, 2016.

11. J. McCally, *Capitation for Physicians* (Chicago: Irwin Professional Publishing, 1996), 176.

12. HCFO & RWJF, "Learning from Medicare."

13. Centers for Medicare and Medicaid Services, "Table 3 National Health Expenditures; Levels and Annual Percent Change, by Source of Funds: Selected Calendar Years 1960-2019," https://www.cms.gov /Research-Statistics-Data-and-Systems/Statistics -Trends-and-Reports/NationalHealthExpendData /NationalHealthAccountsHistorical, accessed June 4, 2021.

14. Ibid.

15. Centers for Medicare and Medicaid Services, "Forecast Summary," https://www.cms.gov/Research -Statistics-Data-and-Systems/Statistics-Trends-and -Reports/NationalHealthExpendData/Downloads /ForecastSummary.pdf, accessed June 4, 2021.

16. H. Larkin, "ACO or No?" *Hospitals & Health Networks, 88*, no. 5 (2014): 26–31.

17. S. Shortell, "The Next Frontier: Creating Accountable Communities for Health," *Hospitals & Health Networks, 89*, no. 7 (2015): 12.

18. M. Zeis, "The Certainty of Analytics," *HealthLeaders, 18*, no. 3 (2015): 32–36.

19. Centers for Medicare and Medicaid Services, "Estimated Sustainable Growth Rate and Conversion Factor, for Medicare Payments to Physicians in 2015," p. 1, www .cms.gov/medicare/medicare-fee-for-service-payment /sustainablegratesconfact/downloads/sgr2015.pdf, accessed September 17, 2016.

20. Ibid., Table 6, p. 8.

21. Medicare Access and CHIP Reauthorization Act of 2015, Pub. L. No. 114-10 (2015).

22. P. Betbeze, "Building an Effective Physician Enterprise," *HealthLeaders, 18*, no. 3 (2015): 38–42.

CHAPTER 27

Value-Based Health Care and Its Financial and Digital Outcomes

PROGRESS NOTES

After completing this chapter, you should be able to:

1. Describe value-based progress and programs in the private and public sector.
2. Distinguish among different types of value-based education efforts.
3. Understand the basics of value-based legislative reform.
4. Describe quality measurement in the public and private sectors.
5. Recognize various possible digital outcomes.
6. Identify types of financial outcomes.
7. Describe elements of strategic planning in the public and private sectors.

Overview: Value-Based Health Care

The term *value-based* has come to mean a combination of both quality and cost to many financial managers. If you are shopping, whether for a box of cereal or a car, you will probably consider this combination. In the case of low-cost items, like cereal, you might first consider quality (taste and so on) and then cost; with larger purchases, such as a car, you may consider the cost first and then quality. Either way, both cost and quality usually enter into your evaluation and choice.

Healthcare organizations have used a variety of methods to determine cost and to measure the quality of care delivered over the years. Recently, the concept of value-based health care has been employed to recognize both quality and cost, just as you might in your personal life. In healthcare today, the term *value-based* has multiple definitions. The definition depends upon a person's particular focus. For healthcare finance, value-based concepts can be, and are, applied to value-based purchasing, payment adjustments, pricing, strategy, and patient care. When we speak of value-based healthcare financial management, we may be referring to different aspects of all these concepts. We can even view the broad span of value-based population health and the role that financial management can play.

This chapter addresses different facets of the value-based concept in healthcare finance and financial management. The chapter is divided into several parts, and each part builds your understanding of the value-based concept. The remainder of the chapter will discuss the following value-based health concepts:

- Progress in the private sector
- Progress in the public sector
- Legislative reform
- Quality measurement concept
- Public reporting efforts
- Financial and digital outcomes
- Strategic planning approaches

Value-Based Progress in the Private Sector

Leaders in innovation within the private sector have adopted a variety of value and quality efforts.

Implementing Value-Based Approaches

An Organizational System Approach

Mayo Clinic's "Value Creation System" and Office of Value Creation are the direct result of this improvement strategy. The Office of Value Creation was originally tasked with owning the various value-based projects. As time went on, however, responsibility and accountability for quality and value efforts shifted to operational levels. This left the Office of Value Creation to monitor quality and value within the organization. Thus, Mayo's system has been in place long enough that progress has moved to a second, higher value-based level.[1]

A Data-Driven Approach

The Geisinger Health System has implemented an approach to health care that is data driven. As a

Wall Street Journal article commented, Geisinger's "...decades of investment in technology and integration have made it a pioneer in the use of electronic medical records and other data."[2] Geisinger is a pioneer in using data-driven management to increase value through standardization and care coordination.

Value-Based Research Centers

A Center for Value-Based Care Research

The Cleveland Clinic supports its own Center for Value-Based Care Research. The center's researchers focus on identifying high-value health care and disseminating this information. That focus is reflected in the center's mission statement: "to make quality healthcare possible for all Americans by conducting research to identify value in healthcare."[3]

A Comparative Effectiveness Research Center

The Brigham and Women's Hospital has established its own Patient-Centered Comparative Effectiveness Research Center. As its name suggests, the center focuses upon comparative effective research and patient-centered outcomes research at the hospital. This center provides value by studying the comparable effectiveness of treatment options for individual patients and the outcomes of healthcare practices. The center's overall approach is to improve the quality of health care.[4]

Value-Based Collaboration and Affiliation

The High Value Healthcare Collaborative

This collaboration actually began in late 2010 with four organizations: the Mayo Clinic, Denver Health, Intermountain Healthcare, and the Dartmouth Institute for Health Policy and Clinical Practice. The group wanted to achieve high value by improving health care and lowering costs. It also wanted to "move best practices out to the national provider community."[5] Since its formation, the collaborative has expanded to almost 20 health systems.

Network Affiliations

The National Comprehensive Cancer Network (NCCN) is a "not-for-profit alliance of 27 of the world's leading cancer centers devoted to patient care, research and education." The NCCN is dedicated to "improving the quality, effectiveness and efficiency of cancer care so that patients can live better lives."[6] Affiliations of this type provide significant value-based benefits in the areas of evidence-based treatment and quality of care.

Value-Based Progress in the Public Sector

The Centers for Medicare and Medicaid Services (CMS) have seven **value-based programs (VBPs):** These programs tie payment to value and are part of an important trend to tie payment to the quality of patient care.[7] These VBPs are important because they show the way toward increasing value. Their structure has provided an important foundation to build upon. In other words, they helped to make today's rapid changes possible.

Three Hospital Value-Based Programs

Hospital Value-Based Purchasing Program

This program provides incentive payments for acute care hospitals. The payment adjustments are based on quality of care and are part of the Inpatient Prospective Payment System (IPPS). In other words, the Hospital Value-Based Purchasing (HVBP) program links payment to performance. The performance measures are adjusted (and typically increased) yearly. CMS has set a timeline for these adjustments that runs out to the year 2022.[8]

Hospital Readmission Reduction Program

The Hospital Readmission Reduction (HRR) program provides incentive payments in order to reduce hospital readmissions, which are costly and may be unnecessary. Reductions may be accomplished in two ways: improving the coordination of transitions of care to other care settings and improving the quality of care provided.[9]

Hospital Acquired Conditions Program

This program reduces payments instead of making incentive payments. In this case, those hospitals whose patients develop the most Hospital-Acquired Conditions (HAC) are penalized (i.e., hospitals that rank worst in HACs have their payments reduced).[10]

Four Other Value-Based Programs

Physician Value-Based Modifier Program

This program for physicians is one of the original value-based programs to be implemented by CMS. The program payments began in 2015 and were paid to ever-expanding groups of physicians over 2016 and 2017. The program expanded to include other clinicians in 2018.

As the title implies, when an eligible claim is submitted, the payment is adjusted, or modified, based on particular quality and cost measures performance. In other words, when the modifier is applied to payment, it rewards physicians for lower costs and/or higher quality. Note that the Physician Value-Based Modifier (PVBM) Program is also known as the **Value Modifier (VM)** Program.[11]

Skilled Nursing Facility Value-Based Program

This program provides incentive payments to skilled nursing facilities (SNFs). The payments reward SNFs based on the quality of care provided.

In other words, payment is received for quality of care, not quantity of care. At the time of this writing, the Skilled Nursing Facility Value-Based Program (SNFVBP) continues to develop. This development is expected to progress in stages.[12] However, the **IMPACT Act** is moving post-acute care facilities (PACs) toward standardization and interoperability. This legislation, which includes SNFs, may affect certain aspects of the SNF value-based program due to standardization efforts.

Home Health Value-Based Program

This program was implemented on January 1, 2016, as a Home Health Value-Based Program (HHVBP) model in nine states. Payment for those participating in the model is based on quality performance. In an interesting concept, the participating home health agencies (HHAs) will compete on value in order to receive quality performance incentive payments. The HHVBP continues to develop and is expected to progress in stages.[13] However, as with SNFs, the HHA value-based program may be impacted by legislative efforts toward standardization and interoperability.

End-Stage Renal Disease Quality Initiative Program

The End-Stage Renal Disease (ESRD) Quality Initiative Program is a disease-specific program. It concerns outpatient dialysis or ESRD facilities and was one of the original programs to be implemented by CMS. This program provides incentive payments for better quality of care and reduces payments to those facilities that do not meet expected standards of performance. In other words, this program links payment to performance.[14]

Value-Based Payments

The traditional method to pay for services is based on the number of services delivered (i.e., volume). CMS is now paying for value and quality and announced two related goals for Medicare fee-for-service payments.

Goal One

"Thirty percent of Medicare payments are tied to quality or value through alternative payment models...by the end of 2016, and 50% [will be] by the end of 2018."[15] Various types of alternative payment models are described elsewhere in this chapter. According to CMS estimates, the 2016 timeline was exceeded.[16]

Goal Two

Eighty-five percent of all traditional Medicare fee-for-service payments have been tied to quality or value by the end of 2016, and 90% will be by the end of 2018. This goal was accomplished through certain CMS programs, including the HVBP and the HRRP.[17] These programs are described elsewhere in this chapter.

Value-Based Legislative Reform

The following summary of legislative progress helps you see the step-by-step progress toward value-based reform.

Initial "Digitizing" Steps

The early efforts toward "digitizing" health care covered a period of several years. One of the more important developments during this time was requiring Medicare providers to submit their claims for payment electronically. We consider this the first real step toward "digitizing," as every CFO wants to get claims paid, and the conversion to electronic claim forms was thus established throughout the country.

HITECH Legislative Funding

The Health Information Technology for Economic and Clinical Health (HITECH) Act was part of the American Recovery and Reinvestment Act that was signed into law on February 17, 2009. The HITECH Act promoted the adoption and use of health information technology (HIT) and **electronic health records (EHRs)** through payment incentives. CMS described these EHR Incentive

Programs in a single sentence: "The Medicare and Medicaid EHR Incentive Programs provide incentive payments to eligible professionals, eligible hospitals and critical access hospitals (CAHs) as they adopt, implement, upgrade or demonstrate **meaningful use** of certified EHR technology."[18]

The HITECH Act's legislative funding provided approximately $17 billion in incentives for hospitals and physicians. This law will impact future healthcare information management for many years to come.

Value-Based Legislative Reform: The MACRA Act

A further legislative reform to the Medicare payment structure is now in place through the Medicare Access and CHIP Reauthorization Act of 2015 (MACRA). This act ends a method of payment to physicians that has been in place since the beginning of the Medicare program in the 1960s.

More Value-Based Legislative Reform: The IMPACT Act

Yet another legislative reform is now in place through the Improving Medicare Post-Acute Care Transformation (IMPACT) Act of 2014. This act requires interoperability between and among the four types of post-acute facilities.

Facts About Physicians and MACRA, MIPS, and APMs

MACRA reforms Medicare payments to physicians and certain clinicians via the following:

- Repealing the Sustainable Growth Rate (SCR) method of payment
- Replacing the SGR method with a new payment framework that emphasizes "giving better care, not just more care"
- Combining existing quality reporting programs into the single new payment framework[19]

For the first two years, the individuals affected by the MACRA Act included physicians, physician assistants, nurse practitioners, clinical nurse specialists, and certified registered nurse anesthetists. Groups that include these eligible professionals are also included. In a second phase (from the third year onward), the secretary can add more eligible professionals such as social workers, certified audiologists, and others.

The MACRA reforms help CMS to move toward the value-based goal of paying for both value and for better care. Physicians and other **eligible professionals (EPs)** can choose one of two quality programs: the **Merit-Based Incentive Payment System (MIPS)** or the **Alternative Payment Models (APMs)**. Both MIPS and APMs will go into effect over a period from mid-2015 through 2021 and beyond.[20]

What Is MIPS?

MIPS is a value-based program combining parts of existing quality reporting programs. The programs involved included the Physician Quality Reporting System (PQRS), the Value Modifier (VM; also known as the Value-Based Payment Modifier) Program, and the Medicare Electronic Health Record (EHR) Incentive Program. These stand-alone programs will be ended when they are combined into the new value-based program.

Physicians and other eligible professionals will be measured in four areas: quality, resource use, meaningful use of certified EHR technology, and clinical practice improvement. The first three areas come from the existing quality reporting programs, but the clinical practice improvement area is new.

The MIPS payment method included an automatic base increase for the period 2015 through 2019, followed by an additional increase applied from 2026 onward. Eligible providers were also at risk for positive or negative performance adjustments to their payments beginning in 2019.

What Are APMs?

APMs provide new methods of payment from Medicare to physicians and other eligible professionals. The MACRA Act considers the following entities to be APMs that are generally eligible for incentive payments:

- CMS Innovation Center Models
- Shared Savings Program Tracks
- Certain statutorily required demonstrations[21]

Specific types of entities within these general categories are then set out annually in a rule published by CMS. These "Advanced APMs" are considered to be advanced because they accept financial risk along with rewards (i.e., the incentive payments).

The APM payment methods include a lump-sum incentive payment for some participating providers for the period 2019 to 2024. In addition, beginning in 2026, some providers can receive higher annual payments. In the future, we can expect increased transparency of such physician-focused payment models (PFPMs) and development of additional PFPMs.

Meaningful Use Is Not Dead but Is Evolving

Meaningful use still exists. At a healthcare conference in the spring of 2016, CMS Acting Administrator Andy Slavitt said that "the meaningful use program, as it has existed, will now be effectively over and will be replaced with something better."[22] However, various media sources reported only that meaningful use was dead, which is incorrect.[23] What Slavitt meant was that meaningful use is being incorporated into the MACRA Act's programs. Thus, meaningful use still exists, but its role has evolved.

Facts About Post-Acute Care and the IMPACT Act

The IMPACT Act of 2014 requires that standardized patient assessment data be reported by four types of post-acute care facilities: SNFs, HHAs, inpatient rehabilitation facilities (IRFs), and long-term care hospitals (LTCHs). Note that hospice, another type of post-acute care facility, is not included in these requirements.

Data Interoperability

The act specifies that "certain data elements must be standardized and interoperable to allow for the exchange and use of data among these PAC and other providers."[24] This will facilitate coordinated care and will "improve the long-term outcomes of beneficiaries receiving post-acute services across different care settings."[25] Standardized data ensure that wording is comparable for purposes of assessment and scoring. Interoperability makes transmitting data across different systems possible.

Transparency and Public Reporting

Transparency and public reporting is another important element in the IMPACT Act. The act stipulates that there must be public reporting of PAC provider performance on both value-based aspects: quality measures and resource use.[26]

Quality Measurement

As one of the two foundations of value-based care, quality must be able to be studied and quantified. The other foundation is cost. Types of quality measures can vary, and developing quality measures is not just the first step in the process but an ongoing project. We hope that, in the future, public–private alignment will become commonplace.

Quality Measures in the Private Sector

The California-Based Integrated Healthcare Association

The Integrated Healthcare Association (IHA), working with health plans and physician organizations, launched a statewide pay-for-performance initiative over 15 years ago. This initiative includes "a common set of measures and benchmarks, health plan incentive payments, public reporting and public recognition awards."[27]

The IHA Value-Based Pay-for-Performance (P4P) program measures quality, cost, and resource use. The program's common measure set is evidence based and includes four major elements:

- Clinical quality
- Patient experience
- Meaningful use of HIT
- Resource use and total cost of care

To put the size of this program into perspective, participation in the Value-Based P4P includes "10 health plans and 200 California physician organizations with 35,000 physicians caring for 9 million Californians enrolled in commercial health maintenance organization (HMO) and point of service (POS) products."[28]

The National Committee for Quality Assurance

The National Committee for Quality Assurance (NCQA) is a not-for-profit organization that accredits health plans and provides annual statistics on the quality of care delivered by these plans. The committee has developed quality standards and performance measures for an array of healthcare organizations.

According to the NCQA website:

- Health plans earning NCQA accreditation at the present time must address an array of more than 60 standards and report on their performance in over 40 areas.
- Health plans are accredited in every state, the District of Columbia, and Puerto Rico.
- These plans cover 109 million Americans or 70.5% of all Americans in health plans.[29]

Quality Measures in the Public Sector

Value and quality are often intertwined when discussing value-based efforts. Certain quality measures have already been established for specific providers. These measures must first be recorded by the provider and then reported to CMS. CMS quality reporting programs include:

- Hospital Inpatient Quality Reporting (HIQR) Program
- Hospital Outpatient Quality Reporting (HOQR) Program
- Physician Quality Reporting System (PQRS)
- Long-Term Care Hospital (LTCH) Quality Reporting Program (QRP)
- Inpatient Rehabilitation Facility (IRF) Quality Reporting Program (QRP)

- Home Health Quality Reporting Program (HHQRP)
- Hospice Quality Reporting Program (HQRP)[30]

Upgrading efforts are ongoing for these programs to provide greater transparency and ease of access.

Challenges in Quality Measure Implementation

CMS has identified a number of challenges in quality measure implementation that can be divided into three areas:

- Issues related to patients and providers including engaging patients in the measure development process and reducing provider burden
- Issues related to shortening and streamlining processes including shortening the period for measure development and streamlining data acquisition for measure testing
- Issues related to development including developing meaningful outcome measures, patient-reported outcome measures (PROMS) and appropriate use measures, and measures that promote shared accountability across settings and providers.[31]

Challenges for the Manager

Managers must deal with a variety of issues related to quality measures. Managers face problems and challenges in both the development and implementation of quality measures. By their very nature such measures are metrics and will require digital changes involving:

- Hardware
- Software
- Training
- Staff stability and related turnover
- Reporting

To succeed, managers involved in measure development and implementation need support from the highest levels within the organization including funding for digital infrastructure and staffing.

Value-Based Public Reporting in the Private Sector

Sharing information about quality reporting programs with the public is vital in value-based efforts. In this section, we discuss three different types of value-based public reporting.

Public Reporting Approaches by Providers and Health Plans

Annual Reporting of Program Results

The California-based Integrated Healthcare Association (IHA), in association with the California Office of the Patient Advocate (OPA), publicly reports value-based pay-for-performance results each year. These reports allow comparison between and among various health plans and providers. The intent is to "allow health care purchasers and consumers to make informed decisions about providers based on value."[32] Other reporting efforts by this partnership include reports on total cost of care by physician organizations and the Medical Group Medicare Report Card focusing on "medical groups caring for seniors and people with disabilities enrolled in Medicare Advantage health plans."[33] In addition, each year the IHA recognizes top-performing and most-improved physician organizations. Another IHA public recognition effort is the Excellence in Healthcare Award.[34]

An Overview of Annual Facts and Statistics

Websites containing an overview allow the viewer to acquire specific information on items of interest including value-based efforts. For example, Cleveland Clinic publishes an annual year-end "Facts + Figures" report. The two-page report provides a snapshot of the organization including their mission, vision, and values and a section titled "Quality, Safety, Transparency." This section mentions Quality and Patient Safety accountability that oversees improvement in quality and safety and emphasizes a "relentless focus on monitoring, recording and reporting quality and safety data."[35]

Public Reporting of Quality and Value by Other Organizations

A variety of other organizations also provide public reporting of quality and associated value. They include, among others, the National Quality Forum, the National Committee for Quality Assurance, the Leapfrog Group for Patient Safety, the Informed Patient Institute, and the Commonwealth Fund.[36]

Public Reporting of Physician Credentials and Experience

Another type of public reporting that websites provide is background information on physician groups and on individual doctors. To experiment, we typed our own GP's name into Google, and seven websites came up that contained his credentials and experience. These sites provide value-based information as they provide information on their healthcare professional including specialties, experience, and credentials. You can find whether physicians have any sanctions, malpractice suits, or board actions against them. These sites may also report the results of patient satisfaction surveys or reviews and provide comparative ratings.

Value-Based Public Reporting in the Public Sector

National Reporting Examples

Value-based quality measurement can be readily linked to public reporting. You may be familiar with one of the CMS "Compare" websites that publishes these quality measures. A brief description of four "Compare" sites follows.

Hospital Compare

The Hospital Compare website contains information about quality of care for over 4,000 hospitals in the United States.[37] The site contains a profile of each hospital. Besides general facility information and certain other measures that are reported, the particular measure of interest to us is "Payment and Value of Care."[38] This value-based measure is in three parts: "Medicare spending per beneficiary," "Payment measures," and "Value of care." The "Value of care" part is a combination of payment measures and quality-of-care measures.[39]

Physician Compare

At the time of writing, group practices are present on the "Physician Compare" CMS website. There are plans to add individual physicians and other healthcare professionals in the future. Note that the site only includes physicians enrolled in the Medicare program.[40] The site contains a profile of each physician, including specialties, board certification, medical school and residency, and other information.[41]

If the physician or group practice participates in one or more of the four quality activities, there is a green check mark on the profile page. The site is careful to say that "participation alone does not mean quality care has been achieved. Showing a commitment to quality is the first step in achieving quality care."[42]

Nursing Home Compare

According to CMS, the Nursing Home Compare website contains information about the quality of care and staffing for the 15,000-plus nursing homes in the United States that are Medicare and Medicaid participating.[43] The site provides a five-star quality rating covering quality measures, staffing, and health inspections. Each of these elements is given an individual rating, and the three ratings are then combined to create an overall rating. The star rating ranges from 1 to 5 with 1

being the lowest and 5 the highest score.[44] The site points out that there can be variation among states due to differences in their inspection processes and Medicaid programs. Thus, it is best to compare facilities within a single state.[45]

Home Health Compare

The Home Health Compare website contains information about the quality of care provided by home health agencies throughout the United States that are Medicare certified.[46] The site contains a profile of each agency, including type of ownership and services offered. The items of interest to us include information about quality measures and the "quality of patient care star rating."[47] The star rating ranges from 1 to 5, with 1 being the lowest and 5 the highest score. Scores are based on the performance of a particular home health agency relative to other agencies.[48]

A State Reporting Example

According to *Health Affairs*, just about half of the states in the United States have created some type of public reporting program.[49] As you might suspect, the content of these programs varies state by state. For example, the Utah Department of Health provides a Public Health Outcome Measures Report (PHOM) that includes 109 public health measures in an online format that is easy to use to "promote an understanding of the health status of the Utah population."[50] These measures, or indicators, are taken from another of Utah's websites, "Indicator-Based Information System for Public Health (IBIS-PH)," which contains more detail.

Financial Outcomes

Intermountain Health (IH) provides an example of documented positive financial outcomes as follows. IH is a Utah-based not-for-profit health system with 22 hospitals and 185 clinics in the Intermountain Medical Group, along with health insurance plans from SelectHealth. Intermountain piloted an integration of mental health with primary care a number of years ago. Every primary care patient at the Intermountain Medical Group clinics receives this screening, whether or not they are members of Intermountain's health plan. This value-based coordinated care model has improved outcomes for patients. Furthermore, Intermountain's financial outcomes are positive. Cost per member was $22 higher up front, but annual per-member cost was $115 lower. The overall lower cost was attributed to fewer emergency room visits and other care.[51]

Financial Outcomes as a Value-Based Business Model

The *Harvard Business Review* has published an article titled "Turning Value-Based Health Care into a Real Business Model."[52] The authors begin by saying the shift from volume-based health care to value-based health care is inevitable. While they discuss benefits in patient care, they also point out that short-term financial losses may be part of the shift to a value-based approach. In some cases, the short-term loss may be offset by a long-term gain. The preceding Intermountain example is one of those cases.

The authors conclude that organizations' short-term financial losses were strategic to obtain longer-term benefits in risk management, collaboration, and competitive advantage. Risk management is an integral part of many pay-for-performance alternative payment models, and gaining experience is valuable. Collaboration and alignment with stakeholders and physicians takes time and becomes even more important in moving toward a population-health approach. Competitive advantage is also gained because the organization has already embraced and adapted to a value-based financial approach (the business model) while other organizations are left behind.

Large Interactive Systems Require Investment Dollars

Large healthcare systems need large electronic health record systems that require substantial investments. In this section, we discuss two examples.

Duke University Health System's Investment

North Carolina–based Duke University Health System (Duke) includes three hospitals along with physician practices, home care, hospice care, and support services.[53] In July 2012, Duke began a multiyear information system project to unify electronic medical records across the health system. The new technology was to be implemented in three phases, from mid-2012 to spring 2014.[54] As of spring 2014, the system was operational in all three hospitals and 223 outpatient facilities.[55]

The investment in this project was reported to be $500 million. However, when the Duke chief medical information officer discussed the financial issues, he acknowledged $500 million as the gross cost but said the net cost was approximately $300 million. The $500 million figure represented total ownership costs over a seven-year period. The amount included the cost to maintain and upgrade the system over seven years in addition to the initial costs to acquire and begin to use the technology. If you add up all the costs to maintain and support the 135 existing applications that were being replaced and subtract that cost from the $500 million, you wind up with a net new investment that is "a little bit more than $300 million."[56] Finally, the project should have been eligible to receive tens of millions of dollars in federal funding that would partially cover the costs of the investment.[57]

Kaiser Permanente's Investment

California-based Kaiser Permanente (KP) is a non-profit integrated health plan that includes 38 hospitals and over 600 medical office buildings and other facilities located in eight states plus the District of Columbia. The plan serves almost 10 million people.[58] KP claims that HealthConnect, the plan's comprehensive electronic record, is "one of the largest private electronic health systems in the world."[59] It took 10 years to build and became fully operational in 2010.[60]

InfoWorld interviewed Philip Fasano, the chief information officer of KP, about the plan's EHR systems. The interviewer asked how much it cost to build the system, to which Fasano replied, "About $4 billion, a substantial amount of money, but we have 9 million members [so it costs about $444 per member]."[61] The CIO went on to make another important point: that it is necessary to continuously invest in the system during its lifetime.

Digital Outcomes

Value-based alternative payment models rely upon an array of performance measures that are reported electronically. The electronic submissions represent the record of the provider's performance. Thus, appropriate data collection and submission represents the positive digital outcome that should result in payment advantages.

For example, physicians and other eligible professionals are in the midst of transition to value-based payment models due to MACRA. This transition relies heavily upon electronic submission of performance data. Specifically, the eligible professionals (EPs) who use certified EHRs and/or qualified clinical data registries (QCDRs) should benefit from reduced data collection and reporting burdens and timely performance feedback. **Figure 27.1** illustrates these points.

Value-Based Digital Outcome Examples in Large Healthcare Systems

Duke University Health System

Duke University Health System's information system project cost was discussed in the preceding investment section. In this section, we discuss the project's digital outcomes. The information system project's purpose was to unify electronic medical records across the system. It accomplished this purpose. Value-based outcomes include medical record access that is seamless and real time. Medical information can now be exchanged across all care settings. As the Duke press release states, quality, safety, speed, and efficiency have all been improved with implementation of the new system. In addition, 130 old clinical information systems became obsolete and were eliminated when the new system went online.[62]

The patient experience has been improved via the system's new online tool, "Duke MyChart." The patient can, among other features, view and/or request appointments, view their medical reports, request prescription refills, and send messages to healthcare providers.[63]

Finally, the organization's commitment to the project is underscored by another statistic. Duke provided 173,000 hours of training to faculty and staff to ensure a smooth transition to the new system. The press release reported that neither patient care nor patient billing was significantly

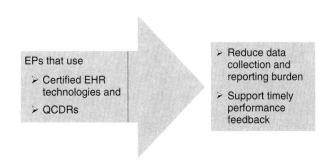

Figure 27.1 MACRA Electronic Specifications Provide Benefits

disrupted during the implementation process of this value-based system.[64]

Kaiser Permanente

The cost of KP's "HealthConnect" project was also discussed in the investment section. In this section, we discuss its digital outcomes. KP covers the spectrum of care, as it is both a health plan (payer) and provider of care and has amassed a huge amount of electronic data that it uses for value-based purposes. For example, HealthConnect is part of KP's online portal called "My Health Manager." This portal allows patients online access to such features as appointment scheduling, refills of prescriptions, messages to care providers, and so on. However, another valuable feature, called the online Patient Action Plan (oPAP), is also available. This web-based system focuses on preventive care that is personalized for the individual patient in a health action plan. Researchers who studied the use of this patient-enabled health management tool found improved patient outcomes for preventive care.[65]

Clinicians also benefit from KP HealthConnect features. They have access to information about latest treatments and preventive care. In one pilot project, this access to information helped physicians reduce coronary artery disease death by 76%.[66]

Electronic Transmission Standards Must Be Updated and Maintained

Electronic transmission standards are important because they directly impact providers, health plans, and other stakeholders. These standards are coordinated with and are the beginning point for certified EHR technology. Both financial and digital outcomes depend upon such technology. Specific versions of the standards are acceptable for certified EHR technology at different points in time. As such, it is imperative that the related standards are updated and maintained at all times.

Value-Based Strategic Planning by the Private Sector

Recognizing That Value-Based Care Is a Long-Term Goal

The Cleveland Clinic has integrated the value-based concept throughout its organization, including research, education, and care delivery. Dr. Tony Cosgrove, president and CEO of Cleveland Clinic, has written that value-based health care is a "breakthrough that will change the face of medicine" and "whether providers like it or not, healthcare is evolving from a proficiency-based art to a data-driven science."[67] One of the Cleveland Clinic's web pages summarizes the organization's strategic positioning as "the ideal result is fewer readmissions, less frequent hospitalization and trips to the ER. Value-based care is a long-term goal."[68]

Taking a Patient-Centered View of Value

At the Mayo Clinic, it seems obvious that the Office of Value Creation must play an important role in value-based strategic planning. However, this office does not operate within a silo. One of the "Quality at Mayo Clinic Update: How the Mayo Value Creation System Is Improving Patient Care" publications a few years says the organization was working to define value with the Office of Value Creation, the Value Program in the Center for the Science of Healthcare Delivery, Government Affairs, and Contracting all working together toward this end. Strategically speaking, "at this point, we are trying to take a patient-centered view of value at the levels of the care pyramid."[69] Their concept at that point in time was a care "pyramid" consisting of complex care, intermediate care, and population health with value definitions and detail for each level.

Value-Based Strategic Planning by the Public Sector

A "national quality strategy" exists and guides planning throughout the U.S. Department of Health and Human Services (DHHS). The value-based and quality programs that are discussed within this chapter are an important part of CMS planning. As CMS is a part of DHHS, these value-based and quality issues are tied into national quality strategy.

National Quality Strategy

The National Quality Strategy (NQS) is led by the Agency for Healthcare Research and Quality (AHRQ) on behalf of the U.S. DHHS,[70] and its three aims are:

- Better care
- Healthy people/healthy communities
- Affordable care[71]

The six NQS priorities and how they interrelate to the CMS quality strategy are discussed in the following section.

Nine Strategic Levers

The NQS created nine "levers" defining core business functions, resources, and/or actions which may be activated to meet quality goals, these strategic elements are:

- Measurement and feedback
- Payment
- Health information technology
- Innovation and diffusion
- Public reporting
- Learning and technical assistance
- Certification, accreditation, and regulation
- Consumer incentives and benefit designs
- Workforce development

The agency has included a phrase for each lever to better describe how the levers work should work. **Table 27.1** illustrates the appropriate phrase for each of the nine levers.[72] The levers are important because they show how all aspects

Table 27.1 How the Strategic Levers Should Work

The Lever	How It Should Work
Measurement and Feedback	Provide performance feedback to plans and providers to improve care
Payment	Reward and incentivize providers to deliver high-quality, patient-centered care
Health Information Technology	Improve communication, transparency, and efficiency for better coordinated health and health care
Innovation and Diffusion	Foster innovation in healthcare quality improvement and facilitate rapid adoption within and across organizations and communities
Public Reporting	Compare treatment results, costs, and patient experience for consumers
Learning and Technical Assistance	Foster learning environments that offer training, resources, tools, and guidance to help organizations achieve quality improvement goals
Certification, Accreditation, and Regulation	Adopt or adhere to approaches to meet safety and quality standards
Consumer Incentives and Benefit Designs	Help consumers adopt health behaviors and make informed decisions
Workforce Development	Investing in people to prepare the next generation of healthcare professionals and support lifelong learning for providers

of value-based and quality programs fit into the national strategic plan. One or more of these nine levers is included in the private and public sector value-based efforts discussed within this chapter.

How Do CMS Quality Strategy and Goals Fit into the National Strategy?

CMS quality strategy coordinates with the national quality strategy's priorities. In other words, the CMS strategy fits into the national strategy because CMS has adopted the NQS priorities as the six CMS goals. A description of this sequence follows.

National Quality Strategy Priorities Are Converted into Domains

To implement these priorities, the priorities are converted into six domains, as described in the CMS Quality Strategy:[73]

- Efficiency and Cost Reduction Domain
- Care Coordination Domain
- Clinical Quality of Care Domain
- Safety Domain
- Person and Caregiver Centered Experience and Outcomes Domain
- Population and Community Health Domain

Detail for each domain is contained in **Table 27.2**.

Strategic Goals for Quality

Linking National and CMS Strategies

CMS has adopted the domains just described as its "framework for measurement" to take this coordination a step further. This methodology is important because it links NQS strategy—and resulting domains—directly and efficiently to CMS strategic goals and their measurement. Thus, each National Quality Priority Domain just described is linked to a specific CMS Quality Strategy Goal. In other words, six domains equal six CMS goals, details for each goal are reported in **Table 27.3**.

Table 27.2 National Quality Domains and Measures

National Priority Domains	Measures
Efficiency & Cost Reduction	Cost Efficiency Appropriateness
Care Coordination	Patient and family activation Infrastructure and processes for care coordination Impact of care coordination
Clinical Quality of Care	Care type (preventive, acute, post-acute, chronic) Conditions Subpopulations
Safety	All-cause harm Hospital acquired conditions (HAC) Hospital acquired infections (HAI) Unnecessary care Medication safety
Person and Caregiver Centered Experience and Outcomes	Patient experience Caregiver experience Preference and goal-oriented care
Population and Community Health	Health behaviors Access Physical and social environment Health status

Table 27.3 National Quality Strategy Domain Links to CMS Quality Strategy Goals

National Priority Domains	CMS Goals
Efficiency & Cost Reduction	Make care affordable
Care Coordination	Promote effective communication & coordination of care
Clinical Quality of Care	Promote effective prevention & treatment of chronic disease
Safety	Make care safer by reducing harm caused while care is delivered
Person and Caregiver Centered Experience and Outcomes	Help patients & their families be involved as partners in their care
Population and Community Health	Work with communities to help people live healthily

WRAP-UP

Summary

This chapter provides an overview of NQS Priorities and Domains and how these domains are linked to CMS goals. Future legislative and regulatory changes will certainly occur. Some are predictable at this time; others are not. We cannot reasonably predict the direction that multiple value-based alternative payment models may take. Likewise, we cannot predict the outcome over the next few years of the current multiple challenges to other aspects of healthcare legislation. One thing is clear: If an organization is to meet its value-based goals, leadership support and encouragement is essential. This quote sums it up very well: "[T]he investment required is as much in leadership as in dollars."[74]

In conclusion, we expect interpretations of the various value-based and health information technology strategic priorities, along with their supporting rules and regulations, to emerge over a considerable period of years. A formidable base of knowledge has been laid as a foundation for these directions. One official was reported to have said we were now on the "glide path" to success in the area of health information technology, meaning that the sailing (or flying) would be smooth from now on. We hope he is correct.

Key Terms

Alternative Payment Model (APM)
Electronic Health Record (EHR)

Eligible Professional (EP)
IMPACT Act
MACRA
Meaningful Use (MU)

Merit-Based Incentive Payment System (MIPS)
Value-Based Program (VBP)
Value Modifier (VM)

Discussion Questions

1. Using your organization as a point of reference, how would you define "value-based care"?
2. If senior management appointed you to chair a committee to adopt "value-based care," whom would you want on your committee?
3. How would you describe a patient-centered view of value?

4. Identify the essential elements of a National Quality Strategy and describe how they are interrelated.

5. Describe key legislative reforms to the Medicare payment structure.

6. Why are value-based digital outcomes important for healthcare providers?

Notes

1. Mayo Clinic, "Quality at Mayo Clinic: 2013 Update: How the Mayo Value Creation System Is Improving Patient Care," http://www.mayo.edu/pmts/mc6300-mc6399/mc6312-33.pdf, accessed April 14, 2016.
2. C. Weaver, "A Health-Care Model in Coal Country," *The Wall Street Journal*, September 27, 2015.
3. Cleveland Clinic, "Center for Value-Based Care Research," https://my.clevelandclinic.org/services/medicine-institute/research/Center-for-Value-Based-Care-Research, accessed April 14, 2016.
4. Brigham and Women's Hospital, "Patient-Centered Comparative Effectiveness Research Center," http://www.brighamandwomens.org/research/centers/pcerc/default.aspx, accessed April 14, 2016.
5. Dartmouth-Hitchcock, "Our Collaborations," http://www.dartmouth-hitchcock.org/about_dh/what_is_population_health.html, accessed April 14, 2016.
6. National Comprehensive Cancer Network, "About NCCN," http://www.nccn.org/about/default.aspx, accessed April 14, 2016.
7. CMS, "CMS' Value-Based Programs," https://www.cms.gov/Medicare/Quality-Initiatives-Patient-Assessment-Instruments/Value-Based-Programs/Value-Based-Programs.html.
8. CMS, "Hospital Value-Based Purchasing," https://www.cms.gov/Medicare/Quality-Initiatives-Patient-Assessment-Instruments/hospital-value-based-purchasing/index.html?redirect=/Hospital-Value-Based-Purchasing/, accessed October 30, 2015.
9. CMS, "Readmissions Reduction Program (HRRP)," https://www.cms.gov/medicare/medicare-fee-for-service-payment/acuteinpatientpps/readmissions-reduction-program.html, accessed April 18, 2016.
10. CMS, "Hospital-Acquired Condition (HAC) Reduction Program," http://www.cms.gov/Medicare/Quality-Initiatives-Patient-Assessment-Instruments/Value-Based-Programs/HAC/Hospital-Acquired-Conditions.
11. CMS, "The Value Modifier (VM) Program," https://www.cms.gov/Medicare/Quality-Initiatives-Patient-Assessment-Instruments/Value-Based-Programs/VMP/Value-Modifier-VM-or-PVBM.html.
12. CMS, "The Skilled Nursing Facility Value-Based Purchasing Program (SNFVBP)," https://www.cms.gov/Medicare/Quality-Initiatives-Patient-Assessment-Instruments/Value-Based-Programs/Other-VBPs/SNF-VBP.html.
13. CMS, "The Home Health Value-Based Purchasing (HHVBP) Model," https://www.cms.gov/Medicare/Quality-Initiatives-Patient-Assessment-Instruments/Value-Based-Programs/Other-VBPs/HHVBP.html.
14. CMS, "End-Stage Renal Disease (ESRD) Quality Incentive Program (QIP)," https://www.cms.gov/Medicare/Quality-Initiatives-Patient-Assessment-Instruments/Value-Based-Programs/Other-VBPs/ESRD-QIP.html.
15. CMS, "What Are the Value-Based Programs?," http://www.cms.gov/Medicare/Quality-Initiatives-Patient-Assessment-Instruments/Value-Based-Programs/MACRA-MIPS-and-APMs.
16. U.S. Department of Health and Human Services, "HHS Reaches Goal of Tying 30 Percent of Medicare Payments to Quality Ahead of Schedule," http://www.hhs.gov/about/news/2016/03/03/hhs-reaches-goal-tying-30-percent-medicare-payments-quality-ahead-schedule.html, accessed March 2016.
17. Ibid.
18. CMS, "EHR Incentive Programs: Getting Started," http://www.cms.gov/Regulations-and-Guidance/Legislation/EHRIncentivePrograms/Getting-Started.html.
19. CMS, "What Are the Value-Based Programs?"
20. Ibid.
21. P.L. 114-10 (April 16, 2015) 129 STAT 121.
22. B. Ahier, "Meaningful Use Isn't Quite Dead Yet," http://www.healthdatamanagement.com/opinion/meaningful-use-isnt-quite-dead-yet, accessed March 1, 2016.
23. Ibid.
24. CMS, "IMPACT Act Spotlights and Announcements," https://www.cms.gov/Medicare/Quality-Initiatives-Patient-Assessment-Instruments/Post-Acute-Care-Quality-Initiatives/IMPACT-Act-of-2014/Spotlights-and-Announcements-.html, accessed August 31, 2016.
25. Ibid.
26. P.L. 113-185 Sec. 2(g)(1) (October 6, 2014).
27. Integrated Healthcare Association, "Fact Sheet: Value Based Pay for Performance in California," http://www.iha.org/sites/default/files/resources/vbp4-fact-sheet-final-20150925.pdf, accessed September 2015.
28. Ibid.
29. National Committee for Quality Assurance, "About NCQA," http://www.ncqa.org/about-ncqa, accessed May 18, 2016.
30. 80 Federal Register (FR) 22067 (April 20, 2015).
31. Adapted from CMS, "CMS Quality Measure Development Plan (MDP)," accessed December 18, 2015, page 8.
32. Integrated Healthcare Association, "Fact Sheet: Total Cost of Care," http://www.iha.org/sites/default/files/resources/fact-sheet-total-cost-of-care-2015.pdf, accessed April 2015.

33. Integrated Healthcare Association, "Results and Public Reporting," http://www.iha.org/our-work/accountability/value-based-p4p/results-public-reporting, accessed May 9, 2016.

34. Integrated Healthcare Association, "Fact Sheet: Total Cost of Care."

35. Cleveland Clinic, "Facts + Figures: 2015 Year-End," https://newsroom.clevelandclinic.org/wp-content/uploads/sites/4/2016/4/16-CCC-332-Facts-and-Figures_04.01.2016.pdf, accessed March 16, 2016.

36. Health Affairs, "Health Policy Briefs: Public Reporting on Quality and Costs," http://www.healthaffairs.org/healthpolicybriefs/brief.php?brief_id=65, accessed March 8, 2012.

37. Medicare.gov, "What Is Hospital Compare?," http://www.medicare.gov/hospitalcompare/About/What-Is-HOS.html, accessed May 10, 2016.

38. Medicare.gov, "What Information Can I Get About Hospitals?," http://www.medicare.gov/hospitalcompare/About/Hospital-Info.html, accessed May 10, 2016.

39. Ibid.

40. Medicare.gov, "About Physician Compare," http://www.medicare.gov/physiciancompare/staticpages/aboutphysiciancompare/about.html, accessed May 10, 2016.

41. Medicare.gov, "Information Available on Physician Compare," http://www.medicare.gov/physiciancompare/staticpages/aboutphysiciancompare/information available, accessed May 10, 2016.

42. Medicare.gov, "About the Data," http://www.medicare.gov/physiciancompare/staticpages/data/aboutthedata.html, accessed May 10, 2016.

43. Medicae.gov, "What Is Nursing Home Compare?," http://www.medicare.gov/nursinghomecompare/About/What-Is-NHC.html, accessed May 10, 2016.

44. Medicare.gov, "What Are the 5-Star Quality Ratings?," http://www.medicare.gov/NursingHomeCompare/About/Ratings.html, accessed May 10, 2016.

45. Medicare.gov, "Strengths and Limitations," http://www.medicare.gov/NursingHomeCompare/About/Strengths-and-Limitations.html, accessed May 10, 2016.

46. Medicare.gov, "What Is Home Health Compare?," http://www.medicare.gov/homehealthcompare/About/What-Is-HHC.html, accessed May 10, 2016.

47. Medicare.gov, "What Information Can I Get About Home Health Agencies?," http://www.medicare.gov/HomeHealthCompare/About/What-Information-Is-Available.html, accessed May 10, 2016.

48. Medicare.gov, "Quality of Patient Care Star Ratings," http://www.medicare.gov/HomeHealthCompare/About/Patient-Care-Star-Ratings.html, accessed May 10, 2016.

49. Health Affairs, "Health Policy Briefs: Public Reporting on Quality and Costs," http://www.healthaffairs.org/healthpolicybriefs/brief.php?brief_id=65, accessed March 8, 2012.

50. Utah Department of Health, "Public Health Outcome Measures Report," http://ibis.health.utah.gov/phom/Introduction.html, accessed April 2014.

51. L. S. Kaiser and T. H. Lee, "Turning Value-Based Health Care into a Real Business Model," https://hbr.org/2015/10/turning-value-based-health-care-into-a-real-business-model, accessed October 8, 2015.

52. Ibid.

53. Duke University Health System, "Duke Human Resources: About Duke University Health System," https://www.hr.duke.edu/jobs/duke_durham/duhs.php, accessed May 10, 2016.

54. Duke University Health System, "Duke Starts to Transfer to Digital Electronic Health Records," http://www.wral.com/lifestyles/goaskmom/blogpost/11364264/?comment_order=forward, accessed September 17, 2016.

55. Duke University Health System, "Duke Medicine Completes Implementation of Electronic Health Records Across All Outpatient Facilities and Duke University Hospital," http://corporate.dukemedicine.org/news_and_publications/news_office/news/duke-medicine-completes-implementation-of-electronic-health-records-across-all-outpatient-facilities-and-duke-university-hospital/view, accessed May 18, 2016.

56. D. Ranii, "Duke Kicks Off Digital Health Records Plan," http://www.ecu.edu/cs-admin/news/clips/upload/071812.pdf, accessed September 17, 2016.

57. Ibid.

58. Kaiser Permanente, "Who We Are," http://www.kaiserpermanentejobs.org/who-we-are.aspx, accessed May 19, 2016.

59. Kaiser Permanente, "About Us: Connectivity," https://share.kaiserpermanente.org/total-health/connectivity/, accessed May 19, 2016.

60. InfoWorld, "How Kaiser Bet $4 Billion On Electronic Health Records—And Won," http://www.infoworld.com/article/2614353/ehr/how-kaiser-bet--4-billion-on-electronic-health-records----and-won.html, accessed May 2, 2013.

61. Ibid.

62. Duke University Health System, "Duke Medicine Completes Implementation."

63. Duke University Health System, "Duke's New Medical Records System Improves Patient Experience," http://corporate.dukemedicine.org/news_and_publications/news_office/news/duke-s-new-medical-records-system-improves-patient-abilities-and-access-to-providers, accessed May 19, 2016.

64. Duke University Health System, "Duke Medicine Completes Implementation."

65. Kaiser Permanente, "Patient Access to Online Health Action Plans Enhances Rate of Preventive Care," https://share.kaiserpermanente.org/article/patient-access-to-online-health-action-plans-enhances-rate-of-preventive-care/, accessed May 19, 2016.

66. Kaiser Permanente, "About Us: Connectivity."

67. Z. Budryk, "How Value-Based Care Will Change Healthcare," http://www.fiercehealthcare.com/healthcare/how-value-based-care-will-change-healthcare/, accessed September 26, 2013.

68. Cleveland Clinic, "Diseases and Conditions: Value-Based Care."

69. Mayo Clinic, "Quality at Mayo Clinic."

70. U.S. Department of Health and Human Services, "The National Quality Strategy: Fact Sheet," http://www.ahrq.gov/workingforquality/nqs/nqsfactsheet.htm, accessed September 2014.

71. Ibid.

72. Ibid.

73. 80 FR 68667 (November 5, 2015).

74. Kaiser and Lee, "Turning Value-Based Health Care into a Real Business Model."

CHAPTER 28

New Payment Methods: MIPS and APM

PROGRESS NOTES

After completing this chapter, you should be able to:

1. Distinguish between the two pay-for-performance choices in the Quality Payment Program.
2. Identify the four MIPS performance categories.
3. Describe how the MIPS Composite Performance Score uses weighted averages.
4. Identify the Advanced APM "significant participation" requirements.
5. Understand the Scoring Standards for APM.
6. Discuss the framework for MACRA Quality Measurement.

Overview: Physician Payment Methods

This chapter explores how new payment methods and quality measures work for physicians and other **eligible professionals (EPs)**. The chapter has several parts, and each part contributes to an understanding of the choices among MIPS, APM, and the related measures that determine payment. The topics include:

- Overview of MACRA and the payment choices
- Choice 1 MIPS incentives: how MIPS is structured, who is eligible for MIPS, and facts about payment and reporting
- Details of the MIPS scoring process and how the scores become payment adjustments for the individual practitioner

- Details about the MIPS performance categories, how the related quality measures are created, and their timelines
- Choice 2 APM incentives: how APM is structured, the various APM models, and facts about payment and reporting
- Details about the Advanced APM participation requirements and scoring standards

Two reference sections are included: one for the three incentive programs as they existed before MIPS and one for existing alternative payment models. This chapter should be read in conjunction with the preceding chapter, "Value-Based Health Care and Its Financial and Digital Outcomes." While this chapter describes how MIPS and APM work, the preceding chapter provides a view of the healthcare industry's overall value-based effort, along with the legislative sequence that came before the MACRA requirements.

Legislative Reform and MACRA: An Overview

The **Medicare Access and CHIP Reauthorization Act of 2015 (MACRA)** was signed into law on April 16, 2015. This chapter reviews the MIPS and APM pay-for-performance programs for physicians and other eligible professionals in Title I.[1]

Repealing the Sustainable Growth Rate

Repeal of the **Sustainable Growth Rate (SGR)** was a true legislative reform, and the history of SGR explains why reform was necessary. The SGR was a formula used to calculate Medicare payments to physicians. Each year, the formula compared increases or decreases in physician spending to increases or decreases in the gross domestic product (GDP). Theoretically, if the increase in GDP exceeded the increase in physician spending, physicians' base rate payment would increase. However, in the real world, the increase in physicians' spending exceeded the increase in GDP, so the base rate payment should have decreased.

An abbreviated SGR timeline looks like this:

1997: The SGR formula came into existence.

2002: The formula results in a 4.8% reduction in the Medicare base payment rate (a wake-up call).

2003: A law blocking the formula's payment reductions was passed.

2004–2005: Congress passes annual "fixes" that disregard the required payment reductions.

2006: Another law was passed that made the annual reductions cumulative.

2009–2010: Congress passes annual "fixes" that disregard the cumulative reduction.

2015: The SGR formula is repealed by law.[2]

The problem with the cumulative annual reduction was the potential excessive cut in payment rates. For example, if last year's blocked cut was 4% and this year's is 5%, then the cumulative reduction of 9% was required, and so on, year after year. The SGR formula was unsustainable. Repealing and replacing the SGR formula with a different approach to physician payment, such as MACRA, is true legislative reform.

New Pay-for-Performance Incentives

MACRA provided new physician pay-for-performance incentives to replace the repealed SGR formula. Providers have a choice of two systems. The first is the **Merit-Based Incentive Payment System (MIPS)**, and the second provides incentive payments when requirements are met to be a qualifying participant in an Advanced **Alternative Payment Model (APM)**.[3] The two payment methods and their related performance measures and/or requirements are described in the following sections.[4]

The new name for this overall payment approach is the Quality Payment Program. Eligible professionals must generally opt for one of the two choices. **Figure 28.1** illustrates the two choices. Note that the start date ("Year 1") for both MIPS and APM incentive payments was 2019.

MIPS—Choice 1

The MIPS payment structure consists of modified inputs from three existing programs plus one new category. The three existing incentive programs whose modified measures were combined into MIPS inputs are described next. The fourth, new category is called "Clinical Practice Improvement Activities." **Figure 28.2** illustrates the four elements that provide inputs for the MIPS payment structure as of 2019.

Three Existing Incentive Programs Combined into MIPS

Many modified features of three existing incentive programs are combined into MIPS. They include

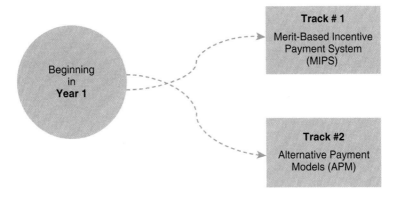

Figure 28.1 Pay-for-Performance Incentive Options

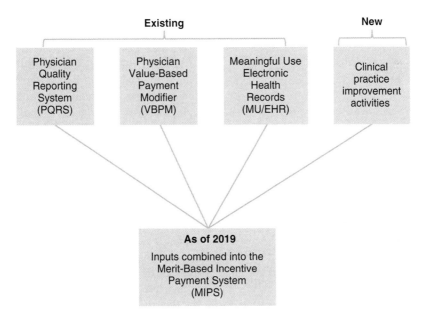

Figure 28.2 Four Pay-for-Performance Inputs Combined into MIPS

the **Physician Quality Reporting System (PQRS) Program**, the **Value Modifier (VM) Program**, and the **Meaningful Use and Electronic Health Records (MU/EHR) Initiative**.

Eligible Professionals for MIPS

This section describes eligible professionals both included and excluded from MIPS. Note the Centers for Medicare and Medicaid Services (CMS) has chosen to use the term **eligible clinicians**

instead of *eligible professionals*. The description that follows uses the term *eligible professionals*.

Eligible Professionals Categories Subject to MIPS Will Increase

Five categories of **eligible professionals (EPs)** were subject to MIPS for the first two payment years. As of the third year, however, the HHS secretary has the right to add other types of eligible professionals, and eight more professional categories have been suggested for addition in the third year.

Exhibit 28.1 **MIPS Eligible Professionals Inclusion Varies by Time**

Years 1 and 2 (2019 and 2020)*

- Physician
- Physician assistant
- Nurse practitioner
- Clinical nurse specialist
- Certified registered nurse anesthetist
- Groups that include such professionals

Third Year Onward (2021)*

- Physical therapists
- Occupational therapists
- Certified audiologists
- Clinical psychologists
- Speech-language pathologists
- Clinical social workers
- Nurse midwives
- Dietitians or nutrition professionals

*Time may change.

Reproduced from SSA Section 1848 (g)(1)(c)(i).

Exhibit 28.2 **Professionals Who May Be Excluded from MIPS**

- A qualifying APM participant
- A partial qualifying APM participant
- Below the low-volume threshold for the performance period
- In the first year of Medicare participation

Reproduced from SSA Section 1848 (g)(1)(c)(ii).

Exhibit 28.1 lists the five EP types included in years 1 and 2, plus the eight types that were suggested for year 3.

Who May Be Excluded from MIPS?

As discussed, physicians and other eligible professionals have a choice between two payment methods: MIPS or APM. Eligible professionals who chose APM may be excluded from MIPS. In addition, some professionals will fall below the low-volume threshold and will be excluded; the low-volume threshold is discussed in more detail in a following section. Finally, an EP in the first year of participation in Medicare may be excluded from MIPS. **Exhibit 28.2** illustrates some reasons for exclusion.

How Are MIPS Physicians and Other Eligible Professionals Paid?

Eligible professionals for MIPS are scored on performance. Their performance is rated on a scale that ranges from maximum positive to neutral to maximum negative. MIPS EPs received an automatic base increase of 0.5% from 2015 through 2019. At the time of this writing, there is zero automatic base increase from 2020 through 2025, with a 0.25% increase applied from 2026 onward.

EPs are then at risk for performance adjustments to their payments beginning in 2019. These payments are budget neutral, meaning the additional dollars paid to successful providers will equal the reduced payments to unsuccessful providers. Thus, the budget-neutral payments range from 4% maximum and minimum in 2019 to a 9% maximum and minimum in 2025, illustrated in **Figure 28.3**.

MACRA also allows an extra bonus for exceptional performance. The bonus amount of $500 million is exempt from budget neutrality and can be paid out over the first five years of the program. Participants are eligible for the bonus based on increases in their MIPS performance scores. The scoring increase for exceptional performance is capped at an additional 10%.[5]

MIPS Composite Performance Score

The MIPS **composite performance score (CPS)** consists of four parts. Each part is a separate performance category within the composite score. Note that some of the titles have changed as indicated.

- Quality
- Advancing Care Information (a.k.a. Meaningful Use of Electronic Health Records)

MIPS Payment Adjustment Timelines							
MIPS	2015–2018*	2019	2020	2021	2022–2024	2025	2026 & Onward
(1) Automatic** Base Increase	0.5%	0.5%	0.0%	0.0%	0.0%	0.0%	0.25%
PLUS (2) Three Levels of Performance Adjustments at **RISK**							
Maximum Positive Adjustment***		+4%	+5%	+7%	+9%	+9%	
Neutral Adjustment		0.0%	0.0%	0.0%	0.0%	0.0%	
Maximum Negative Adjustment***		−4%	−5%	−7%	−9%	−9%	

*Note: PQRS, VM, and EHR remain in effect for the period 2015 to 2018.
**Automatic annual base conversion factor increase of 0.5% also in effect for period 2015–2018.
***Annual totals must be budget neutral.

Figure 28.3 MIPS Payment Adjustments and Timelines

Modified from CMS, "Path to Value: The Medicare Access & CHIP Reauthorization Act of 2015," pp. 9 and 18.

- Clinical Practice Improvement Activities
- Cost (a.k.a. Resource Use)

Each category of the score is discussed in more detail in the following sections.

The payment adjustment illustrated in Figure 28.3 begins with the clinician's (or group's) CPS. The CPS is a unified scoring system that converts measures and/or activities into points, allows partial credit, and provides advance information about what is needed for top-performance scoring.

MIPS Scoring Uses Weighted Averages

MIPS CPS scoring uses weighted averages that will change the categories' weights from year to year. **Figure 28.4** illustrates these changes and shows how the distribution of weighted averages shifted from 2019 to 2021. In other words, the two years in this illustration use a different set of weighted averages among the four categories.

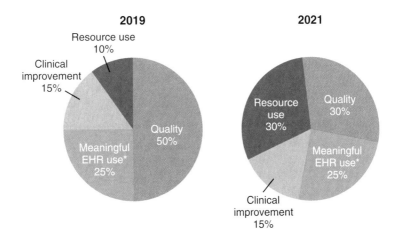

Figure 28.4 Weighted Averages for the MIPS Score Measures as Initially Proposed

MIPS Performance Categories

Each performance category is made up of a series of individual measures. The clinician chooses, within limits, which measures to report within each category. A brief summary about each category follows and is illustrated in **Table 28.1**.

Quality

This category contains streamlined measures from the PQRS and the Quality portion of the VM Program. Required reporting for this category consists of six measures rather than the nine measures previously required by PQRS. There is also more emphasis on outcome measurement. The Year 1 proposed weight of 50% subsequently increased to 60%.

As initially proposed, the EPs are allowed to choose the six measures that best reflect their practice. There are certain limitations to this choice. One must be either an outcome or a high-quality measure, and another has to be a crosscutting measure. A crosscutting measure is one that can be applied across a number of providers and/or specialties. There is another available choice for specialists: They can choose a set of measures related to their particular specialty.[6]

Advancing Care Information

Meaningful use has gained a new name: Advancing Care Information (ACI). The ACI measures, originally derived from the MU/EHR program, have been modified and streamlined for MIPS use. Quarterly reporting has been eliminated, as

has the "all-or-nothing" threshold measurement of EHR technology. Redundant measures and two objectives were eliminated to reduce the reporting burden. The Year 1 weight is 25%.

For purposes of MIPS reporting, EPs can choose the measures that are most important within their practice. These customized choices will represent key measures of interoperability and information exchange. Flexible scoring has been implemented for all measures to promote care coordination and better patient outcomes.[7]

Clinical Practice Improvement Activities

The new Clinical Practice Improvement performance category contains six types of activities for Year 1:

- Expanded Practice Access
- Population Management
- Care Coordination
- Beneficiary Engagement
- Patient Safety and Practice Access
- Participation in an APM

The Year 1 weight is 15%.

The CMS proposed rule sets out measures of more than 90 activities within this category. EPs can choose six measures among these that best reflect goals for the practice, and at least one activity must be chosen to avoid a zero score.[8]

Resource Use (or Cost)

The resource use category will assess all applicable cost measures to the particular clinician or group. This category replaces the cost portion of the VM Program. Over 40 episode-specific measures have been added to address specialty concerns.

Table 28.1 MIPS Performance Categories

Quality	Resource Use
Streamlined measures from PQRS and quality portion of VM	Replaces cost portion of VM
Advancing Care Information	**Clinical Practice Improvement Activities**
Streamlined measures from Meaningful Use EHR program	New category with six activities and 90 options

Year 1 weight proposed at 10% subsequently was reduced to 0%. EPs do not have to report measures for this category. Instead, CMS performs the calculation by comparing resource use across practices that involve similar care episodes and clinical condition groups.[9]

How MIPS Scoring Works

EPs' chosen measures, as reported, are accumulated into annual totals. The clinician's totals from each category's measures as reported are converted into points. The next step is for points earned to become percentage scores. You will recall that there are weighted averages within the composite performance score. Figure 28.4 illustrates these weights for both 2019, which is Year 1 for the Quality Payment Program and MIPS, and for 2021.

Accordingly, the Year 1 maximum score possible for each performance category will equal that category's weight within the overall score (the Composite Performance Score). The Year 1 maximum percentage scores are shown in **Table 28.2**.

Quality = 50%, subsequently increased to 60%

Advancing Care Information = 25%

Clinical Practice Improvement Activities = 15%

Resource Use (Cost) = 10%, subsequently reduced to zero

Points are turned into percentage scores in this manner. First, the clinician earns points by reporting their chosen measures for the first three performance categories listed previously. Recall that the resource use category does not require the reporting of measures because it is calculated by CMS from claims and volume information.

There are a certain number of points needed to reach the maximum score for each of the first three performance categories listed previously. An example follows.

Dr. Brown's Scores: An Example

The points earned by a clinician or group are mathematically converted into the relevant percentage. For example, Dr. Brown's practice earned 60 out of the required 80 on Quality; therefore, his performance category percentage score is 37.5%, $(60 \div 80) \times 50$ (maximum possible score). Some measures for the Advancing Care Information category were not properly reported during the **performance period**, so the practice only earned 50 points of the 100 points needed to reach the maximum score. His percentage score for this category is 12.5%, $(50 \div 100) \times 25$. Dr. Brown earned all 60 points in the Clinical Practice Improvement Activities category, so that portion of his weighted composite performance score is the full 15%, $(60 \div 60) \times 15$. Finally, CMS calculation scored the practice at 80% in the Resource

Table 28.2 MIPS Scoring by Performance Category: An Example

MIPS Performance Category	Maximum Possible Score (%)	Total Points Needed to Reach Maximum Score
Quality	50	80 to 90*
Advancing Care Information (Meaningful Use)	25	100
Clinical Practice Improvement Activities	15	60
Resource Use (Cost)	10	CMS calculates average score

* Depending on group size.

Modified from CMS Quality Program Executive Summary Table 1, p. 10 (May 2016).

Use category, so his percentage score is 8%, 80% × 10. Refer to the left-hand column in Table 28.1 to further understand the maximum possible scores as expressed in percentages. All told, Dr. Brown's four performance category percentage scores looked like this:

Quality = 37.5%

Advancing Care Information = 12.5%

Clinical Practice Improvement Activities = 15.0%

Resource Use = 8.0%

The four performance category composite scores would then be converted into a total composite score using the weighted averages as shown in Figure 28.4. How Dr. Brown's scores affect his payment adjustment is the subject of the next section.

How Do Scores Become Payment Adjustments?

First, the physician or group records and submits selected measures during the performance period. After these data are collected, reported measures are analyzed, and outcomes are calculated. The resulting computations are then converted into scores, and the scores are converted into payment adjustments. While the following section provides a general descriptive overview, the actual computations are quite sophisticated and are beyond the scope of this text.

Five Steps from Measures to MIPS Payment Adjustment

This section provides a general overview of five steps that convert submitted measures into MIPS payment adjustments. For purposes of our description, we will assume that Analyst Jane works for CMS and performs all five steps. This is not realistic, of course, as teams of analysts would be segmenting the process into individual responsibilities.

Step 1: First, Jane analyzes the submitted measures from all over the country.

These represent measures for the Quality, Advancing Care Information, and Clinical Practice Improvement Activities performance categories submitted during the performance period. The national analysis will, of course, include Dr. Brown's submitted measures for the performance period. The team will also compute relevant benchmarks for comparative purposes.

Step 2: Jane then computes costs and certain other outcomes from CMS data sources for the Resource Use category. Note that some of these computations may be based on the prior year's data rather than performance period data.

Step 3: Jane then standardizes the data from the four performance categories and performs a series of statistical analyses. She will compute the national means and medians and divide the results of this analysis into quartiles. Using the quartile results, she will apply standard deviation computations to divide the analysis into three national tiers: high, average, and low.

Step 4: Next, Jane does two things. First, she finds the individual physician or group's composite performance score. In our example, that would be Dr. Brown's composite performance score. Then she assigns the doctor's score to one of the three national tiers (i.e., Dr. Brown's score will be placed in the high, average, or low tier).

Step 5: Now that Jane knows which tier Dr. Brown's score is in, she will compute the doctor's payment adjustment. This payment adjustment will have one of three possible outcomes: It will result in a positive, neutral, or negative payment adjustment for Dr. Brown.[10] **Figure 28.5** illustrates the five-step process just described. This process is repeated each time a performance period ends, and the process may be modified over time.

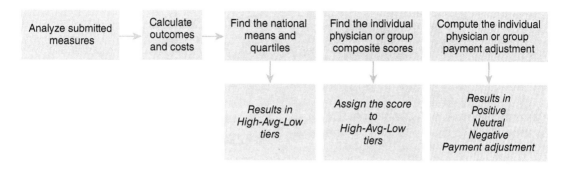

Figure 28.5 An Overview of MIPS Scoring

An EP should be able to view preliminary results, and appeal rights have been established.

MIPS Required Reporting Affects Payment

Reporting on required measures is important because the reported measures directly impact future payments. Complete reporting, reporting every measure that has been previously selected, is necessary for the measures to be recognized when they are submitted. In other words, an incomplete set of measures may not be counted. Accuracy in reporting is equally important.

What Is a Performance Period, and How Does It Affect Payments?

A **performance period** is a designated time span used to capture data. The data that are captured measure how well the clinician or group is performing. The MIPS program performance period covers a one-year period (i.e., a calendar year).[11] The measures reported during a performance period are analyzed to determine a payment adjustment based on quality and value performance. CMS has provided an example of the timeline for the first performance period under MIPS as follows.

The first MIPS performance period was calendar year 2017. CMS used the following year, 2018, for analysis and scoring of the data collected in the 2017. Then the next year, 2019, was when the first MIPS payment adjustments were made. In other words, the performance period reporting made two years ago affects the payment adjustments received in a current year.[12]

Feedback

CMS is expected to provide feedback to the physicians and groups who are MIPS participants. At the time of this writing, the first feedback was anticipated in the middle of the performance period year. This would give an opportunity for adjustments to the participant's reporting process. The second feedback was then anticipated in the middle of the analysis and scoring year (i.e., the year between the performance period and the payment-adjustment year).

Data Submission

Individuals can choose among various options for data submission. The four performance categories differ somewhat in available options. These differences are described as follows.

Individual Performance Reporting

Quality Options

Data submission choices include submission through EHRs or through a Qualified Registry or Qualified Clinical Data Registry (QCDR). Claims submitted by providers are also part of quality data submission, as are administrative claims. "Administrative claims" means CMS will perform any needed computations and no special submission is required from the participant.

Advancing Care Information Options

Submission choices for ACI include through EHRs, a Qualified Registry, or a QCDR. Attestation is another available choice for this category. Administrative claims are also part of the process, but, again, no special submission is required.

Clinical Practice Improvement Activities Options

Submission choices for CPIA also include through EHRs, a Qualified Registry, a QCDR, or attestation. Once again, administrative claims are part of the process, but no action is required on the part of the participant.

Resource Use Options

The Resource Use category entirely uses the administrative claims computation process, so no action is required by the participant.[13]

Group Performance Reporting

Groups have a couple of additional options. In the case of the Quality category, groups may also choose the CAHPS for MIPS Survey option. Groups of 25 clinicians or more may use the CMS Web Interface when submitting data for the Quality, ACI, and CPIA categories.[14]

Reporting by Intermediaries

CMS has proposed to allow certain intermediaries to submit performance data on behalf of eligible clinicians. The allowable intermediaries include health information technology (HIT) vendors who obtain their data from the eligible clinicians' certified EHR technology, CMS-approved survey vendors, Qualified Registries, and QCDRs.[15]

APM-Choice 2

The **alternative payment models (APM)** represent innovations in how to compensate physicians and other eligible professionals.

Advanced APM According to MACRA

MACRA considers the following to be Advanced APM:

- CMS Innovation Center Models under section 1115A (other than a healthcare innovation award)
- Shared Savings Program
- A demonstration under section 1866C
- Demonstrations required by federal law

These APM are considered "advanced" because the participants accept risks along with rewards (i.e., incentive payments). To be eligible for incentive payment, particular criteria about EHR usage and reporting of quality measures must be met.[16]

Eligible Advanced APM Proposed for Year 1

CMS proposes specific criteria for Advanced APM through rulemaking. These criteria fit within MACRA's description of entities as listed previously. The eligible Advanced APM proposed for Year 1 were:

- Comprehensive Primary Care Plus
- Medical Shares Savings Programs—Tracks 2 and 3
- Next Generation ACO Model
- Comprehensive End-Stage Renal Disease Care Model
- Oncology Care Model

It is important to note that the Comprehensive End-Stage Renal Disease Care Model is a large dialysis organization arrangement. Likewise, the Oncology Care Model is a two-sided risk arrangement. **Figure 28.6** summarizes these models. It is important to note that changes to the proposed Year 1 models may occur before actual implementation.

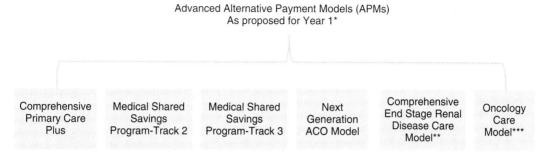

*Other models may subsequently be included.
**A large dialysis organization arrangement.
***A two-sided risk arrangement.

Figure 28.6 Advanced Alternative Payment Models (APM) as Proposed for Year 1

The eligibility for Advanced APM will be reviewed annually. Thus, while these models are proposed for Year 1, we are still at the beginning of this transition to **value-based performance** payment models. We expect a series of modifications, expansions, and revisions as time goes on. We can therefore expect that the choices among future multiple payment approaches will increase along with transparency through public reporting as these models develop and mature.[17]

Other Payer Advanced APM: An Upcoming Option

Another interesting option expected to be in effect for payment in 2021 is Other Payer Advanced APM. As the name suggests, data from payers other than Medicare (e.g., private insurers or state Medicaid programs) could be taken into account when determining a provider's participation status.

Participation requirements for these Other Payer Advanced APM would be as follows:

- Use certified EHR technology.
- Provide payment based on quality measures that are comparable to measures in the MIPS quality performance category.
- Bear more than a nominal amount of risk for monetary losses (or be a particular comparable type of Medicaid Medical Home Model).[18]

Eligible Professionals Within APM

EPs for APM fall into one of two categories: qualifying (QEPs or QPs) and partial qualifying (PQEPs). This distinction is important because APM payment adjustments and their related timelines vary between QEPs and PQEPs. While MACRA refers to eligible professionals, CMS proposes to use the term *eligible clinicians* within its rulemaking.

Qualifying Eligible Professionals (a.k.a. Qualifying Eligible Clinicians) Defined

Qualifying Eligible Professionals (QEPs) meet all thresholds (as defined in the scoring section of this chapter) and are at risk, meaning the EP bears financial burden based on performance.

Partial Qualifying Eligible Professionals (or Clinicians) Defined

Partial qualifying EPs (PQEPs) meet slightly reduced thresholds and are at risk. It is important to understand that EPs within an Advanced APM entity may collectively meet the necessary threshold for participation. In other words, everyone who is eligible within a particular

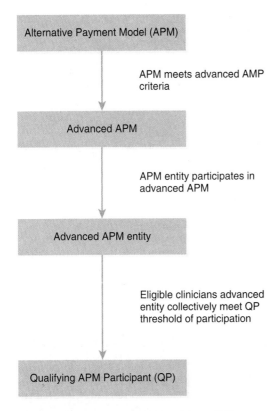

Figure 28.7 Qualifying APM Participant (QP) Pathway

Modified from 81 Federal Register 28295 Figure B (May 9, 2016).

Advanced APM may receive the same score and thus same payment adjustment. The sequence of progression, or pathway, for EPs toward becoming a qualifying APM Participant (QP) is illustrated in **Figure 28.7**.[19]

Four Steps to Find Whether the EP Will Become a Qualifying APM Participant

CMS has published four steps that illustrate whether an EP within an Advanced APM will become a QP. Remember that these clinicians will be collectively meeting the necessary thresholds. The four steps are as follows:

1. QP determinations are made at the Advanced APM Entity level.
2. CMS calculates a threshold score for each Advanced APM Entity.
3. The threshold score for each method is compared to the corresponding QP threshold.
4. All the eligible clinicians in the Advanced APM Entity become QPs for the payment year.[20]

The result: If the threshold scores for the Advanced APM Entity are above the appropriate threshold, then all the eligible clinicians in the Advanced APM Entity will become QPs for that particular payment year. However, if the threshold scores for the Advanced APM Entity are below the corresponding QP threshold, then none of the clinicians will become QPs for that payment year. In other words, the determination is all or nothing at the time of this writing.

It is also important to understand that the threshold scores are derived each year from a calendar year performance period. The performance period will be two years prior to the payment year and is thus aligned with the MIPS performance period.[21]

How Are Advanced APM EPs Paid?

If QEPs meet their thresholds, they receive an annual lump sum incentive payment of 5.0% from 2019 through 2024. These QEPs will also be excluded from MIPS adjustments. At the time of this writing, beginning in 2026, qualifying participants may receive higher fee schedule updates.[22] A timeline payment summary appears later.

QEP Incentive Payment Base Period Versus QP Performance Period

It is important to understand the difference between base period and performance periods for Advanced APM qualifying EPs. The performance period is two years prior to the payment year and is aligned with MIPS performance periods.

The incentive payment base period is for a different purpose. It is used to calculate how much the 5% incentive lump sum will be. To do so, the relevant payments for services are added

Table 28.3 APM Proposed Payment Adjustments and Timelines

APMs Payment Adjustments	2015–2018*	2019	2020	2021	2022–2024	2025	2026 Onward
Qualifying EPs (QEPs; meet all thresholds and are at risk) Annual Lump Sum Payment				5.0%			Higher fee schedule updates starting in 2026
Partial Qualifying EPs (PQEPs; meet slightly reduced thresholds and are at risk)	No lump sum payment; can choose to participate in MIPS **OR** No lump sum paid; can opt out of MIPS and be held harmless						To be determined

*Note: PQRS, VM & EHR remain in effect for the period 2015 to 2018.

Modified from CMS, "Path to Value: The Medicare Access & CHIP Reauthorization Act of 2015," p. 18.

up; then 5% of that figure equals the 5% incentive lump sum to be received. The relevant payments to be added up are based on "the estimated aggregate payments for professional services furnished the year prior to the payment year, e.g., the 2019 APM Incentive Payment will be based on 2018 services."[23]

This cycle is repeated each year. For example, the first cycle is 2017, QP performance period, 2018 is the incentive payment base period to calculate the 5%, and 2019 is the year when the payment adjustment is received. Then the second cycle starts; 2018 is the QP performance period, 2019 is the incentive payment base period, and 2020 is the payment year. The cycle keeps repeating for the duration of the 5% incentive payments.[24]

Partial Qualifying Eligible Professionals Payments

Some EPs may be participating in an Advanced APM that does not meet the standard threshold as previously described. Instead, this Advanced APM meets a slightly reduced threshold, and the EPs are considered to be PQEPs.

The PQEPs receive no lump sum incentive payment. They can choose to either participate in MIPS or opt out of MIPS. If they choose to participate in MIPS, they will receive favorable weights in the MIPS scoring. If they opt out, they will be held harmless (i.e., receive no favorable MIPS payment adjustment or be subject to a negative adjustment).[25]

APM Payment Adjustments and Their Timelines

The APM payment adjustments commenced in 2019. As previously discussed, these APM payment adjustments are based upon the results of reporting for a performance period two years prior to 2019. Thus, measures reported in 2017 represent the performance period for Year 1 (2019) APM incentive payments. **Table 28.3** summarizes both the payment information and the timelines as discussed.

What Is the "Intermediate Option" for Payment Adjustment Choices?

"Intermediate Option" is the term for flexibility of choice between the MIPS and APM tracks. First, as we have previously described, partially qualifying EPs can choose whether they want to receive the MIPS payment adjustment. Second, the APM/MIPS participants would get credit toward their score within the category of Clinical Practice Improvement Activities. CMS has proposed aligning MIPS standards and APM standards in order to "make it easy for clinicians to move between them."[26]

How Significant Participation Works

Significant participation is expressed in terms of ever-increasing percentages. In other words, participation

Table 28.4 Advanced APM: Required Participation by Year

Payment Years

Required participation through an Advanced APM*	2017	2018	2019	2020	2021	2022 & Later
Percentage of payments	25%	25%	50%	50%	75%	75%
OR						
Percentage of patients	20%	20%	35%	35%	50%	50%

* Requirements for percentage of significant participation, by year.

Modified from CMS Quality Payment Program Overview Fact Sheet Table 1, p. 5 (October 14, 2016).

must be met in each applicable payment year in either of the following two ways: percentage of payments through an Advanced APM or percentage of patients through an Advanced APM.

At the time of this writing, participation percentages for APM payments range from 25% to 75% over a six- to seven-year period. Likewise, participation percentages for APM patients range from 20% to 50% over the same six- to seven-year period. **Table 28.4** illustrates the progression of these timelines. It is to be expected that specific requirements will be edited and modified as time goes on. In addition, "CMS will continue to modify models in coming years to help them qualify as Advanced APMs."[27]

Advanced APM Participation Standards

The initial proposed standards for Advanced APM include three particular areas, as follows.

Financial Risk

The financial risk standards involve the reimbursement at risk. If financial risk requirements are not met, then CMS could take action in several ways. These actions include requiring repayment, withholding current payments due, or reducing future rates to equal the required repayment

penalty. In other words, the APM provider would lose money. Of course, if the APM provider exceeds the standards, they would gain through incentive payments. The proposed initial financial risk standards must be met in three ways: total risk, marginal risk, and a minimum loss rate.

Comparable Measures

This standard requires that APM measures be comparable to MIPS measures within the quality category. As you will recall, to be comparable, the measures must be valid and reliable. They must also be evidence-based, and at least one of the measures must be an outcome measure (assuming an appropriate measure is available).

Certified EHR Technology (as Proposed)

This standard requires that in the first year of the performance period, 50% of the APM clinicians must use certified EHR technology. In the second year, 75% of the APM clinicians must use certified EHR technology.[28]

Required Reporting for the First Year

CMS has proposed that all EPs report through MIPS in the first year. This requirement is imposed because it wants to determine whether the particular EP can actually meet the Advanced APM requirements.

Accurate and complete reporting of measures is always important. However, complete reporting is especially important when the provider is attempting to qualify for participation as an Advanced APM. Scoring standards for APM are the subject of the following section.

Scoring Standard for APM

The APM scoring standard implements uniformity across the various types of APM. Goals include reducing reporting burdens while maintaining the goals and objectives of the individual APM entity. Meeting the requirements for this standard can also be viewed as a necessary first step toward becoming an Advanced APM.

Criteria for Eligibility

Eligibility criteria for APM entity scoring standards include:

- The APM participates in an agreement with CMS.
- The APM bases its payment incentives on performance, using quality and cost-utilization measures.
- The APM includes at least one eligible MIPS clinician on a CMS participation list.

Note that the eligible clinician's name must be on an APM participation list by the end of the MIPS performance year. If not, the clinician has to report under standard MIPS methods.[29]

Types of APM Entities That Qualify

At the time of this writing, the following types of APM entities qualified for the APM scoring standard:

- Comprehensive Primary Care Plus (CPC+)
- Medical Shares Savings Programs (all tracks)
- Next Generation ACO Model

- Comprehensive End-Stage Renal Disease Care (CEC) Model
- Oncology Care Model (OCM)
- All other APM that meet the criteria for the scoring standard

The Standard Aggregates Scores

Under the standard, all MIPS scores for eligible clinicians are combined, weighted, and averaged to arrive at a single score at the level of the APM entity. This means that all the eligible clinicians within that APM will receive the exact same MIPS composite performance score. The standard has streamlined both reporting and scoring; wherever possible, the scoring standard uses performance measures related to that APM.

Performance scores under the standard use the same performance categories as MIPS. At the time of this writing, it appears that the Resource Use category will not be applicable and thus will not contribute to the score. The remaining three categories—Quality, ACI, Advancing Care Information (ACI) and CPIA—will be weighted when computing the final composite score based on the type of APM entity.

Creating Physician-Focused Payment Models (PFPMs)

The underlying legislative intent is to encourage the creation of **physician-focused payment models (PFPMs)** as per the following quotation: "[APMs] provide incentive payments for certain eligible professionals (EPs) who participate in APMs, by exempting EPs from the MIPS if they are qualifying APM participants, and by encouraging the creation of physician-focused payment models (PFPMs)."[30]

A New Committee

The overall phrase used to describe these models is "physician-focused payment models" or PFPMs. The Physician Focused Payment Model Technical

Advisory Committee will have the responsibility for reviewing and assessing possible new models.[31]

Building the Measurement Development Plan for MIPS and APM: Developing New Quality Measures

Measuring quality and value are important for MIPS and APM because quality and value are the foundation of the new payment system for EPs. Since MIPS measures are more fully developed than APM, there are difference implementation timelines for MIPS and APM. MIPS measures are more developed than APM and hence are ready for the first stages of implementation. Our focus on measuring quality and value centers upon MIPS for that reason.

What Is the Measure Development Plan (MDP)?

The **Measure Development Plan (MDP)** has been created in response to a MACRA requirement. The law requires that a draft plan for the development of quality measures be developed and posted on the CMS.gov website.[32] A final plan is then to be posted at a later date. The final plan is supposed to take comments regarding the draft plan into consideration. The plan's full title is "CMS Quality Measure Development Plan: Supporting the Transition to the Merit-Based Incentive Payment System (MIPS) and Alternative Payment Models (APMs) (Draft)."[33] The introduction states that the law provides both a mandate and an opportunity for the CMS to leverage quality measure development as a key driver to further the aims of its Quality Strategy:

- Better Care,
- Smarter Spending, and
- Healthier People.[34]

The purpose of the MDP is twofold: "to meet the requirements of the statute and serve as a strategic framework for the future of clinician quality measure development to support MIPS and APMs."[35]

Creating New Quality Measures for MIPS

New quality measures are an important part of the MIPS payment structure. The basic sequence for creating these new measures is:

- First, start with existing measures. These are contained in the PQRS, in the VM program, and in the MU/EHR program.
- Next, align and harmonize these measures. In other words, the existing measures may be combined, expanded, and/or enhanced.
- Then add new measures. New measures will be needed to fill gaps. A process is in place to identify these "identified measure and performance gaps."[36] When adding the new measures, stakeholder comments may be considered. Such comments may be gathered in response to a Request for Information (RFI). In addition, measures that private payers are using may be considered.

New MIPS quality measures will result from this process. **Figure 28.8** illustrates the process just described. Note that any quality measures developed for APM must be comparable.

Timelines for Developing Quality Measures

MACRA called for the initial draft of the MDP to be published as of January 1, 2016. A comment period followed. Then the final MDP was published in May 2016. The Act further called for updates to the MDP to be published annually or otherwise as appropriate.[37] Thus, we expect to see updates, as required, published on a regular annual schedule. Any updates that might be otherwise appropriate, of course, are unpredictable.

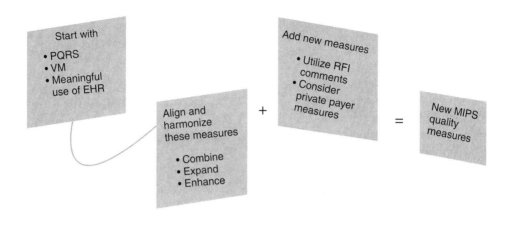

I. Building the MDP for MIPS

Start with

- PQRS
- VM
- Meaningful use of EHR

Align and harmonize these measures

- Combine
- Expand
- Enhance

+

Add new measures

- Utilize RFI comments
- Consider private payer measures

=

New MIPS quality measures

II. Quality measures to be developed for APMs must be comparable

Figure 28.8 Building the MDP for MIPS and APM: Creating New Quality Measures

Procedural Timelines

CMS has another set of procedural timelines to comply with. A final rule about quality measure development will be published each year by CMS no later than the first of November.[38] Within the regulatory rulemaking process, a Call for Measures will be published in the first half of each year. This allows stakeholders to submit their input. After the Call for Measures ends in June of each year, a proposed rule will most probably be published with a multi-month comment period. Only then will the final rule be ready to be published on the first of November.

A Framework for MACRA Quality Measurement

The MDP required by MACRA has been described in a previous section of this chapter. MACRA further requires that the MDP take four priorities into account when creating the quality measures including:

- Outcome measures including patient reported outcome and functional status measures

- Patient experience measures
- Care coordination measures
- Measures of appropriate use of services including measures of overuse[39]

MACRA-Identified Quality Domains

MACRA also sets out specific quality domains for use in quality measure development. MACRA says, "The term quality domains means at least the following domains":

- Clinical care
- Safety
- Care coordination
- Patient and caregiver experience
- Population health and prevention[40]
- A sixth quality domain, efficiency and cost reduction, is under consideration.

The addition is permissible, as the legislative wording is "at least the following." The addition of an efficiency and reduction domain is especially logical because it ties into the National Quality Strategy (NQS) domains. In other words, with this addition, these six domains mirror the six NQS domains that are the subject of the next section.

A Framework for Quality Measurement

CMS has published a Framework for MACRA quality measurement that is linked to NQS domains. The framework is mapped to the six National Quality Strategy (NQS) domains as follows. Note that the details following each domain's title are a part of CMS's framework and some domain titles vary slightly as they were expanded from the NQS titles as listed previously.

Clinical Quality of Care

- Care type (preventive, acute, post-acute, and chronic)
- Conditions
- Subpopulations

Safety

- All-cause harm
- Hospital-acquired conditions (HACs)
- Hospital-associated infections (HAIs)
- Unnecessary care
- Medication safety

Care Coordination

- Patient and family activation
- Infrastructure and processes for care coordination
- Impact of care coordination

Person- and Caregiver-Centered Experience and Outcomes

- Patient experience
- Caregiver experience
- Preference- and goal-oriented care

Population and Community Health

- Health behaviors
- Access
- Physical and social environment
- Health status

Efficiency and Cost Reduction

- Cost
- Efficiency
- Appropriateness[41]

We have illustrated this linkage in **Figure 28.9**. CMS has published two more comments concerning the framework:

- Measures should be patient-centered and outcome-oriented whenever possible.
- Measure concepts in each of the six domains that are common across providers and settings can form a core set of measures.[42]

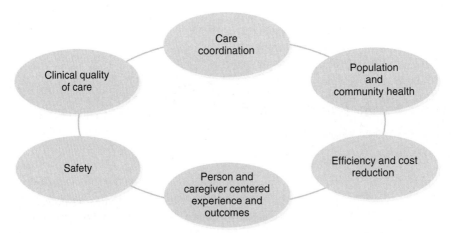

Figure 28.9 CMS Framework for Measurement Mapped to National Quality Strategy Domains

Modified from 80 FR 68668 (November 5, 2015).

Benefits and Costs of the Quality Payment Program

One benefit of the new MIPS program is an increase in the attention to quality of care. The measures' metrics provide information that may be used for internal comparative performance purposes. Another benefit concerns the program feedback about cost of care. The cost of care as computed by CMS may provide financial information based on a national benchmark.

Comparing this national baseline financial information to the provider's own costs, computed by CMS, may be valuable for future financial planning.

Costs of program participation include costs of new software plus potential hardware upgrades and staff training. The potential time lag in cash flow during implementation should also be recognized. Public reporting can be considered either a benefit or a cost depending upon the organization's public image and the results posted to the public reporting venue.

WRAP-UP

Summary

This chapter used a four-part sequence to show how CMS develops quality measures. First, the Measurement Development Plan for MIPS was described (Figure 28.8). Second, the priorities for quality measures, outcomes, patient experience, care coordination, and use of services were described. Third, the quality domains that are identified and required by MACRA legislation were described, and fourth, how the CMS framework for measurement ties back into the six NQS domains was explained (Figure 28.9).

Success of this value-based program begins with proper measure choices and continues with measure development and implementation. Proper implementation first means the right choices. Another crucial element is sufficient training of a focused staff who understand implications.

Success also depends upon complying with all digital requirements involving use of qualified electronic transmission standards. Funding must be made available for sufficient hardware and software, along with proper training of staff. Timely updates on software and staff training are essential. In addition, an electronic disaster plan should be in effect and up-to-date.

Leadership must be responsible for seeing that quality and financial incentives align properly. Such alignment could well result in a move away from so-called "silo," or vertical, departmental responsibilities. Assigning responsibilities differently, not departmentally, could potentially result in horizontal networks of responsibility that are organized around patient groups with similar needs. Finally, leadership must recognize that the digital age has arrived. It is here, and the inevitable change that it brings must be recognized and dealt with to achieve success.

Key Terms

Advancing Care Information (ACI)

Alternative Payment Model (APM)

Composite Performance Score

Eligible Professional (EP) (a.k.a. Eligible Clinician)

Medicare Access and CHIP Reauthorization Act of 2015 (MACRA)

Meaningful Use and Electronic Health Records (MU/EHR)

Measure Development Plan (MDP)

Merit-Based Incentive Payment System (MIPS)

Partial Qualifying Eligible Professional (PQEP)

Performance Period

Physician-Focused Payment Models (PFPMs)

Physician Quality Reporting System (PQRS) Program

Qualifying Eligible Professionals (QEPs)

Sustainable Growth Rate (SGR)

Value Modifier (VM) Program

Discussion Questions

1. Describe how the Merit-Based Incentive Payment System (MIPS) and the Advanced Alternative Payment Model (APM) are illustrative of "pay-for-performance."

2. Put on your physician's hat. How would you determine which of the two incentive payment programs to participate in?

3. How did the sustainable growth rate (SGR) work, and why was it ultimately repealed?

Notes

1. 80 Federal Register 59102 (October 1, 2015).
2. B. Wynne, "May the Era of Medicare's Doc Fix (1997–2015) Rest in Peace. Now What?," http://healthaffairs.org/blog/2015/04/14/may-the-era-of-medicares-doc-fix-1997-2015-rest-in-peace-now-what, accessed April 14, 2015; also M. A. Carey, "Congress Is Poised to Change Medicare Payment Policy. What Does That Mean for Patients and Doctors?," http://khn.org/news/congress-doc-fix-sustainable-growth-rate-sgr-legislation, accessed January 16, 2014.
3. Centers for Medicare and Medicaid Services (CMS), "Proposed Policy, Payment, and Quality Provisions Changes to the Medicare Physician Fee Schedule for Calendar Year 2016," http://www.cms.gov/newsroom/mediareleasedatabase/fact-sheets/2015-fact-sheets-items/2015-07-08.html, accessed July 8, 2015.
4. 80 FR 59102 (October 1, 2015).
5. CMS, "Fact Sheet: Quality Payment Program Executive Summary," p. 5, https://www.cms.gov/Medicare/Quality-Initiatives-Patient-Assessment-Instruments/Value-Based-Programs/MACRA-MIPS-and-APMs/NPRM-QPP-Fact-Sheet.pdf, accessed May 23, 2016.
6. CMS, "The Medicare Access and CHIP Reauthorization Act of 2015: Quality Payment Program," https://www.cms.gov/Medicare/Quality-Initiatives-Patient-Assessment-Instruments/Value-Based-Programs/MACRA-MIPS-and-APMs/Quality-Payment-Program/MACRA-NPRM-Slides.pdf, accessed June 6, 2016.
7. Ibid.
8. Ibid.
9. Ibid.
10. The computation steps overview as described was generalized from the composite score steps used to calculate the 2016 Value Modifier. CMS, "CMS Fact Sheet: Computation of the 2016 Value Modifier," http://www.cms.gov/Medicare/Medicare-Fee-for-Service-Paymen

/PhysicianFeedbackProgram/downloads/2016-VM-Fact-Sheet.pdf, accessed September, 2015.
11. CMS, "Hospital Value-Based Purchasing," http://www.cms.gov/Outreach-and-Education/Medicare-Learning-Network-MLN/MLNProducts/downloads/Hospital_VBPurchasing_Fact_Sheet_ICN907664.pdf, accessed September, 2015.
12. CMS, "MIPS: Advancing Care Information Performance Category," p. 41, http://www.cms.gov/Medicare/Quality-Initiatives-Patient-Assessment-Instruments/Value-Based-Programs/MACRA-MIPS-and-APSs/Advancing-Care--Information-Presentation.pdf, accessed June 7, 2016.
13. CMS, "MACRA: Quality Payment Program," pp. 39–40.
14. Ibid.
15. 81 FR 28280 (May 9, 2016).
16. P.L. 114-10-(April 16, 2015) 129 STAT.121.
17. MACRA, "Delivery System Reform, Medicare Payment Reform: What's the Quality-Payment Program?," https://www.cms.gov/Medicare/Quality-Initiatives-Patient-Assessment-Instruments/Value-Based-Programs/MACRA-MIPS-and-APMs/MACRA--MIPS-and-APMs.html, accessed March 17, 2016.
18. 81 FR 28165 (May 9, 2016).
19. Ibid., 28295.
20. CMS, "MACRA: Quality Payment Program," pp. 63 and 68.
21. Ibid.
22. Ibid., pp. 70–71, and CMS, "Qualifying Eligible Professionals (QEPs) Payments," http://www.cms.gov/Medicare/Quality-Initiatives-Patient-Assessment-Instruments/Value-Based-Programs/MACRA-MIPS-and-APMs, accessed March 17, 2016.
23. CMS, "MACRA: Quality Payment Program," pp. 70–71.
24. Ibid.
25. Ibid., p. 86.
26. CMS, "Fact Sheet: Quality Payment Program ES," p. 4.

27. Ibid., p. 3.
28. Ibid., p. 11.
29. CMS, "MACRA: Quality Payment Program," pp. 87–92.
30. 80 Federal Register (FR) 63485 (October 20, 2015).
31. P.L. 114-10 (April 16, 2015) 129 STAT. 115.
32. P.L. 114-10 Sec 102 (April 16, 2015).
33. CMS, "CMS Quality Measure Development Plan: Supporting the Transition to the Merit-based Incentive Payment System (MIPS) and Alternative Payment Models (APMs)," (Baltimore, MD: Author, 2015), https://www.cms.gov/Medicare/Quality-Initiatives-Patient-Assessment-Instruments/Value-Based-Programs/MACRA-MIPS-and-APMs/Final-MDP.pdf.
34. Ibid., p. 3; also, CMS, "CMS Quality Strategy 2016."
35. Ibid., p. 3.
36. Ibid., p. 4.
37. Sec 1848(s)(1)(A).
38. Ibid.
39. MACRA Sec.102(1)(D).
40. MACRA Sec. 102(1)(B).
41. 80 FR 68668 (November 5, 2015).
42. Ibid.

CHAPTER 29

Standardizing Measures and Payment in Post-Acute Care

PROGRESS NOTES

After completing this chapter, you should be able to:

1. Identify five purposes of the IMPACT Act.
2. Identify four types of facilities affected by the IMPACT Act.
3. Understand three reasons for focusing attention on post-acute care settings.
4. Understand the concept of a core set of measures within domains.
5. Describe standardized data.
6. Define interoperability.

Overview: New Directions for Post-Acute Care

The Improving Medicare Post-Acute Care Transformation (IMPACT) Act of 2014 was signed into law on October 6, 2014. The **IMPACT Act** describes five purposes for the legislation:

- Enable comparable data and quality across **post-acute care (PAC)** settings
- Improve Medicare beneficiary outcomes
- Facilitate coordinated care by allowing provider access to longitudinal information

- Improve hospital discharge planning
- Provide data for research[1]

The purposes reach beyond the post-acute settings; for example, "Provide data for research" implies research that will extend over many years.

Requirement of the IMPACT Act: Standardizing Measures

The act requires the reporting of standardized patient assessment and quality measure data. The act further requires that the **standardized data** be interoperable. Such standardized data enables electronic-related uniformity, exchangeability, and

Table 29.1 IMPACT Act Requirements

Electronic-Related	All Other
• Data element uniformity • Exchangeability of data • Comparing data & quality across all PAC settings	• Quality care and improved outcomes • Coordinated care • Improved discharge planning

Modified from CMS, "The IMPACT Act of 2014 and Data Standardization," *MLN Connects*, p. 4 (October 21, 2015).

comparability across PAC settings. Standardized assessment data allows additional **cross-setting** outcomes. Such outcomes include:

• Quality care
• Improved outcomes
• Coordinated care
• Improved discharge planning[2]

Table 29.1 lists both electronic-related and other benefits.

Facilities Affected by the IMPACT Act

This legislation concerns four care settings that provide care after acute care treatment (thus "post-" or "after-" acute care):

• Skilled nursing facilities (SNFs)
• Home health agencies (HHAs)
• Inpatient rehabilitation facilities (IRFs)
• Long-term care hospitals (LTCHs)

Other Provisions of the Act

Implementing verifiable and auditable data collection about staffing in skilled nursing facilities (SNFs) has been funded in the amount of $11 million. Facilities are required to "electronically submit...direct care staffing information, including information for agency and contract staff, based on payroll and other verifiable and auditable data in a uniform format," which may then be audited to verify staffing information.[3] See Managing Staffing and Salaries, Chapter 9 for details.

Among other provisions, hospice facilities are to be inspected every three years.[4] In addition, both hospitals and PAC providers are affected by

regulations to be promulgated about the discharge planning process.[5]

Why Focus Attention on Post-Acute Care?

The Centers for Medicare and Medicaid Services (CMS) points out three valid reasons for turning attention to post-acute care facilities:

• Escalating PAC costs
• PAC data standards and/or data interoperability are lacking
• Meeting the goal of setting payment rates by individual patient characteristics instead of by care setting[6]

Note that physicians and other eligible professionals are not part of this legislation but hospitals are due to the need for better discharge planning. The costs are substantial, as illustrated in **Table 29.2**. Medicare spent $58.9 billion in 2014 across the four types of facilities.[7] These costs are projected to continue to increase.

Set Data Standards and Ensure Digital Interoperability

Value-based programs need accountability to work, and accountability results from recording and reporting standard measures. Setting uniform standards across all four care settings allows accountability. Ensuring that digital information can be transmitted across these settings (interoperability) is another element toward standardization.

Table 29.2 Post-Acute Care Statistics

Provider	Facilities	Beneficiaries	Medicare Spending (Billions)
Nursing Homes	15,000	1,700,000	$28.7
Home Health Agencies	12,311	3,400,000	18.0
Inpatient Rehabilitation Facilities	1,166	373,000	6.7
Long-Term Care Hospitals	420	124,000	5.5

Modified from http://www.cms.gov/Medicare/Quality-Initiatives-Patient-Assessment-Instruments.html.

Create an Alternative Post-Acute Care Payment Model

Setting payment rates by individual patient characteristics is an important goal. This goal can be accomplished by creating an alternative post-acute care payment model that reaches across the four care settings. As Table 29.2 illustrates, almost 29,000 facilities and 5.6 million beneficiaries could be affected by creating such a "cross-setting model."

A New Alternative Payment Model for Four Care Settings

The new Alternative Post-Acute Care Payment Model proposes to do two things. First, the model would establish a unified payment system across the four care settings. Second, the model would eliminate the present payment methods for the four care settings and set payment rates in accordance with characteristics of individual patients instead of the type of care setting.

Why the New Payment Model Is Possible

The new model is possible because each of the four care settings has some type of patient assessment instrument: SNFs use the Minimum Data Set (MDS), HHAs use the Outcome and Assessment

Information Set (OASIS), IRFs use the IRF-Patient Assessment Instrument (PAI), and LTCHs use the Continuity Assessment Record and Evaluation (CARE). Therefore, since information exists in some form on each assessment, standardizing the data makes the new model possible.

SNFs and HHAs have the most annual assessment submissions. In 2014, HHAs reported 35 million OASIS submissions and SNFs 20 million MDS submissions. The 55 million submissions from these two care settings far overshadow IRF and LTCH submissions. IRFs reported 492,000 PAI and LTCH 76,000 CARE slightly more than 1% of the 55 million submissions received from SNFs and HHAs[8] (**Figure 29.1**).

First Steps: Implementing Uniform Measures in Three Phases

This PAC reform depends upon uniform measures across four care settings. Phase I covers specifications of applicable measures, followed by data collection and analysis of the uniform measures (**Figure 29.2**).[9] In Phase II, providers in the four care settings receive confidential feedback. The feedback reveals how they have performed on the uniform measures they reported. In Phase III, public reporting is implemented (i.e., individual provider performance information is open to the public). Note that providers may receive preview reports before their information is made public.

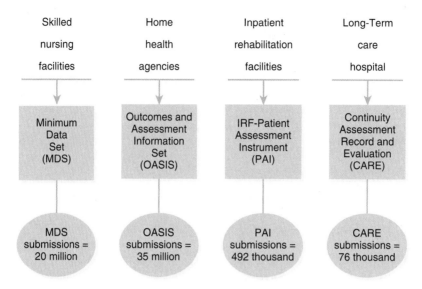

Figure 29.1 Post-Acute Care Assessment Instrument Submissions

Data from http://www.cms.gov/Medicare/Quality-Initiatives-Patient-Assessment-Instruments.html.

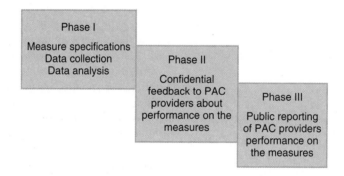

Figure 29.2 PAC Measurement Implementation Phases

Standardized Data and Interoperability: The Keys to PAC Reform

Legislative reform has introduced "cross-setting" to post-acute care while each type of PAC facility has its own set of assessment information—SNFs have the MDS, HHAs have OASIS, and so on. This "silo" of electronic data does not, and typically cannot, cross over into different types of facilities. In "cross-setting," information barriers are eliminated by standardized data. In other words, standardized data enables electronic-related uniformity, exchangeability, and comparability across the various post-acute care settings.

Table 29.1 previously listed three electronic-related elements that are enabled by standardizing assessment data. They include the following: data element uniformity, exchangeability of data (interoperability), and comparability of data and quality across all PAC settings. These requirements are possible because of the improvement in digital technology in health care. The adoption of **electronic health record (EHR)** nationwide was the key that allows today's improvements to recording and submitting electronic data.

What Is Standardized Data?

To standardize is to make uniform (i.e., data that are uniform and comparable). For example, each of the four types of PAC facilities has some type of assessment instrument that it is already using. Certain data elements from each of these assessment instruments have been selected to be standardized. These uniformly reported items will then be comparable across each type of facility.

One example used in a CMS training session was "eating." All four instruments had some type of "eating" assessment item, but the wording was different for each.[10] Standardized data would make sure that the wording and intent of the assessment were the same for each. "Mobility" is another example; of the 17 mobility items listed, eight, or just over half, were present on the instruments for SNFs, IRFs, and LTCHs.[11] Even though individual wording may be different from assessment to assessment, the opportunity for standardization is present.

What Is Interoperability?

Interoperability means the ability to operate or transmit data across the different systems used by organizations. Thus, certain elements of a skilled nursing home's data should be in a standard format that is comparable to the format for those elements used in other organizations. The IMPACT Act requires that such data be interoperable because data needs to be transmitted back and forth across the various care settings. This interoperability, along with standardization, is the key to achieving the anticipated outcomes.

Standardizing Assessment and Measure Domains for PAC Providers

The CMS has developed a framework for measurement that serves as a basic structure for measurement criteria. The criteria within this framework can be applied to measurements required within the IMPACT Act legislation, as follows. Measures utilized for the PAC reform should have two basic characteristics: They should be patient-centered and outcome-oriented.[12] Note that an outcome-oriented measure should be used whenever possible; however, not every measure will or can measure outcomes.

A Core Set of Measures

The CMS measurement framework hinges upon domains. Certain domains can be commonly identified across the four PAC settings and their respective providers. Thus, it is possible to create a core set of measures within these domains. This point is important because it is a basic concept underlying PAC reform.

Note that the IMPACT Act specifically identifies assessment and measure domains that are required under this law. Therefore, it is important to recognize them and their underlying concept. **Figure 29.3** illustrates the measures discussed previously and the "core set" concept. A discussion of required domains for assessments and measures follows.

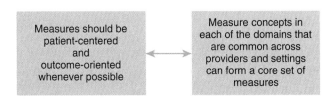

Figure 29.3 Two Structural Elements in the CMS Framework for Measurement

Adapted from 80 FR 68668 (November 5, 2015).

Assessment Domains That Must Be Standardized

The IMPACT Act specifies five assessment domains that must be standardized including:

- Functional status
- Cognitive function and mental status
- Special services, treatments, and interventions
- Medical conditions and comorbidities
- Impairments[13]

Note that additional domains may be added.

Measure Domains That Must Be Standardized

The IMPACT Act also specifies eight measure domains that must be standardized. These eight domains can be divided into three groups, generally based on the intent behind the information to be gained.

The first and largest group of measure domains consists of patient care information, including:

- Various functional status and cognitive function measures for the individual patient
- Skin integrity, etc., typically centering upon pressure ulcers and/or their prevention
- Reconciliation of the patient's various medications
- Number of major falls the patient has experienced

The second group of measure domains consists of information about a patient moving between care settings and/or discharged from care, including:

- Information transfer and care preferences as an individual patient moves from one care setting to another
- Information about the individual patient being discharged from any care setting (i.e., "into the community")
- Information about hospital readmission rates, in particular readmissions that may be preventable[14]

The final "group" is actually a single item that measures resource use, typically a value-based measure. As such, the grouping is expected to utilize estimated Medicare spending per beneficiary. Certain methodology adjustments for resource use may be aligned as necessary, including spending per beneficiary and time period(s), plus geographic and other relevant adjustments.[15]

The reporting of these quality measures is to occur "through the use of a PAC assessment instrument." Therefore, the relevant assessment instruments are to be modified "as necessary" to enable their use for such reporting.[16]

Electronic Reporting Timelines for PAC Providers

CMS estimates that developing quality measures will take six months to two years. The development process includes public and stakeholder input along with guidance from the Measure Applications Partnership (MAP).[17] It is therefore possible that some timelines may be revised. The MAP is a multi-stakeholder partnership that guides the selection of performance measures for federal health programs.[18]

PAC Provider Timelines

Certain standardized assessment domains were implemented for SNF, IRF, and LTCH providers as of October 1, 2018, and for HHAs as of January 1, 2019. There is variation among the four providers as to the specific domain items they must initially report on these dates.

It is important to understand that SNF and LTCH providers should already have begun reporting certain quality and resource use measures two years earlier as part of their new value-based programs. Thus, SNF and LTCH providers may simply add new measures required on October 1, 2018. This contrasts with IRF providers, who will be reporting their required measures for the first time as of October 1, 2018, and HHA providers who will be reporting their required measures for the first time as of January 1, 2019. Beginning in fiscal year 2018, SNF payment rates may be reduced if applicable data is not submitted. The payment rate reduction amounts to 2%.[19]

PAC Action Requirements

The most important action requirements for PAC providers are submission dates. According to CMS, "providers must submit standardized assessment data through PAC assessment instruments under applicable reporting provisions. The data must be submitted with respect to admission and discharge for each patient, or more frequently as required."[20] IMPACT-required measures must begin to be submitted no later than October 1, 2018, for SNF, IRF, and LTCH providers. IMPACT-required measures for HHAs must begin to be submitted no later than January 1, 2019.[21]

Public Reporting: IMPACT Act Requirements

The IMPACT Act requires public reporting of PAC provider performance, including both quality measures and resource use measures. Note that public reporting includes not only reporting the measures themselves but also the provider associated with those measures. The relevant data and information are to be made publicly available no later than two years after the measure's application date.[22] The act stipulates that providers have an opportunity to review information that will be made available to the public. Thus, providers will be able to submit corrections, if needed, prior to public reporting of the data.[23]

Required Improvements to the 5-Star Rating System

CMS has implemented certain improvements to the *Nursing Home Compare* website's five-star rating system. This website provides information about every nursing home that participates in Medicare and/or Medicaid. *Nursing Home Compare* rates facilities using a five-star rating system.

Each facility is rated on a five-point scale for each of three domains—health survey, nurse staffing, and quality measures—plus a composite scale that combines the ratings for the three domains.[24]

Several revisions are directly tied to the act, such as using payroll-based staffing reports and providing additional quality measures. A related improvement is a revised scoring methodology for the five-star rating system that will take advantage of the data and information received from the payroll-based reporting and additional new quality measures.[25]

Two additional improvements are the following: First, CMS and states have implemented focused survey inspections nationwide to verify staffing and quality measure information. Second, CMS has strengthened the requirements that states must maintain a user-friendly website and complete nursing home inspections in a timely manner so the current survey information can be included in the five-star rating system.[26]

IMPACT Act Benefits and Costs

The IMPACT Act's benefits center upon requirements for quality improvement and a focus upon future payment reform. Quality improvement benefits include:

- Facilitate coordinated care among PACs
- Achieve improved outcomes
- Allow overall quality comparisons
- Allow "patient-centeredness"

Payment reform is anticipated through the creation of one or more Alternative Post-Acute Care Payment models. This type of model is based upon the individual patient's care and outcomes instead of the facility-based payment system now in place. Thus, this quality- and value-based type of payment system has the potential to become a significant benefit for post-acute care.

PAC providers will encounter transitional costs, including the following:

- Required changes to hardware and software
- Related staff training
- Potential disruption of cash flow
- Planning costs for leadership

Most of the required changes are phased in over time, so implementation costs may also be phased in instead of occurring all at once.

Challenges

The act's requirements face a challenge in implementing interoperability. A couple of years ago, the Office of the National Coordinator for Health Information Technology (ONC) made its annual report to Congress and noted that national interoperability had increased but widespread interoperability remained a challenge. The challenge included unchanged provider practice patterns and a lack of standardization among EHRs.[27] We believe the IMPACT Act's requirements address both of these challenges as related to post-acute care providers.

Meeting Strategic Goals

The CMS goals for quality strategy are to support the three aims of National Quality Strategy (NQS): "better health; better healthcare; lower costs."[28] The three NQS aims were converted into six NQS priorities, and CMS has adopted these priorities as strategic goals for quality.

The CMS Quality Strategy Goals

As described previously, CMS has adopted a revised version of the NQS priorities as its quality strategy goals. The CMS goals appear as follows with the NQS domain phrase for each follows in parentheses.[29]

- Promote effective communication and coordination of care (Care Coordination)
- Promote effective prevention and treatment (Clinical Quality of Care)
- Make care affordable (Efficiency and Cost Reduction)
- Strengthen person and family engagement (Person- and Caregiver-Centered Experience and Outcomes)
- Make care safer (Safety)

- Work with communities to promote best practices of healthy living (Population/Community Health)[30]

More about goals and the National Quality Strategy can be found in Chapter 27.

The Road Map to Interoperability

The ONC is "the principal federal entity charged with coordination of nationwide efforts to implement and use the most advanced health information technology and the electronic exchange of health information."[31] It created a 10-year Road Map to Interoperability that outlines goals for both governance and certification standards that calls for consistency at federal, state, and private levels—an "unprecedented collaboration."[32] If such widespread interoperability can be accomplished, then technology could seamlessly support patients' health. The IMPACT Act is an important step toward that goal of seamless digital technology.

Innovation in the Digital Age

Innovation may be defined as "the introduction of something new; a new idea, method, or device," while "to innovate" is defined as "to effect a change in; to make changes."[33] In light of this, the scope of reforms proposed for PAC settings, along with the digital conversions involved, would certainly qualify as innovations. How do leaders of an organization approach an innovative project? E. M. Rogers, a communication and innovation researcher, comments upon reaction to an innovation as follows:

> An innovation presents an individual or an organization with a new alternative or alternatives, with new means of solving problems. But the probabilities of the new alternatives being superior to previous practice are not exactly known by the individual problem solvers. Thus, they are motivated to seek further information about the innovation to cope with the uncertainty that it creates.[34]

We visualize this type of information-seeking information approach as a sequential decision process, as discussed in the following section.

The Process of Leadership Decisions Affects Innovation

Leadership decisions are often made in a series of stages. **Figure 29.4** illustrates three decision stages that may lead to adoption, for example, of a particular approach to PAC reform digital choices. The three-stage decision process is as follows:

1. *Gathers information*: This stage seeks enough information to attain knowledge.
2. *Forms an opinion*: This stage uses the knowledge gained to reach an understanding that leads to an opinion.
3. *Makes a decision*: This stage uses the opinion that has been formed to make a decision.

The last stage, "Makes a decision," should result in one of two outcomes: The decision will either be positive (Yes: adopt and implement) or negative (No: do not adopt). There could be a third possible outcome on the last stage; a boss may refuse to say "yes" or "no" but rather say, "Take no action either way." We should note that a positive or negative decision might not always be final, as it could be reversed at a later date.

Bringing About Innovation

How can managers help bring about an innovative concept such as the legislative reforms that are the subject of this chapter? They can help first to understand and then to diffuse.

Understanding the Required Framework and Diffusing the Information

You as a manager can gather information and use it to understand the required framework or gather it for senior management. You as a manager can also build understanding about the innovative concept throughout your part of the organization by specific assignment or informal information sharing. In either case, you would assist in diffusing information to individuals who need to know.

Management and the Impact of Leadership Changes

Internal and external leadership changes may well impact the strategy and progress of healthcare technology management. It seems obvious to say that leadership change within a healthcare organization may well result in a change in strategic direction. A leadership change may alter current initiatives and increase the level of sources provided. Conversely, current initiatives may have their funds and staffing cut or eliminated. It is important for managers to be aware of this possibility and be ready to defend their projects with current, well-organized information. Leadership change within legislative bodies can have a similar impact on projects in progress especially in regard to current and future funding.

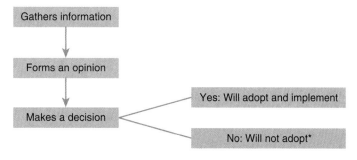

*Negative decisions may not be final.

Figure 29.4 Process Flow: Leadership Decision Stages

WRAP-UP

Summary

The rate of change has accelerated in the digital age of health care. The IMPACT Act's reform legislation resonates across these four provider settings and beyond. It sets an interoperable quality- and vision-based vision of reform. While change is inevitable, it seems these PAC provider changes are in step with future patient-centered goals.

Key Terms

Cross-Setting
Electronic Health Record
 (EHR)

Interoperability
IMPACT Act
Post-Acute Care (PAC)

Standardized Data
Value-Based Program

Discussion Questions

1. Are you familiar with a post-acute care facility?
2. If so, how do you think these legislative requirements have affected that facility?
3. Do you think the requirements to standardize data and achieve interoperability are a good idea?

Notes

1. P. L. 113-185 Sec. 2(a); also Centers for Medicare and Medicaid Services (CMS), "The IMPACT Act of 2014 and Data Standardization," *MLN Connects* (October 21, 2015), p. 5.
2. "The IMPACT Act of 2014 and Data Standardization," p. 4.
3. 80 Federal Register 46462 (August 4, 2015).
4. P. L. 113-185 Sec. 3(a)(1-2).
5. SSA Title XVIII Sec. 1899B (i)(1-3).
6. "The IMPACT Act of 2014 and Data Standardization," p. 5.
7. Ibid., p. 6.
8. Ibid., p. 6.
9. Sec. 1899B (e)(1)(A-C).
10. "The IMPACT Act of 2014 and Data Standardization," p. 10.
11. Ibid.
12. 80 FR 68668 (November 5, 2015).
13. Sec. 1899B (b)(1)(B).
14. Sec. 1899B (c)(1)(A-E).
15. Sec. 1899B (d)(2)(A-C).
16. Sec. 1899B (c)(2)(A).
17. "The IMPACT Act of 2014 and Data Standardization," p. 37.
18. National Quality Forum, "Measure Applications Partnership," http://www.qualityforum.org/setting_priorities/partnership/measure_applications_partnership.aspx.
19. Sec. 1888 (e)(6)(A)(i).
20. "The IMPACT Act of 2014 and Data Standardization," p. 33.
21. Ibid.
22. Sec. 1899B (g)(1-4).
23. Ibid.
24. CMS, "Fact Sheet: Nursing Home Compare Five-Star Quality Rating System," http://www.cms.gov/medicare/provider-enrollment-and-certification/certificationandcomplianc/downloads/consumerfactsheet.pdf, accessed July 8, 2016.
25. CMS.gov, "CMS Announces Two Medicare Quality Improvement Initiatives," http://www.cms.gov/Newsroom/MediaReleaseDatabase/Press-releases/2014-items/2014-10-06.html, accessed October 6, 2014.
26. Ibid.
27. D. Bowman, "ONC Interoperability Road Map Draft," p. 2, http://www.fiercehealthit.com/story/onc-interoperabiliity-road-map-draft-outlines-governance-certification-stand/2014-10-14, accessed October 14, 2014.
28. "The IMPACT Act of 2014 and Data Standardization," p. 18.
29. 80 FR 68668 (November 5, 2015).
30. "The IMPACT Act of 2014 and Data Standardization," p. 19.
31. HealthIT.gov, "Newsroom: About ONC," http://www.healthit.gov/newsroom/about-onc, accessed July 7, 2016.
32. "ONC Interoperability Road Map Draft," p. 1.
33. *Merriam Webster's Collegiate Dictionary*, 10th ed., s.v. "Innovation."
34. E. M. Rogers, *Diffusion of Innovations*, 4th ed., (New York: The Free Press, 1995), xvii.

CHAPTER 30

ICD-10: Finance and Strategic Challenges

PROGRESS NOTES

After completing this chapter, you should be able to:

1. Describe the difference between ICD-9 and ICD-10.
2. Explain the six benefits of ICD-10.
3. Understand how the change to ICD-10 codes is a technology problem and provide three types of implementation costs.
4. Describe how key performance indicators are used.

Overview: The ICD-10 Coding System

The International Classification of Diseases, 10th Revision (ICD-10) is designed to "promote international comparability in the processing classification and presentation of mortality statistics."[1] The ICD is the international standard diagnostic classification for all general epidemiological issues, health management purposes, and clinical use.[2] This classification system was developed by collaboration among the World Health Organization (WHO) and 10 international centers. ICD-11 is slated to be effective January 1, 2022, use in the United States continues to be studied.

ICD-10-CM and ICD-10-PCS Codes

The National Center for Health Statistics (NCHS) was one of the international centers collaborating with the WHO in the development and revisions of the ICD. The NCHS is an agency within the Centers for Disease Control and Prevention (CDC) and is responsible for use of the ICD-10 in the United States.

WHO owns the ICD-10 copyright and has "authorized the development of an adaptation of ICD-10 for use in the United States for U.S. government purposes."[3] The NCHS has developed a clinical modification of the ICD-10, termed

"ICD-10-CM." The ICD-10-CM replaces the ICD-9-CM. The ICD-10-CM diagnosis classification system has been developed for use in all types of healthcare treatment settings in the United States.[4]

Meanwhile, the Centers for Medicare and Medicaid Services (CMS) has developed a procedure classification system, termed the "ICD-10-PCS," for use in inpatient hospital settings within the United States. ICD-10 was first endorsed in 1990, and it was implemented in the United States on October 1, 2015.

Providers and Suppliers Impacted by the ICD-10 Transition

The change from ICD-9 to ICD-10 had a ripple effect that impacted nearly every corner of the healthcare industry in the United States. The companies and organizations impacted by the ICD-10 transition include inpatient providers, outpatient providers, and an array of support services and suppliers.

Figure 30.1 illustrates the entities affected by the ICD-10 transition. Inpatient providers impacted include both hospitals and nursing facilities. Outpatient providers include, at a minimum, physician offices, outpatient care centers, medical diagnostic and imaging services, home health services, other ambulatory care services, and durable medical equipment providers.

Support services and suppliers include health insurance carriers and third-party administrators, along with the vendors who provide computer system design and related services.[5] Note that pharmacies, both chain and independent, are substantially impacted by the required electronic transaction standards updates for pharmacies, while ICD-10 adoption is generally more of a peripheral issue for pharmacies.

E-Record Standards and the ICD-10 Transition

Version 5010 of electronic transmission standards includes infrastructure changes that were necessary to prepare for the adoption of ICD-10. A whole array of sequential rules and regulations has evolved over the past two decades to create electronic transaction standards and require their adoption. A full description of the rules and regulations is beyond the scope of this text;[6] however, two items are of interest:

1. It was necessary to update many electronic transaction standards to accommodate the new **ICD-10 codes**. The groups, or sets, of codes (termed "standard medical data code sets")[7] to be used in those electronic transactions also had to be updated.

2. When the CMS staff compute transition costs, they divide some of these costs

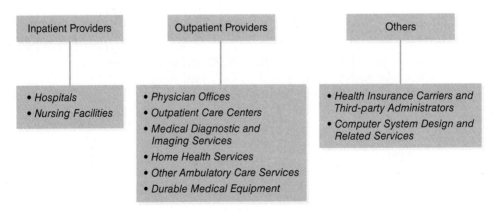

Figure 30.1 Providers and Suppliers Impacted by the ICD-10 Transition

between the updating of transaction standards such as Version 5010, which they argue would have to occur anyway, versus the cost of adopting and implementing the ICD-10 codes. We will be referring to this cost-splitting in a later discussion of implementation costs.

ICD-10 Benefits and Costs

The ICD-10 transition process will require management decisions that take both costs and benefits into account. A brief summary follows.

Benefits

Managers will need to account for what their own organization will realize in conversion savings as benefits. CMS identified six benefits of transitioning to ICD-10:

- More accurate payments for new procedures
- Fewer rejected claims
- Fewer improper claims
- Improved disease management
- Better understanding of health conditions and healthcare outcomes
- Harmonization of disease monitoring and reporting worldwide[8]

The conversion to Version 5010 also recognizes three types of benefits, including operational savings (better standards), cost savings (increase in electronic claims transactions), and operational savings (increase in use of auxiliary transactions).[9]

Managers should also decide what potential governmental financial assistance might be available to their organization. The ICD-10 conversion is, of course, part (but not all) of this adoption process. It is therefore logical for management to consider part of the financial incentives offered as relating to this system conversion when analyzing benefits. The ARRA legislation described in previous chapters provides financial incentives for the timely adoption of electronic health records.

Costs

Management must make decisions about major costs incurred in the ICD-10 transition including adoption and cash flow disruption costs. Some costs will be one-time costs, while other costs will be recurring costs, and both should be considered in the decision-making process.[10]

Three Types of ICD-10 Adoption Costs

CMS acknowledges that transition costs from ICD-9-CM to ICD-10 code sets are unavoidable and will be incurred in addition to the **Version 5010 standards** conversion costs.[11] Three recognized costs of ICD-10 adoption costs are the following:

1. System changes
2. Training costs
3. Productivity losses

CMS believed that large providers and institutions will most likely need to make system changes and software upgrades. However, CMS also believed small providers may only need software upgrades.[12] This belief is based upon findings that the majority of small providers have simplistic systems.[13] Details about training costs and productivity losses are addressed within this chapter. Thus, systems conversion to Version 5010 recognizes two similar types of cost: system implementation costs and transition costs.[14]

Cash Flow Disruption Costs

Code set transition has a learning curve for all users. It is to be expected that a greater proportion of claims will be rejected during this implementation that will reduce cash flow and should be taken into account when decisions are made about implementation costs and benefits. If certain contracts contain stipulations as to ICD-9 codes, these contracts may have to be renegotiated. The much greater specificity of the ICD-10 codes may make such renegotiation necessary in certain cases, and cash flow from contracts may be disrupted in the interim.

ICD-10 Implementation: Systems and Technology Issues

ICD-10 implementation affected numerous computerized systems and created complex technology issues. The ICD-10 technology changes that we will discuss in the following section impacted a broad variety of systems and applications. It is important for the manager to fully understand the breadth and depth of change required by the technological transition from ICD-9 to ICD-10. **Figure 30.2** illustrates the types of systems and applications that had to change.

Twenty-five different examples of systems and applications are contained in Figure 30.2, divided into three categories as follows:

1. Necessary revisions to vendor software and systems
2. Systems that use ICD data to model or calculate patient needs, staffing, and so on
3. Specifications that need to be revised[15]

Necessary Revisions to Vendor Software and Systems for Transition from ICD-9 to ICD-10 include:

Ambulatory systems
Billing systems
Patient accounting systems
Physician office systems
Practice management systems
Quality measurement systems

Emergency department software
Contract management programs
Reimbursement modeling programs

Financial functions such as:
Code assignment
Medical records abstraction
Claims submission
Other financial functions

Systems used to model or calculate are also impacted by the use of ICD-10 code sets:

Acuity systems
Decision support systems and content
Patient care systems
Patient risk systems
Staffing needs systems
Selection criteria within electronic medical records
Presentation of clinical content for support of plans of care

Specifications that will need to be revised for ICD-10 use include specifications for:

Data file extracts
Reporting programs and external interfaces
Analytic software that performs business analysis
Analytic software that provides decision support analytics for financial and clinical management
Business rules guided by patient condition or procedure

Figure 30.2 Systems and Applications Affected by the ICD-10 Change

Reproduced from 74 Federal Register 3348-9 (January 16, 2009).

Understand Technology Issues and Problems

Examining the details of ICD-10 code set changes will help you more fully understand the technological problems that management faced in this transition. The scope of change is illustrated in the next three exhibits. There were approximately 13,000 ICD-9-CM diagnosis codes; ICD-10-CM has approximately 68,000 diagnosis codes, more than a 500% increase. ICD-9-CM diagnosis codes had three to five characters in length, while ICD-10-CM's codes are three to seven characters. The increase means input fields had to be lengthened to accommodate seven characters. In addition, ICD-9-CM's first digit may be alpha (E or V) or numeric and digits two to five are numeric, while ICD-10-CM's first digit is alpha, digits two and three are numeric, and digits four to seven are alpha or numeric. This change means reprogramming was required for many applications. **Exhibit 30.1** sets out a comparison of

Exhibit 30.1 Comparison of ICD-9-CM and ICD-10-CM Diagnosis Codes

ICD-9-CM Diagnosis Codes	ICD-10-CM Diagnosis Codes
3–5 characters in length	3–7 characters in length
Approximately 13,000 codes	Approximately 68,000 available codes
First digit may be alpha (E or V) or numeric; Digits 2–5 are numeric	Digit 1 is alpha; digits 2 and 3 are numeric; Digits 4–7 are alpha or numeric
Limited space for adding new codes	Flexible for adding new codes
Lacks detail	Very specific
Lacks laterality	Has laterality
Difficult to analyze data due to nonspecific codes	Specificity improves coding accuracy and richness of data for analysis
Codes are nonspecific and do not adequately define diagnoses needed for medical research	Detail improves the accuracy of data used for medical research
Does not support interoperability because it is not used by other countries	Supports interoperability and the exchange of health data between other countries and the United States

Reproduced from 73 Federal Register 49803 (August 22, 2008).

ICD-9-CM versus ICD-10-CM diagnosis codes. The exhibit includes six benefits of the new code set in addition to the three differentials previously discussed in this paragraph.[16]

Comparison of ICD-9-CM and ICD-10-PCS Procedure Codes

There were approximately 3,000 ICD-9-CM procedure codes; ICD-10-PCS has approximately 87,000 procedure codes, or 29 times more. ICD-9-CM procedure codes were three to four numbers in length, while ICD-10-CPS's characters are alpha-numeric and seven characters. This again means input fields had to be lengthened to accommodate seven characters and possibly reprogrammed to accept alpha characters. **Exhibit 30.2** sets out a comparison of ICD-9-CM versus ICD-10-PCS procedure codes. The exhibit includes seven benefits of the new code set in addition to the two differentials previously discussed in this paragraph.[17]

Comparison of Old and New Angioplasty Codes

Exhibit 30.3 sets out one example of the proliferation of codes. In the ICD-9-CM, angioplasty had one code (39.50). In ICD-10-PCS, angioplasty has 1,170 codes.[18] *The Wall Street Journal* used this example in a headline: "Why We Need 1,170 Angioplasty Codes."[19] The original 1,170 codes were subsequently reduced to 874, as shown in Exhibit 30.3.

ICD-10 Implementation: Training and Productivity Costs

CMS identified three types of individuals who would require varying levels of training on ICD-10: coders, **code users**, and physicians.

Coders

It was vital that coders received adequate training on the ICD-10 coding changes. CMS, therefore,

Exhibit 30.2 Comparison of ICD-9-CM and ICD-10-PCS Procedure Codes

ICD-9-CM Procedure Codes	ICD-10-PCS Procedure Codes
3–4 numbers in length	7 alpha-numeric characters in length
Approximately 3,000 codes	Approximately 87,000 available codes
Based upon outdated technology	Reflects current usage of medical terminology and devices
Limited space for adding new codes	Flexible for adding new codes
Lacks detail	Very specific
Lacks laterality	Has laterality
Generic terms for body parts	Detailed descriptions for body parts
Lacks description of methodology and approach for procedures	Provides detailed descriptions of methodology and approach for procedures
Limits DRG assignment	Allows DRG definitions to better recognize new technologies and devices
Lacks precision to adequately define procedures	Precisely defines procedures with detail regarding body part, approach, any device used, and qualifying information

Reproduced from 73 Federal Register 49803 (August 22, 2008).

Exhibit 30.3 Comparison of Old and New Angioplasty Codes

ICD-9-CM Angioplasty Code: 39.50 (1 code)
ICD-10-PCS Angioplasty Codes: 854 codes specifying body part, approach, and device, including:
047K04Z Dilation of right femoral artery with drug-eluting intraluminal device, open approach
047K0DZ Dilation of right femoral artery with intraluminal device, open approach
047K0ZZ Dilation of right femoral artery, open approach
047K34Z Dilation of right femoral artery with drug-eluting intraluminal device, percutaneous approach
047K3DZ Dilation of right femoral artery with intraluminal device, percutaneous approach

Reproduced from CMS, "ICD-10-CM/PCS: The Next Generation of Coding," ICN #901044 (June 2015).

estimated training costs for both full-time and part-time coders. In producing cost estimates, CMS assumed that full-time coders were primarily dedicated to hospital inpatient coding and that part-time coders worked in outpatient ambulatory settings. The difference is based on the job setting for a reason. CMS further assumed that all coders will need to learn ICD-10-CM, while the coders who work in the hospital inpatient job setting will also need to learn ICD-10-PCS.[20]

Code Users

CMS refers to the American Health Information Management Association (AHIMA) definition of code users as "anyone who needs to have some level of understanding of the coding system, because they review coded data, rely on reports that contain coded data, etc., but are not people who actually assign codes."[21] These users can be people who are outside healthcare facilities (individuals such as researchers, consultants, or auditors) or inside a healthcare facility but not coders. Such facility users might include upper-level management, business office and accounting personnel, clinicians and clinical departments, or corporate compliance personnel.[22]

Physicians

CMS believed that the majority of physicians did not work with codes and thus would not need training. The initial assumption was that only one in 10 physicians would require such knowledge. CMS also believed that physicians would probably obtain the needed training through continuing professional education courses that they would attend anyway.[23]

Costs of Training

ICD-10 training costs were estimated for each category described previously: coders, code users, and physicians.

Coder Training Costs

CMS initially assumed:

1. There were 50,000 full-time hospital coders who would need 40 hours of training per coder on ICD-10-CM and ICD-10-PCS. The 40 hours of training was estimated to cost $2,750, including lost work time of $2,200, plus $550 for the expenses of training, for a total of $2,750 per coder.
2. Training of full-time coders would start the year before ICD-10 implementation. It was further assumed that 15% of training costs would be expended in this initial year, 75% would be expended in the year of implementation, and the remaining 10% would be expended in the year after implementation.
3. There were approximately 179,000 part-time coders who would require training only on ICD-10-CM (and not on ICD-10-PCS). The part-time coders' training expense would amount to $110 for the expenses of training, plus $440 for lost work time, for a total of $550.[24]

Code Users Training Costs

CMS estimated there were approximately 250,000 code users, of which 150,000 would work directly with codes. Each code user was estimated to need eight hours of training at $31.50 per hour or approximately $250 apiece.[25]

Physician Training Costs

CMS estimated there were approximately 1.5 million physicians in the United States, of which one in 10 would require training. Each physician was estimated to need four hours of training at $137 per hour or approximately $548 apiece.[26]

Costs of Lost Productivity

CMS used a productivity loss definition as follows: "The cost resulting from a slow-down in coding bills and claims because of the need to learn the new coding systems."[27] Thus, the productivity loss slowdown reflects the extra staff hours that are needed to code the same number of claims per hour as prior to the ICD-10 conversion. For instance, Jane normally codes 24 inpatient claims per day; during the first month learning the new system, she slows down to 22 claims per day.

CMS estimated that inpatient coders would incur productivity losses for the first six months after ICD-10 implementation; it further estimated that productivity would increase (and losses thus decrease) month by month over the initial six-month period until by the end of six months, productivity had returned to its former level. It was estimated that inpatient coders would take an extra 1.7 minutes per inpatient claim in the first month. At $50 per hour, 1.7 minutes equates to $1.41 per claim; $50.00 per hour divided by 60 minutes equals $0.8333 per minute times 1.7 minutes equals $1.41 per claim.

CMS assumed the same six-month productivity loss period for outpatient coders. CMS further assumed that outpatient claims require much less time to code. In fact, the initial assumption was that outpatient claims would take one-hundredth of the time for a hospital inpatient claim. Thus, one-hundredth of the inpatient 1.7 minute productivity loss equals 0.017 minutes. At the same $50 per hour, one-hundredth of the $1.41 inpatient loss equals $0.014 per claim, or about 1.5 cents. The reasoning for this small amount of coding time per claim is that physician offices "may use preprinted forms or touch-screens that require virtually no time to code."[28]

Key Performance Indicators for ICD-10

Key performance indicators (KPIs) reveal problems regarding ICD-10 implementation and maintenance. The problems may affect productivity and/or cash flow.[29] The ICD-10 KPIs are typically used for two purposes: The KPIs track opportunities for improvement and progress in transitioning, maintaining, and updating ICD-10 within the organization.

Using KPIs to Improve Performance

Improvements include system revisions and/or enhancements, plus staff training to increase productivity and/or reduce errors.[30] The following KPIs are grouped into six categories; the first two categories contain "essential indicators" all organizations should track.[31]

Four Essential Claims Indicators

These four indicators should be available to you as they report claim submission and payment performance:

Days to final bill: The number of days from time of service until the provider generates and submits claims

Days to payment: The number of days from the time the claim is submitted until the provider is paid

Claims acceptance/rejection rates: The percentage of claims that are accepted or rejected during payer "front-end" edits. Front-end edits are those a payer performs before the claim is entered into the payer's adjudication system.

Claims denial rate: The percentage of claims accepted into the payer's adjudication system that are denied

Two Essential Payment and Reimbursement Indicators

These KPIs can provide a picture of payment amounts received per service and the rate of reimbursement against amounts billed.

Payment amounts: Payment amounts that your organization receives for specific services, especially high-volume and resource-intensive services

Reimbursement rate: Cents on the dollar that your organization receives on claims versus the amount billed

Four Coder Productivity Indicators

Productivity is measured by various methods as follows:

Coder productivity: The number of medical records coded per hour. This indicator should be reviewed separately for each coder.

Volume of coder questions: The number of records that coders returned to clinicians with requests for more documentation needed to support proper code selection. Again, reviewing this indicator separately for each coder may reveal whether a problem exists with an individual coder or with a particular professional or department generating the source records.

Requests for additional information: The number of requests from payers asking for additional information required to process claims. Reviewing this indicator separately by payer may highlight specific coding issues.

Daily charges or claims: The number of charges or claims submitted per day.

This is a pure productivity indicator for the department.

Three Internal Error Indicators

These indicators concern the individuals or departments that generate the initial information that coders use:

Incomplete or missing charges: The number of incomplete or missing charges, analyzed either by the week or by the month. Again, separate reviews of particular departments will highlight problems to be solved.

Incomplete or missing diagnosis codes: The number of incomplete or missing ICD-10 diagnosis codes on orders. If ICD-10 implementation is running smoothly, this indicator should be close to zero. Problems, on the other hand, could be with either individuals generating the information or the software they are using.

Use of unspecified codes: The volume and frequency of unspecified code use. The use of unspecified codes may be perceived as a time-saving maneuver, but it should be tracked and corrected. Unspecified codes cause revenue losses.

Four External Error Indicators

These indicators concern actions by entities outside your own organization:

Clearinghouse edits: This indicator can be approached in two ways: First, obtain and review the number and content of edits that are required by clearinghouses. Second, obtain and review the number of claims either accepted or rejected by clearinghouses.

Payer edits: The number and reason for edits required by payers

Return to provider (RTP)/fiscal intermediary shared system (FISS) volumes: The number of rejections in the RTP/FISS volumes

Medical necessity pass rate: The rate of acceptance (or rejection) of claims with medical necessity content

A Positive Usage Indicator

This indicator reveals best practices within the coding field:

Use of ICD-10 codes on prior authorizations and referrals: The number of orders and referrals that include ICD-10 codes

Using KPIs to Track ICD-10 Implementation Progress

The first step in assessing ICD-10 implementation is to choose the particular KPIs that you intend to use. You may choose from the KPIs listed in **Exhibit 30.4**. Your next steps are as follows.[32]

Establish Baselines

It is necessary to establish baselines, or points of comparison, for each of your chosen indicators. These baselines should be pre-implementation—that is, from a period shortly before your organization implemented ICD-10 codes. If so, you will be able to compare pre- and post-implementation results for your assessment purposes.

Track Your Chosen Indicators

To properly assess KPIs, it is desirable to track your chosen indicators on a periodic preset schedule, for example, monthly, quarterly, or semiannually. The schedule should be reasonable as to the timing of assessment dates.

Compare Against Baselines

Comparison of pre–ICD-10 implementation versus post–ICD-10 implementation is an essential

Exhibit 30.4 **Checklist for Assessing ICD-10 Progress: Key Performance Indicators**

- Number of days to final bill
- Number of days to payment
- Claims acceptance/rejection rates
- Claims denial rate
- Payment amounts
- Reimbursement rate
- Coder productivity
- Volume of coder questions
- Payer requests for additional information
- Daily charges or claims
- Incomplete or missing charges
- Incomplete or missing diagnosis codes
- Use of unspecified codes
- Clearinghouse edits
- Payer edits
- RTP/FISS volumes
- Medical necessity pass rate
- Use of ICD-10 codes on prior authorizations & referrals

Modified from CMS, "ICD-10: Next Steps for Providers—Assessment & Maintenance Toolkit."

to identify transition problems. Comparisons should also review early transition outcomes to later outcomes to gauge improvement. You might find significant improvement in some areas and virtually no improvement or deterioration in other areas.

Review Results

Some revisions may be desirable after tracking has been in place for several cycles. You may find that you are able to break results into smaller segments for more detailed results. For example, you may decide to keep separate track of authorization denials versus coding denials. Detail about reviewing such results appears in the following section.

Reviewing KPI Results

Taken together, the four essential indicators about claims and the two payment and reimbursement indicators provide a snapshot of your ICD-10 implementation progress and ongoing performance. When these six performance indicators from your baseline pre-implementation are compared to results post-implementation, problem areas that require action should be highlighted. It is also good practice to compare indicators such as "days to final bill" and "days to payment" against national or regional standards. If your organization is part of a multi-facility system, it is also a good practice to compare facility-specific results within the system.

Review Coder Productivity and Internal Error Indicator Results

The four coder productivity indicators provide an overview of the internal department or division responsible for coding. If your organization uses an outside billing service, then the important indicator would be "requests for additional information." The outside billing service's requests for more information would be coming back to somewhere in your organization and would indicate a problem.

The three internal error indicators relate to places and people within the organization other than coders. If a claim has incomplete or missing charges and/or diagnosis codes, then the coders cannot complete the claim and submit it for payment. In other words, the problem exists elsewhere, segmenting the review by departments assists in identifying problem area(s).

Review External Error Indicator Results

Claims are sent back by either payers or clearinghouses for further edits. These indicator results may be a people or computer system issue. In either case, the result is unpaid claims, and the reason or reasons need to be addressed. The financial impact of external errors should be quantified, and the review should be segmented by department to explore ways of reducing rejections.

Allow for Feedback

Build a formal system for feedback regarding performance indicator results. One proven method is to create an "issues list" that resides in a single location. Responsibility for providing the related feedback must then be formally designated.

Creating Action Plans to Deal With Problems

The KPIs are likely to reveal a series of different problems that will vary in severity. Thus, it makes sense to create a set of action plans to deal with this variety.

What Is an Action Plan?

An action plan consists of a series of steps (actions) that are intended to bring about positive change. Each step should be able to answer the following questions:

- What actions or changes will occur?
- Who will carry out these actions or changes?
- When will they take place, and for how long?
- What resources (such as funding and staff) are needed to carry out the actions or changes?
- How will information regarding the actions or changes be communicated (who should know what)?[33]

What Makes a Good Action Plan?

To be successful, your action plan needs to be complete, clear, and current. "Complete" means that the plan lists all the relevant action steps required to accomplish the desired actions or changes. "Clear" means that the plan clearly answers the "who, when, what, and communication" questions. "Current" concerns whether the plan actually contains current work.[34] In other words, has the plan anticipated and addressed recently emerging issues, or is it already behind the times by the time it is released?

Building Specific Action Plans to Correct Deficiencies

Action plans typically point toward solutions. Different KPIs are designed to measure performance in different areas that impact productivity, payment, and cash flow, the following issues all require some type of solution.[35]

Isolate Internal Coding Problems

- What codes are causing the most difficulty? What is the particular difficulty, and where within the organization does it originate?
- Who selects diagnosis codes, and who makes sure the codes adhere to guidelines (clinicians, billers, certified coders, others)?
- Would chart audits support selection of a particular ICD-10 code?
- When KPIs expose coding productivity issues, who is responsible for initiating supplemental training and subsequent tracking to assess improvement? If such improvements are not forthcoming, what is the next step?

Isolate Internal Systems Problems

- Are system deficiencies regarding the ICD-9/ICD-10 transition not yet corrected?
- Are adjustments for annual ICD-10 updates not yet in place (i.e., overdue)?
- Have all systems implemented all available upgrades?
- Are there departmental "silo" issues? (In other words, do IT and coding supervisors regularly communicate?)

External Coding and Payer Action Plan Issues

Action plans provide structure while working to resolve issues with your payers and your external systems vendors. Producing the relevant data from your KPI process will serve to reinforce the concerns that you are expressing.

Isolate External Coding and Payer Problems

- Is code selection driven by vendor templates? If so, is this acceptable? Can it be changed? If not, why not? Who is responsible for finding out?
- Is the external systems vendor slow to install coding updates to your system? If so, who is responsible for pressuring the vendor to comply? What is the plan if such efforts fail?
- If KPIs expose a reoccurring claim edit and/or rejection problem with a particular payer, who is responsible for addressing and resolving the issue with the payer? Under what time frame?
- If KPIs expose consistently slow payments from a particular payer, who is responsible for researching and resolving the issue? If such efforts fail, what is the next step?

Isolate External Systems Problems

- If KPIs expose productivity problems due to an outside systems vendor, is that vendor responsive to your organization's problems? If not, why not?
- Do contractual obligations with the system vendor hinder making changes? Is there a reasonable solution? Who is responsible for negotiating such a solution?
- Does the outside systems vendor provide experienced professionals to work with your staff or is your organization a training ground for the vendor's new employees? Is vendor support a problem significant enough to justify inclusion in an action plan?

Untangling Internal Versus External Performance Problems: An Example

It is sometimes difficult to determine whether the root cause of a performance problem is inside or outside the organization. This example centers upon the KPI for claims acceptance/rejection rates. For instance, certain problem areas can be isolated by computing the number of days in your accounts receivable for each payer. Problem areas can best be revealed by tracking the age of claims for each payer in 30-day intervals (e.g., how many of payer 1's claims are 0–30 days old, 31–60 days, 61–90 days, 91–120 days, and over 120 days? What about payer 2 and so on?).

In our experience, receiving payment for claims older than 90 days is questionable; these old claims should be red flags in your assessment. If you break down your aging assessment by payer, the culprits' red flags should be very evident. It may be that these old claims sitting in your accounts receivable are claims rejected by your payer. On the one hand, does this payer have an extraordinary number of rejected claims, and if so, why? Who is responsible for revising and refiling rejected claims in the organization? How many claims cannot be resubmitted as the date for doing so has passed?

Another possibility is that the old claims residing in your accounts receivable are actually denied claims. Again, does the payer have an extraordinary number of denied claims, and if so, why? Should secondary payers be pursued? If they haven't been pursued, who is responsible, and why haven't they been doing so? Finally, managers should determine if the claims are viable, and if not, they should be written off the books as bad debts.

Understanding the Lines of Authority

As in the preceding example, it is helpful to clearly understand the lines of authority concerned with your issues. In other words, what department, office, division, or individual is in charge of the procedures that you are attempting to improve? What is the chance that this department, office, division, or individual will cooperate? It is likely that some member of the task force or one of your supervisors should be able to help define the applicable lines of authority that are relevant.

WRAP-UP

Summary

ICD-10 has been implemented, but managers should still understand the benefits and costs of implementation of new systems as ICD-11 may be right around the corner. The chapter also highlights the need for managers to implement effective claim review processes to monitor implementation progress and improve day-to-day performance post-implementation.

Key Terms

Code Users
ICD-10 Codes

Key Performance Indicator (KPI)

Version 5010 of Standards

Discussion Questions

1. Describe the difference between ICD-9 and ICD-10.
2. Explain the six benefits of ICD-10.
3. Describe how the change to ICD-10 codes was a technology problem and provide three types of implementation costs.
4. Describe how key performance indicators (KPIs) can be used to assess system implementation and upgrades and ongoing performance.

Notes

1. National Center for Health Statistics, International Classification of Diseases, Tenth Revision (ICD-10), http://www.cdc.gov/nchs/about/major/dvs/icd10des.htm.
2. World Health Organization, Classifications, http://www.who.int/classifications/icd/en/
3. National Center for Health Statistics (NCHS), About the International Classification of Diseases, Tenth Revision, Clinical Modification (ICD-10-CM), http://www.cdc.gov/nchs/icd/icd10cm.htm.
4. CMS, "ICD-10-CM-PCS Fact Sheet."
5. 74 Federal Register (FR) 3357 (January 16, 2009).
6. CMS, "New Health Care Electronic Transactions Standards Versions 5010, D.0, and 3.0," Medicare Learning Network Fact Sheet ICN #903192 (January 2010).
7. 74 Federal Register (FR) 3328 (January 16, 2009).
8. 73 Federal Register (FR) 49821 (August 22, 2008).
9. Ibid., 49769.
10. Ibid., 49811.
11. Ibid., 49813.
12. Ibid., 49818.
13. Ibid., 49829.
14. Ibid., 49769.
15. 74 Federal Register (FR) 3348-9 (January 16, 2009).
16. 73 Federal Register (FR) 49803 (August 22, 2008).
17. Ibid.
18. CMS, "ICD-10-CM-PCS Fact Sheet."
19. J. Zhang, "Why We Need 1,170 Angioplasty Codes," *Wall Street Journal*, November 11, 2008.
20. 73 Federal Register (FR) 49814-5 (August 22, 2008).
21. Ibid., 49815-6.
22. Ibid., 49815.
23. Ibid., 49816.
24. Ibid., 49815.
25. Ibid., 49816 and 74 Federal Register (FR) 3346-7 (January 16, 2009).
26. Ibid., 49816.
27. M. Libicki and I. Brahmakulam, *The Costs and Benefits of Moving to the ICD-10 Code Sets* (Santa Monica, CA: RAND Corporation, 2004), http://www.rand.org/pubs/technical_reports/2004/RAND_TR132.pdf.
28. 73 Federal Register (FR) 49817 (August 22, 2008).
29. CMS, "ICD-10 KPIs at a Glance," http://www.cms.gov/Medicare/Coding/ICD10/Downloads/ICD10KPIs20160309.pdf, accessed March 9, 2016.
30. CMS, "ICD-10 Next Steps for Providers: Assessment & Maintenance Toolkit," https://www.cms.gov/Medicare

/Coding/ICD10/Downloads/ICD10Next
StepsToolkit20160226.pdf, accessed February 26, 2016.

31. Certain KPI information within this section may be modified and/or condensed from "ICD-10 Next Steps... Assessment & Maintenance Toolkit."

32. Ibid.

33. Work Group for Community Health and Development at the University of Kansas, "Developing an Action Plan," http://ctb.ku.edu/table-of-contents/structure/strategic -planning/develop-action-plans/main, accessed July 14, 2016.

34. Ibid.

35. Some concepts within this section may be modified and /or condensed from "ICD-10 Next Steps."

PART VIII

Case Studies

The cases are designed to test the reader's mastery of the concepts and tools provided in multiple chapters to extract actionable information from the provided data and convey their findings effectively to others (i.e., given the information and situation, what should be done?). The cases go beyond the chapter problems in that the reader will have to develop multiple inputs to reach a conclusion and provide recommendations. Each case provides students with a set of tasks to complete that builds in a step-by-step manner to address the key issue in the case and the necessary data to complete the required work. In most cases, a template is provided for calculations and to record findings.

The cases provide the issue under consideration, historical financial information and assumptions, and needed deliverables (i.e., the required analyses and the analyst's interpretations and conclusions). The case studies attempt to bridge the gap between real-world applications and the classroom. The end-of-chapter problems were designed to be straightforward, providing all the data needed to complete required analyses in a short period of time. The case studies require a more comprehensive understanding of finance to develop the inputs needed to complete them, explain the financial situation, and justify the recommended action, so they are more time-consuming. The cases require the ability to identify key variables, recognize how these variables can affect the outcome, and convey the riskiness of the recommended action to decision-makers.

The cases are designed to provide a "real-world experience" without getting bogged down in data acquisition problems that are often the hardest part of any analysis. As such, the cases often lack the specific information needed to make definitive recommendations on action, such as adding, expanding, contracting, or eliminating a specific service. When you encounter a lack of information problem, whether in the real world or in a case study, one of your recommendations should be to collect more information. This recommendation should be specific (i.e., exactly what information do you need, and how will you use it?).

Note to instructors: Given the availability of information on the internet, I recommend that key variables such as output, reimbursement, and/or expenses be altered to create unique solutions for each case.

CHAPTER 31

Break-Even Analysis

Background and Issue

The trend in physician services has been toward consolidation into hospital-led integrated delivery systems, and physicians who desire to remain independent are increasingly building larger, multi-physician practices. Pat Harrison is a physician and the managing partner of Harrison Medical Practice, an independent three-physician multispecialty practice with admitting privileges at both major hospitals in their area. All three doctors are middle-aged and living comfortable lives. They are contemplating opening another three-physician practice on the other side of town. They have directed you, the office manager, to prepare a financial analysis for the new practice. The new practice will be structured similarly to the existing practice (i.e., same staffing and services), so your starting point is the current and past income statements of the practice. The issue is should the doctors invest in the new practice, and can the new practice provide enough patient visits to justify investment?

Financial Data and Assumptions

Table 31.1 provides the income statement for the last completed fiscal year and shows that the existing practice is profitable. The $82,350 net income is shared equally among the three doctors,

potentially increasing their salary by $27,450 each. Decisions on distributing net income or retaining it to improve the current practice and/or invest in new endeavors are based on unanimity among the doctors (i.e., each must approve of the use of funds before action is taken). All the physicians believe investments should increase practice income in the long run but recognize that short-term losses may be required when adding services and equipment or building a new practice.

Patient Volume

The existing practice has provided roughly 18,000 patient visits per year over the past several years, and the doctors expect the proposed practice most likely should provide 16,000 visits in its first startup year. The best-case projection is 17,000 visits, and the worst-case projection is 15,000 visits. The most likely estimate assumes some patients of the existing practice will go to the new location as it will be located closer to their homes, but all lost patient visits at the existing practice will be replaced by new patients and/or more visits by existing patients. You estimate the probability of reaching 16,000 at the new practice is 70%, best-case probability is 20%, and worst-case probability is 10%.

After the first year, patient visits in the proposed practice are expected to increase by 500 per year until 18,000 patients are served in year 5 (**Table 31.2**). Like the existing practice,

Table 31.1 Income Statement

	FY 2023
Revenue	$1,162,350
Expenses	
Staff salaries and benefits	$300,000
Physician salaries and benefits	540,000
Supplies	150,000
Equipment and facility expenses	60,000
Other expenses	30,000
	$1,080,000
Profit	$82,350
Patient visits	18,000

Table 31.2 Projected Patient Visits

Year	Projected Patient Visits
1	16,000
2	16,500
3	17,000
4	17,500
5	18,000

the physicians believe 18,000 patients per year is the optimal patient load based on time and space constraints.

Reimbursement

The existing practice charges $105 per visit and collected $1,362,350 in total revenue or $64.58 per patient visit in 2023. **Table 31.3** shows the current reimbursement rates, percent of patients reimbursed by payer, and projected payer mix at the new practice. The new practice will be opened in an older and less affluent section of town, and the percentage of Medicare and Medicaid patients is expected to be higher with a corresponding decrease in managed care and commercial patients.

Table 31.3 Reimbursement and Payer Mix

Payer and Reimbursement		Existing Payer Mix %	Projected Payer Mix %
Medicare	$52.50	50%	55%
Managed Care	$73.50	35%	30%
Commercial	$105.00	10%	5%
Medicaid	$42.00	5%	10%
	$68.25	100%	100%

Operating Expenses

Four out of the five operating expenses for the current practice—staff and physician salaries and benefits, supplies, equipment and facility expenses, and other expenses—are considered fixed. While physician salaries and benefits are considered fixed costs, the three doctors being practice owners share any net income or loss from the practice. The only variable cost is supply expenses.

The proposed practice's expenses are shown in **Table 31.4**. Physician salaries are expected to be lower than the existing practice as it is anticipated that three newly graduated doctors will be hired at a lower base salary than the partners. It is

Table 31.4 Projected Practice Expenses

Expenses	Startup Year 1	Year 2
Staff salaries and benefits	$300,000	$300,000
Physician salaries and benefits	480,000	480,000
Supplies	133,333	137,500
Equipment and facility expenses	80,000	60,000
Other expenses	40,000	30,000
	$1,033,333	$1,007,500

anticipated that two of the new doctors will work in the new clinic and one will work in the existing practice as one of the partners will shift to the new clinic to provide oversight as it will be located closer to his residence. Equipment and facility and other expenses are expected to be higher during the first startup year and then be the same as the existing practice in following years.

Deliverables

1. Calculate the weighted average reimbursement for a patient visit in the proposed clinic.
2. Calculate the variable cost per patient visit in the proposed clinic.
3. Calculate startup year 1 break-even quantity (BE$_Q$).
4. Calculate startup year 1 net income if actual patient visits are 16,000 (most likely), 15,000 (worst case), and 17,000 (best case).
5. Calculate startup year 1 expected net income if the most likely probability is 70%, best case 20%, and worst case 10%.
6. Calculate year 2 net income assuming patient visits increase to 16,500, staff and physician salaries are unchanged, equipment and facility expense decreases by $20,000, and other expenses decreases by $10,000.
7. Prepare the recommendation for the three partners including a discussion of best and worst possible outcomes.

Optional: Incorporate expected increases in reimbursement, +2%, and expenses, physician salaries increase by $5,000 per year, supplies, equipment, and other 3%, into future years.

CHAPTER 32

Ratios and Operating Indicators

Background and Issue

Barton Medical Center is a 309-bed nonprofit teaching hospital located in a major urban area. The board of directors is concerned that the low profitability of the medical center will not provide sufficient capital for future expansion and improvements. The board has asked the CFO for a review of the last four years of operations for the board meeting next month. The CFO has delegated the task to you and provided income statements, balance sheets, and operating statistics for fiscal years 2019 through 2022 and benchmarks for 2022. The key issue is how Barton is performing relative to its peer group and, if improvements are needed, where actions be taken.

Financial Data

Table 32.1 shows that Barton earned $5.5 million in net income in 2019, suffered a large drop in 2020, and almost completely recovered by 2021. In 2022, net income increased to $7.2 million; however, since 2020, other revenue has exceeded net income.

Table 32.2, the balance sheet, shows that total assets have declined by $4.1 million since 2019. The decrease could be alarming but for the fact that liabilities fell by $18.4 million over the same time period. Overall, net worth has increased by $14.3 million since 2019.

Table 32.3, operating statistics, shows decreasing discharges and patient days but an increasing CMI. Outpatient revenue per encounter and the number of encounters are increasing. Total FTEs are increasing, and inpatient FTEs are decreasing.

Table 32.4 provides peer group benchmarks based on Barton's location and teaching status.

Table 32.5, "Expenses by Department," provides the total expenses from 2019 through 2022 by department.

Table 32.1 Barton Medical Center Income Statement (millions)

Revenue	2019	2020	2021	2022
Inpatient revenue	$125.4	$119.7	$121.9	$118.9
Outpatient revenue	121.9	120.9	129.2	138.6
Other revenue	2.9	3.1	8.2	10.5
Total Revenue	$250.2	$243.7	$259.3	$268.0
Expenses				
Salaries	$105.6	$107.2	$109.6	$111.9
Fringe benefits	22.3	21.8	23.2	24.0
Supplies	51.1	49.5	53.0	54.5
Rent	3.4	3.3	3.5	3.6
Depreciation	10.8	10.5	11.2	11.6
Interest	7.8	7.3	6.8	6.5
Other expense	43.7	42.4	46.6	48.7
Total Expense	$244.7	$242.0	$253.9	$260.8
Net Income	$5.5	$1.7	$5.4	$7.2

Table 32.2 Barton Medical Center Balance Sheet (millions)

Assets	2019	2020	2021	2022
Cash	$11.8	$11.7	$12.3	$12.7
Accounts receivable	40.2	39.5	44.7	42.7
Inventory	18.7	18.6	19.3	21.1
Property, plant, and equipment	215.0	213.2	225.5	235.7
Investments	135.0	133.2	108.7	97.3
Other assets	53.2	52.6	56.8	60.3
Total Assets	$473.9	$468.8	$467.3	$469.8
Liabilities				
Accounts payable	$38.30	$41.20	$44.30	$45.10
Long-term debt	155.9	146.2	136.2	130.7
Total Liabilities	$194.20	$187.40	$180.50	$175.80
Net Worth	$279.70	$281.40	$286.80	$294.00

Table 32.3 Barton Medical Center Operating Statistics

	2019	2020	2021	2022
Licensed beds	309	309	309	309
Total discharges	12,645	12,066	12,385	12,406
Patient days	65,754	63,949	64,400	63,272
CMI	1.43	1.45	1.46	1.49
Medicare discharges	27,682	27,178	27,756	27,523
Medicaid discharges	3,682	3,709	3,928	3,923
Net outpatient revenue	$250.00	$709.00	$282.94	$318.60
Outpatient encounters	554,091	565,173	576,476	588,006
Total FTEs	1,778	1,801	1,821	1,845
Inpatient FTEs	902	896	884	852

Table 32.4 2022 Peer Group Benchmarks

Financial Ratios	Median	25th Percentile	75th Percentile
Total margin	4.4%	−0.2%	9.7%
Operating margin	3.8%	−0.8%	9.1%
Return on equity (ROE)	8.4%	1.2%	18.0%
Return on assets (ROA)	4.5%	−0.1%	10.4%
Days in accounts receivable	56.1	46.8	70.5
Equity financing	57.5%	35.2%	79.2%
Times interest earned	4.7	0.9	13.1
Total asset turnover	1.2	0.8	1.7
Current asset turnover	3.7	2.4	5.1
Fixed asset turnover	2.7	1.9	4.3
Operating Indicators	**Median**	**25th Percentile**	**75th Percentile**
Occupancy	60.1%	40.4%	70.1%
Discharges per bed	36.2	21.7	49.5
ALOS	4.7	4.1	7.2
Medicare % discharges	40.5%	31.0%	53.2%
Medicaid % discharges	5.6%	1.9%	12.9%
Outpatient revenue %	58.4%	44.2%	71.5%

(continues)

Table 32.4 2022 Peer Group Benchmarks   (continued)

Financial Ratios	Median	25th Percentile	75th Percentile
Salaries per FTE	$58,180	$55,222	$61,859
I/P FTEs per occupied bed	4.2	3.2	4.5
Salaries as % of total expense	41.8%	34.6%	44.7%
Deductible ratio	63.7%	49.8%	71.5%
Net price per discharge	$11,054	$9,004	$14,339
Cost per discharge	$10,162	$7,789	$14,673

Table 32.5 Expenses by Department (millions)

Expenses	2019	2020	2021	2022
Administration	$29.4	$29.7	$31.2	$32.7
Finance	$13.7	$13.5	$14.0	$14.5
Housekeeping	$11.0	$10.5	$10.8	$11.2
Material management	$8.6	$8.7	$9.0	$9.2
Laundry	$7.3	$6.9	$7.2	$7.4
Med/surg nursing units	$53.8	$53.2	$59.1	$58.7
Intensive care	$17.1	$16.9	$17.3	$17.9
OB-nursery	$7.3	$7.5	$7.4	$7.6
Operating and recovery rooms	$12.2	$12.1	$12.5	$12.9
Laboratory	$14.7	$14.5	$14.8	$15.3
Radiology	$17.1	$16.8	$17.3	$17.7
Pharmacy	$19.6	$20.2	$21.1	$22.5
Emergency department	$13.5	$13.7	$13.9	$14.1
Respiratory therapy	$9.8	$9.6	$9.9	$10.2
Physical and occupational therapy	$8.6	$8.2	$8.4	$8.9
Total Expense	$244.7	$242.0	$253.9	$260.8

Deliverables

1. Calculate the financial ratios and operating statistics and comment on the ratios and operating indicators that have increased or decreased by 10% or more since 2019.

Financial Ratios	Benchmark	2019	2020	2021	2022
Total margin	4.4%	_____	_____	_____	_____
Operating margin	3.8%	_____	_____	_____	_____
Return on equity (ROE)	8.4%	_____	_____	_____	_____
Return on assets (ROA)	4.5%	_____	_____	_____	_____
Days in accounts receivable	56.1	_____	_____	_____	_____
Equity financing	57.5%	_____	_____	_____	_____
Times interest earned	4.7	_____	_____	_____	_____
Total asset turnover	1.2	_____	_____	_____	_____
Current asset turnover	3.7	_____	_____	_____	_____
Fixed asset turnover	2.7	_____	_____	_____	_____
Operating Indicators	**Benchmark**	**2019**	**2020**	**2021**	**2022**
Occupancy	60.1%	_____	_____	_____	_____
Discharges per bed	36.2	_____	_____	_____	_____
ALOS	4.7	_____	_____	_____	_____
Medicare % discharges	40.5%	_____	_____	_____	_____
Medicaid % discharges	5.6%	_____	_____	_____	_____
Outpatient revenue %	58.4%	_____	_____	_____	_____
Salaries per FTE	$58,180	_____	_____	_____	_____
I/P FTEs per occupied bed	4.2	_____	_____	_____	_____
Salaries as % of total expense	41.8%	_____	_____	_____	_____
Deductible ratio	63.7%	_____	_____	_____	_____
Net price per discharge	$11,054	_____	_____	_____	_____
Cost per discharge	$10,162	_____	_____	_____	_____

2. Calculate and evaluate the compound growth rates for revenue, expense type, and department expenses from 2019 through 2022.
3. Compare Barton's 2022 financial ratios and operating indicators with the benchmarks provided in the template provided in part 1 and discuss any ratio or indicator where hospital performance deviates by +/–10% or more from the benchmarks. Create graphs to highlight important factors, trends, and large changes.
4. Identify areas for improvement and prepare recommendations.

CHAPTER 33

Budgeting

Background and Issue

The CEO of Barton Medical Center has rejected the recently assembled incremental budget as she does not believe it accurately projects resource needs. Specifically, she notes inpatient discharges are expected to decline and outpatient encounters are expected to increase so an incremental budget may provide too many or too few resources to caregivers. The CEO has requested the CFO prepare two flexible budgets, one for inpatient and one for outpatient services. The CEO knows the board of directors is concerned about the low profitability of inpatient and outpatient services and wants suggestions of how to increase profitability. The issue or goal is to construct a budget that supplies the appropriate level of resources based on output produced.

Financial Data and Assumptions

The initial and rejected 2023 budget was created by annualizing the year-to-date (YTD) actual revenues and expenses, the first six months of 2022, and inflating these amounts for expected increases in output and inputs prices (**Table 33.1**). The incremental budget projected a $6.8 million net income due primarily to $11.2 million in

non-patient revenues. The projected net income is considerably lower than planned in the 2022 budget but is comparable to 2022 YTD net income.

Inpatient services were budgeted to generate a $46,000 net income in the first six months of 2022 but declining discharges, 99 or 1.58% fewer discharges than budgeted, lower revenue, and higher expenses produced a loss of $2.081 million (**Table 33.2**). If performance for the rest of the year follows the first six months, the total loss for inpatient services will be $4.162 million. Similarly, outpatient services experienced a more modest decline in encounters, 338 or 0.11% fewer than budgeted, but had higher revenue and higher expenses, resulting in a loss of $319,000 versus an expected net income of $54,000.

Deliverables

The CFO has delegated to you the responsibility for creating the flexible budget and provided an income statement that separates inpatient and outpatient revenues and expenses (Table 33.2). You need to do the following:

1. Explain why actual net income is $2.081 million under budget.
2. Create the preliminary flexible budgets for inpatient and outpatient areas based on 12,200 forecasted discharges and 611,072

Table 33.1 Barton Medical Center Rejected 2023 Incremental Budget (millions)

Revenue	2022 Budget	2022 YTD Actual	2023 YTD Budget	2022 YTD Actual Annualized	2023 Inflation Factor	2023 Incremental Budget
Inpatient revenue	$123.656	$60.500	$61.828	$121.000	2.0%	$123.420
Outpatient revenue	145.530	73.400	72.765	146.800	4.0%	152.672
Other revenue	11.550	5.400	5.775	10.800	4.0%	11.232
Total Revenue	$280.736	$139.300	$140.368	$278.600		$287.324
Expenses						
Salaries	$115.257	$58.900	$57.600	$117.800	3.0%	$121.334
Fringe benefits	24.720	13.300	12.540	26.600	6.0%	28.196
Supplies	56.135	27.600	28.100	55.200	2.0%	56.304
Rent	3.708	1.900	1.900	3.800	0.0%	3.800
Depreciation	11.948	5.900	6.000	11.800	0.0%	11.800
Interest	6.695	3.200	3.300	6.400	2.0%	6.528
Other expense	50.161	25.500	25.100	51.000	3.0%	52.530
Total Expense	$268.624	$136.300	$134.540	$272.600		$280.492
Net Income	$12.112	$3.000	$5.828	$6.000		$6.832
Discharges	12,530	6,166	6,265	−99	−1.58%	12,200
O/P encounters	599,766	299,545	299,883	−338	−0.11%	611,072

outpatient encounters and the inflation factors used in the rejected incremental budget (Table 33.1). After the flexible budgets are created, roll them up with the other revenue estimate from Table 33.1 to create the master budget for Barton.

3. Compare the preliminary flexible budget with the initial incremental budget and explain the major changes.

4. Draft suggestions for enhancing profitability including changes in volume, revenue enhancements, and/or cost reductions.

5. Restate the flexible budget for actual volumes assuming the 2023 fiscal year has ended and actual inpatient discharges and outpatient encounters are 12,260 and 610,233.

Table 33.2 YTD Financial Performance by Revenue Line (millions)

	YTD 2022 I/P Actual	YTD 2022 I/P Budget	YTD 2022 O/P Actual	YTD 2022 O/P Budget
Total Revenue	$60.500	$61.828	$73.400	$72.765
Expenses				
Salaries	$27.043	$26.446	$31.857	$31.154
Fringe benefits	6.107	5.779	7.193	6.761
Supplies	12.672	12.902	14.928	15.198
Rent	0.872	0.872	1.028	1.028
Depreciation	2.709	2.755	3.191	3.245
Interest	1.469	1.515	1.731	1.785
Other expense	11.708	11.524	13.792	13.576
Total Expense	$62.581	$61.794	$73.719	$72.746
Net Income	−$2.081	$0.034	−$0.319	$0.019
Profit margin	−3.44%	0.07%	−0.44%	0.07%
Discharges	6,166	6,265		
O/P encounters			299,545	299,883

CHAPTER 34

Variance Analysis

Background and Issue

Financial performance for Barton Medical Center is running lower than expected for the first six months of 2022. Two members of the board of directors want to understand the causes of the lower performance and what can be done to increase net income. The CFO has delegated the task to you and provided income statements and operating statistics for the medical center. Supplemental financial reports have been created for inpatient and outpatient services so a better understanding of the performance of the two primary business lines can be achieved (i.e., are the lower financial results due to changes that affect inpatient, outpatient, or both revenue lines?). You should note that the budgeted net income, $5.9 million, was due almost entirely to the $5.8 million budgeted other revenues. Inpatient and outpatient services were budgeted at break-even. The issue is to identify why net income is lower than budgeted and determine how financial performance can be improved.

Financial Data and Assumptions

Tables 33.1 and **33.2** provide the year-to-date income statement for Barton and the supplemental report on the profitability of the inpatient and outpatient areas.

Deliverables

1. Calculate price (revenues), cost (expenses), and volume variances for the medical center using discharges as the output variable.
2. Calculate price, cost, and volume variances for inpatient services using discharges as the output variable.
3. Calculate price, cost, and volume variances for outpatient services using outpatient encounters as the output variable.
4. Describe the changes in output, revenue, and expenses for inpatient and outpatient services.
5. Prepare recommendations for increasing net income.

Table 34.1 Year-to-date Income Statement (millions)

Revenue	2021	YTD Actual 2022	YTD Budget 2022	$ Variance	% Variance
Inpatient revenue	$118.9	$60.5	$61.8	–$1.3	–2.1%
Outpatient revenue	138.6	73.4	72.8	0.6	0.8%
Other revenue	10.5	5.4	5.8	–0.4	–6.9%
Total Revenue	$268.00	$139.30	$140.40	–$1.10	–0.8%
Expenses					
Salaries	$111.9	$58.9	$57.6	$1.3	2.3%
Fringe benefits	24.0	13.3	12.5	0.8	6.1%
Supplies	54.5	27.6	28.1	–0.5	–1.8%
Rent	3.6	1.9	1.9	0.0	0.0%
Depreciation	11.6	5.9	6.0	–0.1	–1.7%
Interest	6.5	3.2	3.3	–0.1	–3.0%
Other expense	48.7	25.5	25.1	0.4	1.6%
Total Expense	$260.8	$136.3	$134.5	$1.8	1.3%
Net Income	$7.2	$3.0	$5.9	–$2.9	–48.5%
Discharges	12,406	6,166	6,265	–99	–1.6%
O/P encounters	588,006	299,545	299,883	–338	–0.1%

Table 34.2 Year-to-Date Income Statement for Inpatient and Outpatient Services (millions)

	2022 YTD I/P Actual	2023 YTD I/P Budget	$ Variance	2022 YTD O/P Actual	2023 YTD O/P Budget	$ Variance
Revenue	$60.500	$61.800	–$1.300	$73.400	$72.800	$0.600
Expenses						
Salaries	$27.043	$26.446	$0.597	$31.857	$31.154	$0.703
Fringe benefits	$6.107	$5.739	$0.367	$7.193	$6.761	$0.433
Supplies	$12.672	$12.902	–$0.230	$14.928	$15.198	–$0.270
Rent	$0.872	$0.872	$0.000	$1.028	$1.028	$0.000
Depreciation	$2.709	$2.755	–$0.046	$3.191	$3.245	–$0.054
Interest	$1.469	$1.515	–$0.046	$1.731	$1.785	–$0.054
Other expense	$11.708	$11.524	$0.184	$13.792	$13.576	$0.216
Total Expense	$62.581	$61.754	$0.826	$73.719	$72.746	$0.974
Net Income	–$2.081	$0.046	–$2.126	–$0.319	$0.054	–$0.374
Discharges	6,166	6,265				
O/P encounters				588,006	299,545	299,883

CHAPTER 35

Capital Budgeting

Background and Issue

Barton Medical Center is evaluating whether to build an air ambulance service. One of the positive outcomes of the Vietnam War was the use of helicopters to evacuate wounded soldiers and improve health outcomes. The golden hour is used to describe the higher probabilities for survival when care is rendered within 60 minutes of injury. In the United States, large numbers of people lack quick access to a level 3 trauma center, and investing in helicopter transport is cheaper than building a trauma center within 30 miles of every citizen.

The metropolitan area that Barton serves has two for-profit air ambulance providers, but citizens have voiced strong concerns over the prices charged for service. The board and senior management believe a third nonprofit provider would reduce time to treatment and could put downward pressure on prices thus garnering public support. The board and senior management also believe the investment will raise the public profile for other hospital services. The non-pecuniary benefits are believed to be large, but the financial condition of Barton—that inpatient and outpatient services are losing money—requires that at a minimum the service recover all its costs if not increase the net income of the organization. The issue is to determine if adding an air ambulance service will be financially advantageous for Barton Medical Center.

Financial Data and Assumptions

Barton's capital expenditures are typically evaluated over a five-year horizon, and the board requires that the weighted average cost of capital be used as the discount rate. The following discussion summarizes the thoughts of the finance and planning departments on the expected output of the service, monetary benefits including additional revenues and avoided costs, capital expenditures, and operating expenses.

Expected Monetary Benefits

The largest benefit from an air ambulance service is the revenues generated from transporting patients. Transport fees range from $50 to $250 per mile not including liftoff fees. Management believes an average price of $80 per mile would differentiate the service from the higher-cost services in the area. The $80 charge, however, will not be collected from most patients. Medicare typically pays 60% of billed charges, Medicaid 40%, and little to no reimbursement is collected from the poor and uninsured. The CFO believes a net price of $40 per mile is obtainable given the projected patient mix. In addition, a $400 liftoff fee is charged. The CFO again believes only $200 on average will be collected. Future reimbursement is expected to increase by 2% annually.

The anticipated number of inbound transports is two per day, 365 days per year. The average trip is 50 miles one-way, and the mileage fee is charged one-way. Inbound transports are expected to increase 2% annually.

In additional to the liftoff and mileage fees, expanding the geographic reach of the hospital is expected to generate two additional inpatient discharges that otherwise would have been transported and admitted to other hospitals. Therefore, in addition to transport fees, there are also the revenue and costs of these cases. Currently, the average reimbursement is lower than cost for inpatients, but the CFO notes after considering that rent, depreciation, and interest expense are fixed costs, the marginal cost of inpatient treatment is about $630 less than reimbursement, and this should be included as a monetary benefit. Although reimbursement is expected to increase 2% annually, expenses are expected to increase by 3%, so the net benefit from these additional discharges should decrease by 1% annually.

Currently 120 patients are transferred to other hospitals every year due to lack of service or overcapacity. The hospital must stabilize these patients prior to transfer, receives little revenue for services, and incurs high costs for these patients. Under Medicare regulations, the intake hospital receives the lion's share of reimbursement. The finance department estimates the hospital loses an average of $2,000 for every transfer to another hospital. It is anticipated that roughly 40 transfers per year can be avoided by transporting the patient directly to another hospital when a service is at capacity or the service is not provided at Barton. In addition, another 40 patients are expected to be more quickly transferred from the emergency department (ED) when services are unavailable, reducing the amount of expenses incurred prior to transfer. Finance estimates that faster transfer could save $1,000 per patient. No transport fees are charged for outbound patients. Similar to inbound transports, the number of outbound transports is expected to increase by 2% annually, and the expected cost savings should increase by 3% annually.

Capital Costs and Financing

The purchase price for the helicopter is $2,000,000, plus construction of the helipad is estimated at $400,000. As $110 million is currently held in cash and investments, the purchase will not require any additional debt.

Operating Expenses

The typical flight crew will be a pilot, flight nurse, and paramedic. On occasion, a physician may be required, but given the rarity of this event, no physician salary should be included in the operating expenses. Pilots are expected to earn an average of $75,000 in salary plus 25% for fringe benefits; four pilots will be hired. Flight nurses and paramedics are expected to earn $70,000 and $40,000 plus 25% for fringe benefits. A designated flight nurse and paramedic will be stationed in the ED around the clock, seven days per week, so four of each will be employed. It is assumed 70% of these nurses' and paramedics' time will be spent providing medical services in the ED, so only 30% of their salaries and fringe benefits should be allocated to the air ambulance service.

The cost of medical supplies and onboard equipment is estimated at $50 per inbound transport.

Fuel consumption is estimated at 1/10 gallon per mile at a cost of $5.00 per gallon. Fuel expense should be based on 92,250 total miles, which includes 73,000 inbound miles, 800 outbound miles, and 18,450 miles for training and other purposes.

The helicopter manufacturer offers two maintenance options. The first is an inclusive contract for 15% of the helicopter purchase price covering all needed repairs and maintenance. The second is per service used. Helicopter maintenance expense typically ranges from $2.00 to $4.00 per mile. The CFO believes a cost of $3.00 per mile should be used for the non-contract maintenance expense.

Air ambulances have higher accident rates than other helicopters due to the emergency nature of their cases because they often fly in adverse conditions that ground other helicopters. Insurance is estimated at 7.5% of the helicopter purchase price. The insurance covers the crew, helicopter, and other liability.

Although the purchase will be paid out of cash and/or investments, the CFO believes the air ambulance service should be allocated interest expense based on Barton's current capital structure, the percent of assets funded by debt (total liabilities ÷ total assets), interest expense (interest expense ÷ total liabilities), and the total capital outlay (**Table 35.1**).

No depreciation expense should be included as the cash outlay will occur in year 0 and no tax savings will be received as Barton is a nonprofit organization.

All expenses are expected to increase 3% annually.

Best-Case and Worst-Case Estimates

Table 35.2 reports the best- and worst-case estimates developed by finance and planning for inbound transports, average reimbursement based on payer mix assumptions, operating expenses, and future growth rates.

Table 35.1 Financial Statements

Balance Sheet		Income Statement	
Assets	**2022**	**Revenue**	**2022**
Cash	$12.7	Inpatient revenue	$118.9
Accounts receivable	42.7	Outpatient revenue	138.6
Inventory	21.1	Other revenue	10.5
Property, plant, and equipment	235.7	Total Revenue	$268.0
Investments	97.3		
Other assets	60.3	**Expenses**	
Total Assets	$469.8	Salaries	$111.9
		Fringe benefits	24.0
Liabilities		Supplies	54.5
Accounts payable	$45.1	Rent	3.6
Long-term debt	130.7	Depreciation	11.6
Total Liabilities	$175.8	Interest	6.5
		Other expense	48.7
		Total Expense	$260.8
Net Worth	$294.0		
		Net Income	$7.2

Table 35.2 Best-Case, Most Likely, and Worst-Case Estimates

Estimates	Best Case	Most Likely	Worst Case
In-bound transports	910	730	510
Average reimbursement (per mile)	$50.00	$40.00	$35.00
Total salaries	$480,000	$540,000	$640,000
Supplies (per in-bound transport)	$45.00	$50.00	$60.00
Maintenance (per mile)	$2.00	$3.00	$4.00
Growth rate, output	3.0%	2.0%	1.0%
Inflation rate, output prices	4.0%	2.0%	0.0%
Inflation rate, expenses (not maintenance)	1.0%	3.0%	5.0%

Deliverables

The CFO has delegated preparing the capital budget request to you. You must do the following:

1. Calculate the discount rate, which will be the weighted cost of capital, so ROE and the cost of debt must be calculated.

2. Create a five-year capital budgeting worksheet and calculate the internal rate of return (IRR) and net present value (NPV).
3. Calculate the expected IRRs and NPVs using (1) best-case inbound transports and average reimbursement and (2) worst-case inbound transports and average reimbursement.
4. Prepare recommendations.

Glossary

Accountable Care Organization (ACO) An organization consisting of a group of providers who have joined together voluntarily to provide coordinated, quality care to patients.

Accounting System Records the evidence that an economic event has occurred in the healthcare financial system.

Accrual Basis Accounting Revenue is recorded when it is earned, not when payment is received. Expenses are recorded when they are incurred, not when they are paid. The opposite of accrual basis accounting is cash basis accounting.

Action Plan A detailed plan of operations that shows how one part of a particular objective will be accomplished.

Alternative Payment Model (APM) Provides new methods of payment by Medicare for physicians and other eligible professionals (a.k.a. eligible clinicians).

Amortization Schedule Reports the amount paid on interest and principal in each loan payment.

Annualization To convert data to an annual (12-month) period.

Annuity A series of equal payments made or received over time.

Assets The net value of what an organization owns.

Balance Sheet One of the four basic financial statements. Generally speaking, the balance sheet records what an organization owns, what it owes, and what it is worth at a particular point in time.

Base Year A 12-month unit of time (one year) used as a basis for comparison.

Baseline Period A unit of time (period) used as a basis for comparison.

Benchmarking The continuous process of measuring products, services, and activities against the best levels of performance. Best levels may be found inside or outside of the organization.

Big Data A very large data set that is typically used for analysis to reveal patterns and/or trends.

Bonds A financial instrument where the purchaser expects to receive a certain amount of annual interest and that the bonds will be redeemed on a certain date.

Book Value The book value (also known as net book value) of a fixed asset is a balance sheet figure that represents the remaining undepreciated portion of the fixed asset cost.

Break-Even Analysis A method for determining the number of units of output that must be sold to recoup fixed and variable costs, i.e., the output where net income is $0.

Break-Even Point The point when the contribution margin (i.e., net revenues less variable costs) equals the fixed costs.

Budget The organization-wide instrument through which activities are quantified in financial terms.

Budget Standard The budgeted input cost per output, i.e., the cost standard inflated for expected price increases in the budget year.

Bundled Payment A reimbursement system that combines payment for pre-admission, inpatient, and post-discharge services into a single payment.

Business Plan A document that is typically prepared in order to obtain funding and/or financing.

Buy-or-Lease Decisions A decision aimed at reducing the cost of acquiring equipment by comparing the total cost of owning or leasing the equipment.

Capital Represents the financial resources of the organization. Generally considered to be a combination of debt and equity.

Capital Budget or Capital Expenditure Budget A budget usually intended to plan, monitor, and control long-term financial issues.

Capital Structure Means the proportion of debt versus equity within the organization. The phrase "capital structure" refers to the debt–equity relationship.

Capital Structure Ratios Ratios that reflect the ability of the organization to pay the annual interest and principal obligations on its long-term debt and its reliance on debt.

Capitalized Asset An asset placed on the balance sheet.

Capitation or Capitation Reimbursement A reimbursement system that pays a provider a fixed payment typically per month for all required care.

Case Mix Adjustment A performance measure that has been adjusted for the acuity level of the patient and, presumably, the resource level required to provide care.

Cash Basis Accounting A transaction does not enter the books until cash is either received or paid out. The opposite of cash basis is accrual basis accounting.

Cash Flow Analysis This type of analysis illustrates how the project's cash is expected to move over a period of time.

Cash Flow Statement A financial statement reporting the cash generated and used by operations, investing, and financing activities and the beginning and ending cash balance for an organization.

Census The total number of patients in a hospital typically at midnight.

Certificate of Need (CON) A program to control excess capacity in the form of facility overbuilding.

Chart of Accounts Maps out account titles in a uniform manner through a method of numeric coding.

Code Users Any individual who needs to have some level of understanding of the coding system, but does not actually assign codes.

Column or Bar Chart A column chart places different groups on the x-axis and their number or rate on the y-axis, a bar chart places the groups on the y-axis and their number or rate on the x-axis, both are used to compare groups.

Common Sizing or Vertical Analysis Process of converting dollar amounts to percentages to put information on the same relative basis. Also known as vertical analysis.

Common Stock Stocks represent equity, or net worth, in a company. Common stock typically pays a proportionate share of net income out as a dividend to its investors.

Composite Performance Score See also Composite Score.

Composite Score An overall score assembled from multiple scores, or parts.

Compound Growth Rates the rate of growth for a series over multiple years.

Contribution Margin Called this because it contributes to fixed costs and to profits. Computed as net revenues less variable costs.

Controlling and Directing Making sure that each area of the organization is following the plans that have been established.

Cost The amount of cash expended (or property transferred, services performed, or liability incurred) in consideration of goods or services received or to be received.

Cost-Profit-Volume A method of illustrating the break-even point, whereby the three elements of cost, profit, and volume are accounted for within the computation.

Cost and Volume (Two-Variance) Analysis A variance analysis method that divides total variance between the amount due to changes between budgeted and actual output (volume) and the cost of per output.

Cost Center A responsibility center where output and quality are measurable and the manager controls the mix of inputs used to produce the output; manager should be evaluated on minimizing the cost per output.

Cost Object Any unit for which a separate cost measurement is desired.

Cost Reimbursement A reimbursement system that pays providers their cost of producing the service rather than the price of the service.

Cost Standard The cost per output during the expenditure base (year-to-date actual, budget, or last completed fiscal year).

Cost Variance The amount of the total variance due to changes in the budgeted and actual cost per output.

Cross-Setting Allowing information to flow back and forth among different types of facilities (thus "across settings").

Cumulative Cash Flow The accumulated effects of cash inflows and cash outflows are added and/or subtracted to show the overall net accumulated result.

Current Asset Turnover A financial ratio that assesses the use of current assets. Computed by dividing total revenue by current assets.

Current Ratio A liquidity ratio considered to be a measure of short-term debt-paying ability. Computed by dividing current assets by current liabilities.

Data Analytics The process of mining data to discover patterns, correlations, and other related information, primarily in order to make better decisions.

Data Mining The process used by organizations to turn raw data into useful information.

Days Cash on Hand A liquidity ratio that indicates the number of days of operating expenses represented in the amount of unrestricted cash on hand. Computed by dividing unrestricted cash and cash equivalents by the cash operating expenses divided by number of days in the period.

Days in Accounts Receivable A liquidity ratio that represents the number of days in receivables. Computed by dividing net receivables by net credit revenues divided by number of days in the period.

Debentures Bonds that are unsecured. Debentures are backed by revenues that the issuing organization can earn.

Debt Service Coverage Ratio A solvency ratio universally used in credit analysis to measure ability to pay debt service. Computed by dividing change in unrestricted net assets (net income) plus interest, depreciation, and amortization by maximum annual debt service.

Decile A distribution into 10 classes, each of which contains one-tenth of the whole; any one of the 10 classes is a decile.

Define, Measure, Analyze, Improve, and Control (DMAIC) A structured performance improvement approach that encourages, if not requires, problems and opportunities be thoroughly examined, solutions targeted to the factors most likely to produce the desired results, and performance continually monitored.

Denominator The bottom part of a fraction. The denominator indicates the total number of parts available to be divided. See also Numerator.

Depreciation Depreciation expense spreads, or allocates, the cost of a fixed asset over the useful life of that asset.

Diagnoses A common method of grouping healthcare expenses for purposes of planning and control. Such a grouping may be by major diagnostic categories or by diagnosis-related groups.

Diagnosis-Related Groups (DRGs) A system Medicare uses to classify and reimburse inpatient care.

Direct Costs These costs are incurred for the sole benefit of a particular operating unit. They can therefore be specifically associated with a particular unit or department or patient. Laboratory tests are an example of a direct cost.

Discounted Fee-for-Service (percent of charge) The provider of services is paid according to an agreed-upon contracted discount and after the service is delivered.

Double Declining Balance Depreciation A depreciation method that uses two times the straight-line depreciation rate but only applies the rate to the remaining book value of an asset.

Efficiency Variance The variance that calculates the amount of the total variance caused by differences in the amount of inputs budgeted and actually used to produce output.

Eight Wastes Overproduction, excess inventory, idleness (time waste), unnecessary transport, overprocessing, unnecessary motion, defects, and underutilized talent.

Electronic Health Record (EHR) A health-related electronic record of an individual that includes patient demographic and clinical information and that has the capacity to provide clinical decision support, support physician order entry, capture and query quality information, and exchange and integrate electronic health information. It is possible for this digital record to contain information about a patient's total health status across all providers.

Eligible Clinician Another term for Eligible Professional.

Eligible Professional (EP) In this context, physicians, practitioners, and other professionals who are eligible for payment in certain incentive programs.

Employee Turnover Rate The ratio of employees hired divided by total FTEs.

Equity Claims held by the owners of the business because they have invested in the business; what the business is worth on paper, net of liabilities.

Equity Financing Ratio Used to assess use of debt. Computed by dividing net worth by total assets.

Estimates A judgment that takes the place of actual measurement.

Evaluating The retrospective element of management where managers are assessed on their ability to achieve goals.

Expense Center A responsibility center where output and quality are not easily measured where the manager controls the mix of inputs used to produce the output, manager should be evaluated on their cost compared to similarly sized organizations.

Expenses Actual or expected cash outflows incurred in the course of doing business. Expenses are the costs that relate to the earning of revenue. An example is salary expense for labor performed.

Expired Costs Costs that are used up in the current period and are matched against current revenues.

Federal Deposit Insurance Corporation (FDIC) A federal agency that insures deposits in banks and thrift institutions for $250,000 per depositor.

Fee for Service The provider of services is paid according to the service performed and after the service is delivered.

Finance A set of theories and tools to guide the operation of an organization.

Financial Accounting Is generally for outside, or third-party, use and thus emphasizes external reporting.

Financial Lease A formal agreement that may be called a lease but is actually a contract to purchase. This type of lease must meet certain criteria.

Financial Projection "Projected" prospective financial statements that are often prepared to answer "what-if" questions. The statements "project" a view of future events, projects, or operations using a set of presumed, or hypothetical, assumptions.

First In, First Out (FIFO) The first-in, first-out inventory costing method recognizes the first costs placed into inventory as the first costs moved out into cost of goods sold when a sale occurs.

Fixed Asset Turnover A financial ratio that assesses the use of fixed assets. Computed by dividing total revenue by fixed assets.

Fixed Cell Reference A Excel feature that allows a user to specify that columns and/or rows are not incremented when the cell is copied across or down a worksheet by placing a $ in front of the column letter and/or row number.

Fixed Costs Those costs that do not vary in total when activity levels or volume of operations change. Rent expense is an example of fixed cost.

Flexible (preliminary and final) Budget A budget based on actual rather than forecasted volume. The preliminary flexible budget based on forecasted volume is restated or flexed at the end of the budget period based on actual output.

Flow A Lean six sigma principle seeking continuous movement in a process without delay or wasted motion.

Forecasts Information used for purposes of planning for the future. Forecasts can be short, intermediate, or long range.

For-Profit Organization A proprietary organization that is generally subject to income tax.

Full-Time Equivalent (FTE) A measure to express the equivalent of an employee (annualized) or a position (staffed) for the full time required.

Fund Balance The difference between net assets and net liabilities; a term generally used by not-for-profit organizations.

Future Value Determining the amount of money an investor will have in the future based on the amount invested, amount of time invested, and interest rate.

General Ledger A document in which all transactions for the period reside.

General Services Expenses This type of expense provides services necessary to maintain the patient, but the service is not directly related to patient care. Examples of general services expenses are laundry and dietary.

Goal A statement of aim or purpose that is part of a strategic plan.

Gross Domestic Product (GDP) A measure of the output of goods and services produced by labor and property located in the United States. The Bureau of Economic Analysis (BEA) is responsible for releasing quarterly estimates of the GDP.

Healthcare Analytics Data analytics applied to the healthcare industry.

Healthcare Delivery System A health system containing varying levels of care and multiple sites of service that deliver care under one integrated system.

Histogram A column chart that displays the distribution or frequency of occurrence of an outcome.

Horizontal Analysis The process of comparing and analyzing figures over several time periods. Also known as trend analysis.

ICD-10 Codes The International Classification of Diseases (ICD) is the international standard for diagnostic disease classifications. ICD-10 indicates the tenth revision.

IMPACT Act A legislative act that requires standardized patient assessment data be reported by four types of post-acute care facilities. Its full name is the "Improving Medicare Post-Acute Care Transformation Act of 2014."

Income Statement One of the four basic financial statements, this statement reports the inflow of revenue and the outflow of expense over a stated period of time. The difference is net income (loss).

Incremental (static or fixed) Budget A budget based on a single level of operations, or volume. After it is approved, the revenues and expenses are not adjusted if budgeted and actual output differ.

Indirect Cost These costs are incurred on behalf of the overall operation and therefore cannot be associated with the provision of specific health services. The finance office is an example of an indirect cost. Also known as joint costs.

Inflation An increase in the volume of money and credit relative to available goods and services resulting in a continuing rise in the general price level.

Inflation Factor A factor used in budgeting to increase budget year revenues and expenses for expected changes in prices.

Information System Gathers the evidence that some event has occurred in the healthcare financial system.

Information Technology (IT) Computer and telecommunications technology that organizes, processes, stores, retrieves, secures, and transmits information.

Internal Rate of Return A return on investment method, defined as the rate of interest that discounts future net inflows (from the proposed investment) down to the amount invested.

Interoperability The ability to operate, or transmit, across data systems used by different types of facilities.

Inventory All the items ("goods") that an organization has for sale in the normal course of its business.

Inventory Loss Ratio A ratio that assesses inventory management. Computed as the difference between actual inventory and reported inventory divided by reported inventory.

Inventory Turnover A ratio that shows how fast inventory is sold, or "turns over."

Investment Center A responsibility center where the manager has authority over input mix, product, mix, output prices and capital expenditures, manager should be evaluated on their ability to produce higher net income than other organization.

Jidoka Japanese term for "stop the line," indicates degree of authority given to employees to take action when problems arise.

Joint Costs These costs are incurred on behalf of the overall operation and therefore cannot be associated with the provision of specific health services. The finance office is a typical example of a joint cost. Also known as indirect cost.

Kaizen Japanese term for continuous improvement.

Kanban Japanese inventory system using two bins where the emptying of one bin signals need for replenishing supplies.

Key Performance Indicator (KPI) A step in a process that must be effectively completed to achieve desired goals.

Last In, First Out (LIFO) The last-in, first-out inventory costing method recognizes the latest, or last, costs placed into inventory as the first costs moved out into cost of goods sold when a sale occurs.

Lean Six Sigma A set of visual and statistical tools designed to improve performance and reduce defects.

Lease-Purchase A formal agreement that may be called a lease but is really a contract to purchase where the equipment must be recorded on the books of the organization as an asset on the balance sheet with a corresponding liability.

Liabilities What the organization owes.

Line or Area Chart A chart that displays performance over time with time on the x-axis and performance on the y-axis.

Liquidity Ratios Ratios that reflect the ability of the organization to meet its current obligations. Liquidity ratios are measures of short-term sufficiency.

Load Leveling A Lean concept seeking to ensure workers are neither over- or underworked by matching demand to time available, i.e., effective scheduling.

Loan Costs Those costs necessary to close a loan.

Long-Term Borrowing The use of debt in situation where the debt will not be repaid for more than 12 months.

MACRA A legislative act that reformed Medicare payment to physicians and certain eligible professionals (a.k.a. eligible clinicians). Its full name is the "Medicare Access and CHIP Reauthorization Act of 2015."

Major Diagnostic Categories (MDCs) A method for organizing diagnostic-related groups (DRGs) by body system, used in Medicare inpatient reimbursement.

Managed Care A means of providing healthcare services within a network of healthcare providers. The central concept is coordination of all healthcare services for an individual.

Managed Services Agreements A leasing arrangement where the lessor often bundles hardware, software, and maintenance and allows the lease to upgrade or downgrade equipment and change contract duration.

Managerial Accounting Is generally for inside, or internal, use and thus emphasizes information useful for managerial employees.

Marginal Cost The cost of the next unit produced (versus average cost). Calculated as the change in cost divided by the change in output.

Marketing Plan Specifies current and expected market size, units to be sold, prices, revenues, how customers will be reached, and obstacles to achieving goals.

Master Budget The aggregation of all department budgets, used to ensure an organization will have sufficient resources to complete desired goals.

Mean An average of numbers or values.

Meaningful Use (MU) Providers must show that they are "meaningfully using" their certified EHR technology by meeting thresholds, or minimums, for certain program objectives.

Measure Development Plan (MDP) A plan to develop quality measures that support the transition to new payment methods for physicians and certain other professionals.

Median The median occupies a position in a ranked series of values (numbers) in which the same number of values appears above the median as appear below it (or, in the case of an even number of values, the average of the two middle-ranked values).

Medicaid A federal and state matching entitlement program intended to provide medical assistance to eligible needy individuals and families. The program was established under Title XIX of the Social Security Act.

Medicare A federal health insurance program for the aged (and, in certain instances, for the disabled) intended to complement other federal benefits. The program was established under Title XVIII of the Social Security Act.

Merit-Based Incentive Program (MIPS) A value-based program that combines certain parts of existing quality reporting programs for physicians and certain eligible professionals (a.k.a. eligible clinicians).

Mission Statement A mission statement explains the purpose of the organization. It explains "what we are now."

Mode The number or value that appears the most frequently within a series of numbers or values.

Money Market Funds Investments in conservative instruments such as commercial bank CDs and Treasury bills.

Municipal Bonds Long-term obligations that are typically used to finance capital projects.

Net Present Value The difference between the discounted value of revenue and expenses.

Net Worth See Equity.

Nonproductive Time Paid-for time when the employee is not on duty—that is, not producing. Paid-for vacation days and holidays are examples of nonproductive time.

Nonprofit Organization Indicates the taxable status of the organization. A nonprofit (or voluntary) organization is exempt from paying income taxes.

Not-for-Profit Organization See Nonprofit Organization.

Numerator The top part of a fraction. The numerator indicates the total number of parts of the denominator taken. See also Denominator.

Occupancy The ratio of occupied beds to licensed hospital beds (sometimes staffed beds), calculated as patient days divided by licensed beds times 365 days.

Operating Budget A budget that generally deals with actual short-term revenues and expenses necessary to operate the facility.

Operating Lease A lease that is considered an operating expense and thus is treated as an expense of current operations. This type of lease does not meet the criteria to be treated as a financial lease.

Operating Margin A profitability ratio generally expressed as a percentage, the operating margin is a multipurpose measure. It is used for a number of managerial purposes and also sometimes enters into credit analysis. Computed by dividing operating income (loss) by total operating revenues.

Operations Expenses This type of expense provides service directly related to patient care. Examples of operations expenses are radiology expense and drug expense.

Opportunity Cost The alternative foregone, recognizes that every action requires foregoing other actions.

Organization Chart Indicates the formal lines of communication and reporting and how responsibility is assigned to managers.

Organizing Deciding how to use the resources of the organization to most effectively carry out the plans that have been established.

Original Records Provide evidence that some event has occurred in the healthcare financial system.

Overhead Refers to the remaining expenses of operation that are necessary to produce the service but that are not directly attributable to that service.

Pareto Analysis An analytical tool employing the Pareto principle, also known as the 80/20 rule. The Pareto principle states that 80% of an organization's problems are caused by 20% of the possible causes.

Partial Qualifying Eligible Professional (PQEP) A healthcare provider paid under APM that meet slightly reduced performance thresholds and bear some financial risk.

Patient Mix or Payer Mix A term indicating the mix of payers; thus, whether the individual is a Medicare patient, a Medicaid patient, a patient covered by private insurance, or a private pay patient varies the patient mix proportions. Patient mix information allows estimated payment levels to be associated with the service utilization assumptions.

Pay-for-Performance (P4P) Providers receive payment incentives when meeting performance measures that show they are delivering and promoting improvements in high-quality, efficient care.

Payback Period The length of time required for the cash coming in from an investment to equal the amount of cash originally spent when the investment was acquired.

Payer Mix The proportion of revenues realized from different types of payers. A measure often included in the profile of a healthcare organization.

PEDMAS An Excel acronym showing the order of execution in mathematical calculations, parenthesis (first), exponents, multiplication and division, and addition and subtraction (last).

Per Case Reimbursement A reimbursement system that pays a flat rate per inpatient admission, e.g., Medicare DRG reimbursement.

Per Diem Reimbursement A reimbursement system that pays a flat rate per day of hospitalization.

Perfection A Lean six sigma principle seeking minimum defects by doing it right the first time.

Performance Measures Measures that compare and quantify performance. Performance measures may be financial, nonfinancial, or a combination of both types.

Performance Period A unit of time during which performance is measured.

Period Cost For purposes of healthcare businesses, period cost is necessary to support the existence of the organization itself, rather than actual delivery of a service. Period costs are matched with revenue on the basis of the period during which the cost is incurred. The term originated with the manufacturing industry.

Physician-Focused Payment Models (PFPMs) New reimbursement models for physicians encompassing MIPS and APMs.

Pie or Doughnut Chart A chart designed to show the composition of a variable by dividing a circle into sectors.

Planning Identifying objectives of the organization and identifying the steps required to accomplish the objectives.

Population Health Health care concerned with the outcomes of an entire population instead of a single patient.

Post-Acute Care (PAC) Healthcare services delivered by nursing homes, home health agencies, inpatient rehabilitation facilities, and long-term care hospitals,

Predictive Analytics An advanced analytical method used to extract value from data.

Preferred Stock Stock that has preference over common stock in certain issues such as payment of dividends.

Present Value A concept based on the time value of money. The value of a dollar today is more than the value of a dollar in the future.

Price, Efficiency, and Volume (Three-Variance) Method A variance analysis method that divides total variance between the amount due to changes between budgeted and actual output (volume), the cost of inputs, and the amount of inputs used to produce outputs.

Price Variance The amount of the total variance that is due to differences between the budgeted and actual price of inputs.

Private Sector Organizations Those organizations that are not part of the government.

Procedures A common method of grouping healthcare expenses for purposes of planning and control. Such a grouping will generally be by Current Procedural Terminology (or CPT) codes, which list descriptive terms and identifying codes for medical services and procedures performed.

Product Cost For the purposes of healthcare businesses, product cost is necessary to actually deliver the service. The term originated with the manufacturing industry.

Productive Time Equates to the employee's net hours on duty when performing the functions in his or her job description.

Profit Center A responsibility center where the manager is responsible for both the revenue/volume (inflow) side and the expense (outflow) side of a department, division, unit, or program; manager should be evaluated on the difference between budgeted and actual net income.

Profitability Ratios Ratios that reflect the ability of the organization to operate with an excess of operating revenue over operating expense.

Profit-Volume (PV) Ratio The contribution margin (i.e., net revenues less variable costs) expressed as a percentage of net revenue.

Prospective Analytics A subset of predictive analytics that is used as a decision-making tool.

Public Organization An organization owned and managed by a federal, state, county, or city government.

Pull A Lean six sigma principle aimed at ensuring goods and services are delivered when needed, e.g., hospital admission triggers call for the resources that will be needed for each day of hospitalization and day of discharge.

Qualifying Eligible Professionals (QEPs) Providers that meet all APM performance thresholds and are at financial risk based on performance.

Quartile A distribution into four classes, each of which contains one-quarter of the whole; any one of the four classes is a quartile.

Range A measure of dispersion, calculated as the largest value in a series minus the lowest value.

Rates A measure of the frequency of an event, calculated as number of occurrences divided by the total number of events where it could have occurred.

Reimbursement A method of paying (reimbursing) a healthcare provider for services or procedures provided.

Reporting System Produces reports of an event's effect in the healthcare financial system.

Responsibility Centers Makes a manager responsible for both the revenue/volume (inflow) side and the expense (outflow) side of a department, division, unit, or program. Also known as a profit center.

Retrospective Analytics Identifies trends and problems by looking at historical information and drawing empirical conclusions.

Return on Assets (ROA) A broad measure of profitability in common use, computed by dividing net income by total assets.

Return on Equity (ROE) A measure of the amount of wealth created based on net worth, computed by dividing net income by net worth.

Revenue Actual or expected cash inflows due to the organization's major business. Revenues are amounts earned in the course of doing business. In the case of health care, revenues are mostly earned by rendering services to patients.

Risk/Return Trade-Off An investment fact, in order to obtain higher returns an investor must accept higher risk, i.e., the investment could lose value.

Salvage Value Also known as residual value or scrap value, represents any expected cash value of the asset at the end of its useful life.

Scatter or XY Diagram A graph used to determine the relationship between two variables by graphing points in a two-dimensional space, typically the suspected cause is plotted on the x-axis and the effect is on the y-axis.

Securities and Exchange Commission (SEC) A government agency that oversees stock markets, securities brokers and dealers, investment advisers, and mutual funds.

Semifixed Costs Those costs that stay fixed for a time when activity levels or volume of operations change; rises will occur, but not in direct proportion.

Semivariable Costs Those costs that vary when activity levels or volume of operations change, but not in direct proportion. A supervisor's salary is an example of a semivariable cost.

Short-Term Borrowing The use of debt in a situation where the debt should be repaid in 12 months or less.

Situational Analysis Management tool that reviews, assesses, and analyzes the organization's internal operations for strengths and weaknesses and the organization's external environment for opportunities and threats.

Staffing A term that means the assigning of staff to fill scheduled positions.

Stakeholder A person or entity that has an interest in a service, program, and/or outcome.

Standard Deviation A measure of dispersion, square root of the variance, and is used in conjunction with the mean to identify outliers.

Standardized Data Data that are both uniform and comparable.

Statement of Changes in Net Worth A financial statement that ties net income and nonoperating gains to changes in net worth, in other words, shows the relationship between the income statement and balance sheet.

Stock Warrants Warrants allow the owner of the warrant to purchase additional shares of stock in the company, generally at a particular price and prior to an expiration date.

Straight-Line Depreciation A depreciation method that divides the depreciable value by the expected life of an asset and writes off the value as an expense until the value of the asset is zero or equal to its expected salvage value.

Strategic Objective A strategic objective further defines intended outcomes in order to achieve a goal.

Subsidiary Journals Documents that contain specific sets of transactions and that support the general ledger.

Sum-of-the-Years Depreciation An accelerated depreciation method that adds up the useful years of an asset and calculates the depreciation expense based on the year and total expected years, e.g., an asset with a four-year life has total expected years of 10, $1 + 2 + 3 + 4$, first year expense is $4 \div 10 \times$ depreciable value, year 2 is $3 \div 10$ and so on.

Super Bill A standardized bill for medical services that is widely accepted by third-party payers.

Support Services Expenses This type of expense provides support to both general services expenses and operations expenses. It is necessary for support, but it neither is directly related to patient care nor is it a service necessary to maintain the patient. Examples of support services are insurance and payroll taxes.

Sustainable Growth Rate (SGR) A method to ensure that the yearly increase in expense per Medicare beneficiary does not exceed the growth in the GDP.

SWOT Analysis Acronym for a method of situational analysis assessing an organization's strengths, weaknesses, opportunities, and threats—thus, "SWOT."

Time Value of Money The present value concept, which is that the value of a dollar today is more than the value of a dollar in the future.

Total Asset Turnover A financial ratio that assesses the use of all assets. Computed by dividing total revenue by total assets.

Total Margin A profitability ratio measuring net income and sales, Computed as net income divided by total revenue.

Trend Analysis The process of comparing and analyzing figures over several time periods. Also known as horizontal analysis.

Trend Line An Excel feature that allows a user to insert the best fitting line in a graph, used to detect trends.

Trial Balance A document used to balance the general ledger accounts and to produce financial statements.

Turnover Ratios Ratios that measure the amount of revenue generated for each dollar invested in assets.

Unexpired Costs Costs that are not yet used up and will be matched against future revenues.

Units of Production (Units of Service) Depreciation A depreciation method that calculates the depreciation expense based on the number of units produced during the accounting period divided by total expected units over the life of the assets, factor is then multiplied by the asset's depreciable value

Useful Life of an Asset The useful life of a fixed asset determines the period over which the fixed asset's cost will be spread.

Value A Lean six sigma principle that focuses managers' attention on what customers want and what activities enhance customer satisfaction.

Value-Based Concept In finance, a combination of cost and quality. Value-based concepts may be applied to purchasing, payment, pricing, strategy, and/or patient care.

Value Modifier (VM) A budget-neutral payment adjustment for physicians that increases and decreases Medicare reimbursement based on the quality of care delivered.

Value Stream Mapping A Lean six sigma principle that documents every step taken to design, produce, and deliver a product.

Value-Based Programs (VBPs) A series of program designed to tie reimbursement to the quality of care delivered.

Values Statement Express the philosophy of the organization.

Variable Costs Costs that vary in direct proportion to changes in activity levels of volume of operations. Food for meal preparation is an example of variable cost.

Variance A measure of dispersion calculated as the sum of the square of the differences between each individual value in a data set and the mean divided by the number of observations − 1, used to compute standard deviation.

Variance Analysis A variance is the difference between standard and actual prices and quantities. Variance analysis analyzes these differences.

Version 5010 of Standards The current version of electronic transmission standards at the time of this writing.

Vertical Analysis A process of converting dollar amounts to percentages to put information on the same relative basis. Also known as common sizing.

Vision Statement The vision statement explains "what we want to be." It is a look further into the future.

Volume Variance The amount of the total variance due to changes in the budgeted and actual output produced.

Index

Note: Page numbers followed with *f* and *t* refer to figures and tables